New Advances in Optic Nerve Diseases

New Advances in Optic Nerve Diseases

Guest Editor

Livio Vitiello

MDPI

Basel • Beijing • Wuhan • Barcelona • Belgrade • Novi Sad • Cluj • Manchester

Guest Editor
Livio Vitiello
Eye Unit
"Luigi Curto" Hospital,
Azienda Sanitaria Locale Salerno
Salerno
Italy

Editorial Office
MDPI AG
Grossprteranlage 5
4052 Basel, Switzerland

This is a reprint of the Special Issue, published open access by the journal *Journal of Clinical Medicine* (ISSN 2077-0383), freely accessible at: https://www.mdpi.com/journal/jcm/special_issues/849R9SA152.

For citation purposes, cite each article independently as indicated on the article page online and as indicated below:

Lastname, A.A.; Lastname, B.B. Article Title. *Journal Name* **Year**, *Volume Number*, Page Range.

ISBN 978-3-7258-5333-5 (Hbk)
ISBN 978-3-7258-5334-2 (PDF)
https://doi.org/10.3390/books978-3-7258-5334-2

Contents

About the Editor

Livio Vitiello

Livio Vitiello is a Medical Doctor at the Eye Unit of "Luigi Curto" Hospital in Polla (Salerno, Italy). He is particularly skilled in ocular ultrasound, but he also deals with retinal and optic nerve diseases, areas in which he is particularly dedicated to research.

Journal of
Clinical Medicine

MDPI

Article

Morpho-Functional Assessment of Retinal Ganglion Cells and Visual Pathways in Patients with Optic Disc Drusen: Superficial Drusen Visible Height as a Marker of Impairment

Giulio Antonelli, Lucia Ziccardi *, Lucilla Barbano, Antonio Di Renzo and Vincenzo Parisi

IRCCS—Fondazione Bietti, 00198 Rome, Italy; giulio.antonelli@fondazionebietti.it (G.A.); lucilla.barbano@fondazionebietti.it (L.B.); vincenzo.parisi@fondazionebietti.it (V.P.)
* Correspondence: lucia.ziccardi@fondazionebietti.it; Tel.: +39-06-84009486

Abstract: The aim of this study was to assess the morpho-functional involvement of the retinal ganglion cells (RGCs) and of the visual pathways in patients with superficial (ODD-S) or deep (ODD-D) optic disc drusen. This study enrolled 17 patients with ODD (mean age of 59.10 ± 12.68 years) providing 19 eyes and 20 control subjects (mean age 58.62 ± 8.77 years) providing 20 eyes. We evaluated the following: best-corrected visual acuity, visual field mean deviation (MD), the amplitude (A) of Pattern Electroretinogram (PERG), the implicit time (IT) and A of Visual Evoked Potentials (VEPs), retinal nerve fiber layer thickness (RNFL-T) and ganglion cell thickness (GC-T). In ODD-S eyes, the drusen visible height was measured. ODD-D and ODD-S were detected in 26.3% and 73.7% of ODD eyes, respectively. Significantly ($p < 0.01$) reduced MD, PERG A, VEP amplitude, RNFL-T and GC-T values and significantly ($p < 0.01$) increased VEP IT values were found in the ODD Group as compared to the Control one. In the ODD Group, no significant correlation ($p > 0.01$) between PERG As and VEP ITs was found. In ODD-S, the visible height was significantly correlated ($p < 0.01$) with reduced MD, PERG As and RNFL-T and with increased PSD and VEP IT values. Our findings suggest that ODD might induce morpho-functional changes in RGCs and their fibers and an unrelated visual pathway dysfunction leading or not leading to visual field defects. The observed morpho-functional impairment should be ascribed to an alteration in retrograde (from the axons to the RGCs) and anterograde (from the RGCs up to the visual cortex) axoplasmic transport. In ODD-S eyes, a minimum visible height of 300 microns represented the threshold for the abnormalities, suggesting that "the higher the ODD, the worse the impairment".

Keywords: optic disc drusen; PERG; VEP; OCT; RGCs

1. Introduction

Optic disc drusen (ODD) are congenital acellular deposits of calcium, amino and nucleic acids, and mucopolysaccharides located in front of the lamina cribrosa of the optic nerve [1], with an unknown pathogenesis. The predictive factors of these formations are a narrow scleral canal and a genetic predisposition contributing to axoplasmic metabolism disruption, an extrusion of mitochondria into the extracellular space and an abnormal calcium metabolism [2]. ODD are mainly bilateral, with a female predilection (61–71% of cases) and a prevalence that ranges from 0.4 to 3.7% of the overall population; however, the prevalence of subclinical ODD may be even higher [3,4]. ODD have been associated with several diseases, including retinitis pigmentosa, papilledema, rare types of uveitis, syndromic retinal dystrophies, retinal myelination, benign hamartoma and angioid streaks [4]. Moreover, ODD have been associated with glaucoma, hiding the optic disc cupping typical of glaucoma, leading to a misdiagnosis or a delayed diagnosis [5].

According to the ODD Studies Consortium, ODD can be divided into superficial (ODD-S) and deep (ODD-D), depending on whether the localization is above or below the level of Bruch's membrane opening (BMO) [6]. ODD-D are not easily detectable in a classical routine ophthalmological examination [6]. By contrast, ODD-S, which are thought to represent 40% of cases [7], can be detected by using autofluorescence due to the presence of calcium and by using ocular ultrasound. With the advent of spectral-domain optical coherence tomography (Sd-OCT) and of enhanced depth imaging OCT (EDI-OCT) in clinical practice, the detection rate of ODD has improved for the highest sensitivity near the inner sclera and the excellent visualization of ODD-D [8]. Even if many patients with ODD do not declare visual symptoms, visual field (VF) defects (arcuate defects, enlargement of the blind spot and concentric contraction) [9] are more commonly described in ODD-S than in ODD-D [10], and a progression of the deficit is possible [10].

The impact of ODD on the neural conduction along the visual pathways was studied by using Visual Evoked Potential (VEP) recordings [11,12], often yielding contrasting results, since an increased VEP P100 implicit time was found, ranging from 0% to 83% of ODD cases across studies [13]. Although it is possible to selectively evaluate the neural conduction along small and large axons of the visual pathways by using different visual stimuli [11,12], previous VEP studies have not provided specific information on the impairment of different axons in ODD.

Moreover, the function of the innermost retinal layers (retinal ganglion cells—RGCs—and their fibers), in a cohort of 24 ODD eyes [14], was assessed using Pattern Electroretinogram (PERG) [15], and the findings showed a reduced N95 wave amplitude in almost 79% of ODD eyes.

Regarding the impact of ODD on the thickness of the peripapillary retinal fiber nerve layer (RNFL) [7,16–18], more recent reports uniquely identified a reduction in RNFL thickness [5,10,19].

Regarding the potential correlations between the volume and size of ODD and the morphologic and functional data of visual pathways [20–23], RNFL thinning has been found to be significantly correlated with ODD diameter and number [5], and an association between ODD size and VF defects has also been described [22,24].

Nevertheless, there is a lack of comprehensive data on the effects of ODD on the psychophysics and morpho-function of the inner retina and visual pathways. Therefore, the aim of our study was to evaluate whether the occurrence of ODD may induce changes in visual acuity and/or VF defects, morphological and functional impairments in RGCs and their fibers, and/or a dysfunction of the small and large axons of the visual pathways. In addition, in eyes with ODD-S, it was investigated whether the ODD visible height influences the morpho-functional retinal and visual pathway conditions.

2. Materials and Methods

2.1. Study Design and Participants

In this retrospective case series, based on the inclusion criteria (see below), we included, between June 2021 and October 2022, seventeen patients (mean age of 59.10 ± 12.68 years, range: 42–78 years) with a clear diagnosis of ODD, made via an ophthalmological evaluation and by using autofluorescence/Ss-OCT imaging and/or ultrasonography. Diagnoses were made at our Clinical and Research Center of Neurophthalmology, Genetic and Rare Diseases of IRCCS—Fondazione Bietti, and the ODD Group was selected based on the inclusion criteria.

We studied 19 ODD eyes from 17 patients, showing bilateral ODD in only 2 cases of ODD-S.

Furthermore, 20 normal age-similar subjects (mean age of 58.62 ± 8.77 years, range: 40–78 years), providing 20 eyes, served as Controls.

An extensive ophthalmological examination was performed in all Controls and patients with ODD, and it involved an assessment of best-corrected visual acuity (BCVA), an examination of the anterior segment using slit-lamp biomicroscopy, a measurement of intraocular pressure (IOP) and an evaluation of the optic nerve head using indirect ophthalmoscopy and 30° color photography. In addition, the Controls and patients were tested using the Humphrey 30-2 automated VF test (Humphrey Field Analyzer (HFA)

740; Zeiss, San Leandro, CA, USA), swept-source optical coherence tomography (Ss-OCT) and autofluorescence.

The Controls had an IOP of less than 18 mmHg; a BCVA of 0.0 logMAR with a refractive error between −2.00 and +2.00 spherical equivalent; a 30-2 threshold VF with a mean deviation (MD) > −2.0 dB and pattern standard deviation (PSD) < 2.0 dB [25]; and no evidence of an optic disc (or retinal diseases) in the indirect ophthalmoscopy, color photography, Ss-OCT or B-scan ultrasonography.

The inclusion criteria for the patients with ODD were as follows:

(1) Age ranging from 18 to 80 years;
(2) HFA 30-2 VF with defects that preserved the ability to maintain stable fixation comparable to that of normal subjects (fixation loss rate higher than 4%);
(3) Capacity to clearly distinguish a target of fixation placed in the center of the screen, at a viewing distance of 114 cm, in which the visual stimuli of PERG and VEP were presented (see below);
(4) BCVA between 0.00 and 0.40 logarithm of the minimum angle of resolution (logMAR);
(5) Refractive error (when present) between −3.00 and +3.00 spherical equivalent;
(6) IOP less than 18 mmHg;
(7) Absence of cornea, lens, and retina/macula diseases or detectable spontaneous eye movements (i.e., nystagmus).

We excluded from the present study all eyes showing any sign of optic nerve pathology other than ODD. We also excluded eyes with HFA 30-2 defects consisting of a cecocentral scotoma and or central defects enclosing the physiological blind spot.

In the present retrospective case series study, all procedures adhered to the tenets of the Declaration of Helsinki. The study protocol (NEU_03-2021; 125/21/FB) was approved by the local ethical committee (Comitato Etico Centrale IRCCS Lazio, Sezione IFO/Fondazione Bietti, Rome, Italy), and, upon recruitment, informed consent was obtained from each subject enrolled in the study.

2.2. Procedures

2.2.1. Visual Acuity Assessment

Modified Early Treatment Diabetic Retinopathy Study (ETDRS) Tables (Lighthouse, Low vision products, Long Island City, NY, USA) were used to evaluate BCVA at a distance of 4 m. VA is quantified in LogMAR values.

2.2.2. Visual Field Examination

Static perimetry was performed by using the HFA 30-2 SITA Standard strategy, and MD (in dB) and PSD (in dB) values were obtained. Exams showing a fixation loss rate higher than 4% were discarded.

2.2.3. Electrophysiological Examinations

According to our previously published studies [26–31], simultaneous PERGs and VEPs were carried out by using our previously published methods.

Briefly, visual stimuli were presented monocularly on a TV monitor subtending 23 degrees at a distance of 114 cm, and they consisted of a checkerboard pattern with a contrast of 80% and mean luminance of 110 cd/m^2. In the center of the monitor, a small fixation target was placed. The check edges subtended 60 min (60′) and 15 min (15′) of the visual angle and were reversed in contrast at 2 reversals per second. All electrophysiological procedures followed the International Society for Clinical Electrophysiology of Vision (ISCEV)'s standards [11]. We used two different checkerboard patterns to obtain a predominant activation of larger (60′ checks) or smaller (15′ checks) axons [26,27,29,32].

PERG Recordings

PERG responses were recorded by using two skin Ag/AgCl electrodes placed over the lower eyelid, one as an active electrode on the open stimulated eye and one as a reference electrode on the pathed eye [33]. The ground electrode was in Fpz [34]. The interelectrode resistance was lower than 3000 ohms. The signal was amplified (gain of 50,000), filtered (band pass of 1–30Hz) and averaged with the automatic rejection of artefacts (100 events free from artefacts were averaged for every trial) using CSO (CSO, Firenze, Italy). The analysis time was 250 msec. In the analysis of the PERG responses, we considered the peak-to-peak amplitude between the first positive peak (P50) and the second negative peak (N95). The PERG P50-N95 amplitude (PERG A) was measured in microvolt.

VEP Recordings

VEP responses were recorded by using Ag/AgCl electrodes placed in Oz (active electrode) and in Fpz (reference electrode) [34], and the ground electrode was placed on the left arm. The interelectrode resistance was kept below 3000 ohms. The bioelectric signal was amplified (gain of 20,000), filtered (band pass of 1–100 Hz) and averaged (200 events free from artefacts were averaged for every trial) using CSO. The analysis time was 250 ms. In the analysis of the VEP responses, we considered the implicit time (VEP IT) of the first positive peak (P100) = mea and the peak-to-peak amplitude between the first negative peak (N75) and the P100 peak. The VEP N75-P100 amplitude (VEP A) was measured in microvolt.

For the PERG and VEP responses, we measured the signal-to-noise ratio (SNR) following our previous published works [26–31]. In all subjects and patients, we accepted PERG and VEP signals with a signal-to-noise ratio >2.

2.2.4. Spectral-Domain Optical Coherence Tomography

The peripapillary RNFL thickness and the structural condition of the RGCs were investigated by performing swept-source optical coherence tomography (Ss-OCT) (Topcon DRI OCT Triton, Topcon, Japan) after pupil dilation with tropicamide 1% eye drops. Each scan was carefully reviewed for the accurate identification and segmentation of the retinal layers by two expert graders (L.Z. and L.B.). We followed the APOSTEL recommendations for quality control [35]. The acceptable signal strength index of the acquired scan was at least 40. The macular ganglion cell complex (GCC) was segmented by using the macula 3D scan (V) protocol with the following parameters: an area of 7.0 × 7.0 mm centered on the fovea and a scan density of 512 (vertical) × 128 (horizontal) scans. Only the GC-Inner Plexiform thickness was taken into consideration (GCL+). Peripapillary RNFL was recorded as superior, inferior, temporal, nasale or overall components using a 6.0 × 6.0 mm area centered on the optic nerve with a scan density of 512 (vertical) × 128 (horizontal) scans. In the Ss-OCT results, we assessed the averaged values of RNFL thickness (RNFL-T measured in microns) from superior (RNFL-ST), inferior (RNFL-IT), nasal (RNFL-NT) and temporal (RNFL-TT) quadrants, and the data obtained from the average of all quadrants (average of 4 values) were identified as RNFL overall (RNFL-OT); the GCC thickness (GC) was also measured.

According to The Optic Disc Drusen Studies Consortium [6], we classified ODD as ODD-S or ODD-D by using Ss-OCT. ODD were detected as acellular deposits visualized on B-scan Ss-OCT images. ODD were defined as a mass with a boundary, which contrasted with the normal optic nerve head anatomy; they did not belong to the normal retinal layers above BMO, or they contrasted with the prelaminar tissue beneath BMO. In ODD-S eyes, the ODD visible height was measured as the perpendicular distance of ODD protruding above BMO [21]. With ODD-D being located below BMO, no measurement could be obtained. The B-scan Ss-OCT image with the largest height was used for the measurement.

2.2.5. Statistics

A Gaussian distribution of our data was assumed and assessed using the Kolmogorov–Smirnov test. From a pilot study conducted in 8 ODD eyes from 8 subjects and in 8 eyes from 8 Control subjects, other than those included in the current study (unpublished data), we obtained size estimates. Inter-individual variability, expressed as standard deviation

(SD) data, was estimated for 15′ PERG A. For 15′ PERG A, the mean/SD ratio value was higher for the Control Group (mean: 2.50 microvolt; SD: 0.41 microvolt, 16.4% of the mean) than for the ODD Group (mean: 1.85 microvolt; SD: 0.45 microvolt, 24.3% of the mean).

Assuming the above mean and SD values, a sample size of Controls and patients with ODD was established. A power of 90% (β = 10%) at α = 1% detected a between-group difference of 26% in 15′ PERG A. Thus, a sample size of 14 patients with ODD and 18 Control subjects was obtained.

Based on the t-Student distribution for the PERG, VEP and Ss-OCT parameters, 95% confidence limits (CLs) were obtained from the Control data considering superior CL for VEP IT and inferior CL PERG A, VEP A, RNFL-T and GC (see Table 1).

MD and PSD were considered abnormal for values greater than −2 dB and +2 dB, respectively.

A one-way analysis of variance (ANOVA) was used to assess the differences in the values of the HFA, PERG, VEP and Ss-OCT parameters observed in the ODD and Control Groups. A comparison of electro-functional (PERG A, VEP IT and VEP A), HFA (MD and PSD) and morphological (ODD visible height (in ODD-S eyes), RNFL-T and GC) data was carried out by performing Pearson's test.

A p value lower than 0.01 was considered significant in all statistical analyses.

All statistical analyses were performed using MedCalc V.13.0.4.0 (MedCalc, Mariakerke, Belgium).

Table 1. Individual data of optic disc drusen characteristics (type and visible height), 30-2 Humphrey Field Analyzer mean deviation and pattern standard deviation, 60′ and 15′ Pattern Electroretinogram P50-N95 amplitude, Visual Evoked Potential P100 implicit time and N75-P100 amplitude, and sectorial retinal nerve fiber layer thickness and ganglion cell thickness detected in all 19 studied eyes with optic disc drusen.

	ODD [a]		HFA [b] 30-2		60′ PERG [c]	60′ VEP [d]		15′ PERG [c]	15′ VEP [d]		RNFL [e]					GC-T [f]
	Type	Visible Height (µ [g])	MD [h] (dB [i])	PSD [l] (dB [i])	A [m] (µV [n])	IT [o] (msec [p])	A [m] (µV [n])	A [m] (µV [n])	IT [o] (msec [p])	A [m] (µV [n])	TT [q] (µ [g])	ST [r] (µ [g])	IT [s] (µ [g])	NT [t] (µ [g])	OT [u] (µ [g])	(µ [g])
ODD#1	Deep		**−7.06**	**[illegible].5**	2.7	106	**7.1**	2.2	104	**2.4**	**65**	**68**	**51**	87	[illegible]7.75	**50**
ODD#2	Deep		3.46	1[illegible]81	**1.5**	**109**	**6.2**	**1.9**	**117**	**3.7**	79	138	**73**	152	[illegible]10.50	67
ODD#3	Superficial	559	**−6.57**	**1[illegible]41**	**1.5**	**121**	**4.2**	**1.5**	**124**	**2.7**	**32**	**44**	**20**	**40**	**[illegible]4.00**	**54**
ODD#4	Superficial	625	**−11.22**	**8[illegible]24**	**2.0**	**118**	**8.1**	**1.5**	**118**	8.1	**33**	**37**	**50**	**65**	**[illegible]6.25**	56
ODD#5	Superficial	371	0.53	1[illegible]45	**1.4**	**117**	**7.5**	**1.5**	103	**4.4**	94	**85**	**68**	150	**[illegible]9.25**	**50**
ODD#6	Superficial	121	−0.39	1[illegible]72	3.1	106	11.5	**2.0**	107	11.6	82	147	**77**	155	[illegible]16.24	66
ODD#7	Superficial	358	−1.91	**4[illegible]52**	**1.9**	**114**	**5.2**	**1.8**	101	**6.3**	**59**	**61**	**51**	84	**[illegible]3.75**	58
ODD#8	Superficial	397	**−2.43**	**6[illegible]52**	**1.3**	**120**	14.8	**1.6**	**120**	15.5	**36**	**56**	**45**	**69**	**[illegible]1.53**	**50**
ODD#9	Superficial	635	**−9.36**	**9[illegible]24**	**1.2**	**127**	**8.2**	**1.4**	**131**	10.7	**72**	**68**	**45**	**52**	**[illegible]9.25**	**50**
ODD#10	Superficial	464	0.12	1[illegible]37	**1.3**	**110**	**5.1**	**1.2**	**112**	**5.5**	82	**67**	**43**	**66**	**[illegible]4.52**	**55**
ODD#11	Superficial	436	**−8.9**	**10[illegible]43**	**2.1**	**123**	**4.2**	**1.4**	**119**	**6.1**	**62**	**84**	**55**	82	**[illegible]0.75**	**50**
ODD#12	Superficial	404	**−9.97**	**10[illegible]74**	**2.0**	**108**	15.3	**1.9**	**117**	**7.2**	**45**	133	**72**	86	**[illegible]6.28**	**28**
ODD#13	Superficial	372	−0.45	1[illegible]2	**1.5**	**109**	9.1	**1.4**	106	**3.5**	81	**63**	**65**	95	**[illegible]6.05**	**53**
ODD#14	Superficial	298	−1.54	**4.[illegible]8**	**1.9**	106	**3.2**	2.2	**112**	**4.5**	104	**63**	**30**	100	**[illegible]4.25**	62
ODD#15	Deep		−0.48	**2.[illegible]8**	2.3	107	**4.5**	**2**	108	5.1	100	**79**	**47**	110	**[illegible]4.00**	63
ODD#16	Superficial	319	1.96	1.[illegible]1	2.6	104	16.6	**2.1**	101	12.2	**62**	**56**	**57**	87	**[illegible]5.50**	**52**
ODD#17	Deep		0.78	**2.[illegible]7**	**1.8**	107	11.5	2.6	102	10.5	**64**	**87**	**63**	82	**[illegible]4.00**	**55**
ODD#18	Superficial	230	3.08	[illegible].62	2.4	**108**	18.7	**1.9**	107	10.6	**68**	149	**75**	153	1[illegible]1.25	69
ODD#19	Deep		−1.45	[illegible].38	**1.8**	103	10	**1.1**	**112**	13	**60**	133	**58**	139	**[illegible]7.50**	**55**
95%CL [v]			−2.0	2[illegible]	2.14	107.19	8.38	2.14	109.59	7.48	76.65	109.74	119.13	78.68	1[illegible]4.73	56.00

[a] ODD = optic disc drusen; [b] HFA = Humphrey Field Analyzer, [c] PERG = Pattern Electroretinogram, [d] VEP = Visual Evoked Potential; [e] RNFL = retinal nerve fiber layer; [f] GC-T = ganglion cell thickness; [g] µ = microns; [h] MD = mean deviation, [i] dB = decibel; [l] PSD = pattern standard deviation 60′; 60′ and 15′ = visual stimuli checks subtending 60 and 15 min of visual arc; [m] A = amplitude; [n] µV = microvolt; [o] IT = implicit time; [p] msec = milliseconds; [q] TT = Temporal Thickness; [r] ST = Superior Thickness; [s] IT = Inferior Thickness; [t] NT = Nasal Thickness; [u] OT = Overall Thickness; [v] CL 95%: = confidence limits obtained from Control data considering upper confidence limit for VEP IT and lower confidence limit for PERG A, VEP A, RNFL and GC-T. MD and PSD were considered abnormal for values greater than −2 dB and +2 dB, respectively. The abnormal values with respect to the 95% confidence limits are reported in bold.

3. Results

3.1. Demographic and Clinical Features

Figure 1 presents examples of the VF, PERG and VEP recordings and Ss-OCT scans detected in one representative Control eye (#7) and in one eye with ODD-S (#4).

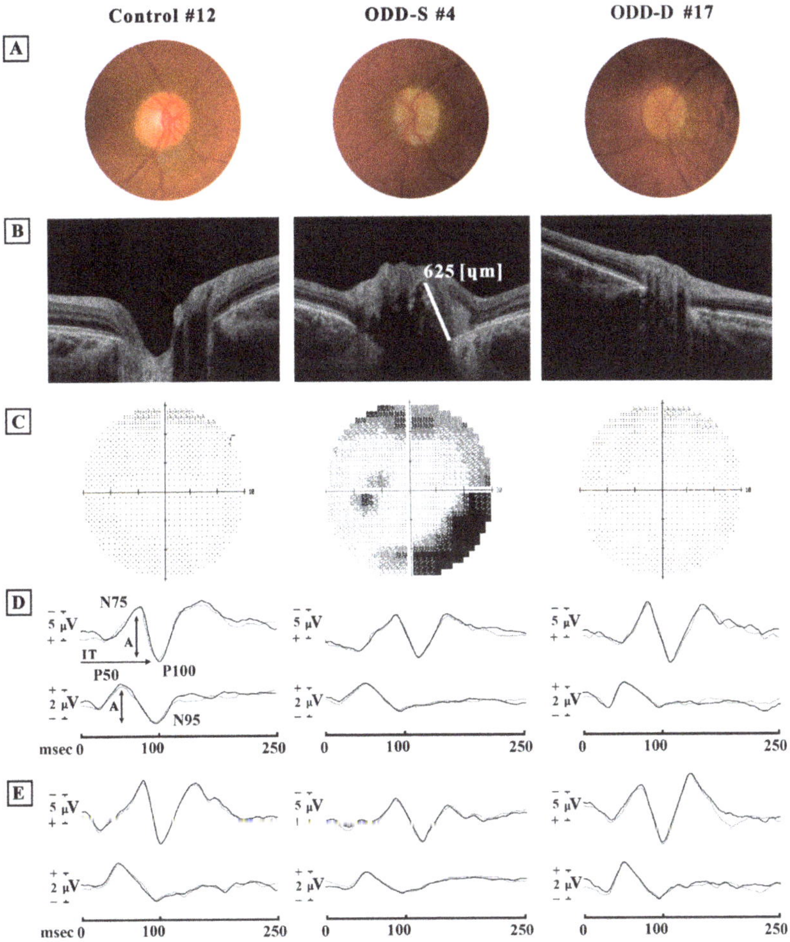

Figure 1. Examples of optic nerve fundus photography (**A**), optical coherence tomography (OCT) B-scan images (**B**), 30-2 Humphrey Field Analyzer (HFA) (**C**), simultaneous recordings of Visual Evoked Potentials (VEPs) and Pattern Electroretinogram (PERG) in response to 60′ (**D**) and 15′ (**E**) visual stimuli checks from one eye of one normal Control subject (Control #12), from one eye with superficial optic disc drusen (ODD-S #4) and from one eye with deep optic disc drusen (ODD-D #17). In ODD-S #4 eye (**B**), the white line indicates the measurement of the ODD visible height (microns). In (**D**,**E**), N75 and P100 refer to the first negative and the first positive peaks of VEP recordings (the implicit time of P100 (→) and the peak-to-peak N75-P100 amplitude (↕) were considered); P50 and N95 refer to the first positive and the second negative peaks of PERG recordings (the peak-to-peak P50-N95 amplitude (↕) was considered). msec = milliseconds; μV = microvolt. When compared to Control eyes, in ODD-S eye, abnormal HFA, reduced 60′ N75-P100 VEP and 60′ and 15′ P50-N95 PERG amplitudes, and delayed 60′ and 15′ P100 VEP implicit times can be observed. By contrast, in ODD-D eye, with respect to Control eye, similar HFA but reduced 60′ P50-N95 PERG amplitude can be found.

In Table 1, individual ODD data items (ODD-D and ODD-S with relative visible height), consisting of the HFA, PERG and VEP and Ss-OCT parameters from all 19 eyes, are presented.

The number and the relative percentage of abnormal values for each psychophysical (HFA 30-2), electrophysiological (PERG and VEP) and morphological (RNFL-T and GC-T) parameter are reported in Table 2. The mean HFA, PERG, VEP, RNFL and GC-T values observed in the Control and ODD Groups and the relative statistical analyses between the Groups are shown in Table 2.

Table 2. Mean values of age, 30-2 Humphrey Field Analyzer mean deviation and pattern standard deviation, 60′ and 15′ Pattern Electroretinogram P50-N95 amplitude, Visual Evoked Potential P100 implicit time and N75-P100 amplitude, sectorial retinal nerve fiber layer thickness (RNFL), and ganglion cell thickness (GC-T) detected in the Control Group and in the Group of eyes with optic disc drusen.

	Controls (N [a] = 20)		**ODD [b] (N [a] = 19)**		**ODD [b] *Ab* [c] (N [a])**	***Ab* [c] %**	**ANOVA [d]: ODD [b] vs. Controls**	
	Mean	1SD [e]	Mean	1SD [e]			f (1,38) =	*p*=
Age (years)	58.62	8.77	59.10	12.68			0.02	0.894
HFA [f] MD [g] (dB [i])	0.82	0.38	−2.69	4.50	7	36.84	12.09	<0.001
HFA [f] PSD [h] (dB [i])	0.68	1.36	4.77	3.85	11	57.89	19.97	<0.0001
60′ PERG [l] A [m] (μV [n])	2.68	0.27	1.92	0.52	14	73.68	33.30	<0.0001
60′ VEP [o] IT [p] (msec [q])	101.29	2.95	111.51	7.00	12	63.15	35.95	<0.0001
60′ VEP [o] A [m] (μV [n])	13.4	2.51	8.97	4.49	11	57.89	14.66	<0.0001
15′ PERG [i] A [l] (μV [n])	2.66	0.26	1.77	0.39	16	84.21	71.00	<0.0001
15′ VEP [o] IT [p] (msec [q])	104.21	2.69	111.53	8.25	10	52.63	14.18	<0.0001
15′ VEP [o] A [l] (μV [n])	12.52	2.52	7.75	3.80	11	57.89	21.55	<0.0001
RNFL [r]-TT [s] (μ)	86.39	4.87	67.83	20.63	12	63.15	15.31	<0.0001
RNFL [r]-ST [t] (μ)	136.22	13.24	86.39	35.60	14	73.68	34.24	<0.0001
RNFL [r]-IT [u] (μ)	142.37	11.62	58.21	20.60	19	100.00	250.24	<0.0001
RNFL [r]-NT [v] (μ)	97.42	9.37	96.63	35.24	5	26.31	0.01	0.923
RNFL [r]-OT [w] (μ)	116.21	5.74	77.87	22.95	16	84.21	52.43	<0.0001
GC-T [x] (μ)	62.4	3.2	54.95	8.74	13	68.42	12.75	0.001

[a] N = number of eyes, [b] ODD = optic disc drusen; [c] Ab = abnormal with respect to 95% confidence limits (MD and PSD were considered Ab for values lower or greater + or −2 dB, respectively); [d] ANOVA = one-way analysis of variance; [e] SD = 1 standard deviation [f] HFA = 30-2 Humphrey Field Analyzer, [g] MD = mean deviation; [h] PSD = pattern standard deviation [i] dB = decibel; 60′ and 15′ = visual stimuli checks subtending 60 and 15 min of visual arc; [l] PERG = Pattern Electroretinogram; [m] A = amplitude; [n] μV = microvolt; [o] VEP = Visual Evoked Potential; [p] IT = implicit time; [q] msec = milliseconds; [r] RNFL = retinal nerve fiber layer; [s] TT = Temporal Thickness; [t] ST = Superior Thickness; [u] IT = Inferior Thickness; [v] NT = Nasal Thickness; [w] OT = Overall Thickness. [x] GC-T = ganglion cell thickness.

3.2. Optic Disc Druse Characteristics

In our enrolled patients with ODD, we considered ODD-D as cases where the prevalent druse deposits visible in SS-OCT were below BMO and ODD-S as cases where the prevalent druse deposits visible in SS-OCT were above BMO. ODD-D were detected in 5/19 (26.3%) eyes, whereas we found ODD-S in 14/19 (73.7%) eyes. The visible height of ODD-S ranged from 121 to 635 μ (mean of 399.21 ± 142.40 μ). Considering selectively ODD-S eyes, the visible height was not significantly correlated with patient age ($r = -0.099$, $p = 0.7362$).

3.3. Best-Corrected Visual Acuity Data

In all enrolled ODD eyes, we observed a BCVA of 0.0 LogMAR.

3.4. Visual Field Changes: HFA Data

None of our patients presented a central scotoma, and, therefore, all of them had a preserved BCVA. Only 7 ODD eyes (36.8%) showed VF defects, whereas in the others (12 eyes, 63.2%), a normal visual field was assessed. The most frequent defects in the ODD eyes with VF defects were reduced peripheral sensitivity (15.8%), peripheral constriction (15.8%) and blind spot enlargement (5.2%).

Reduced values of MD (<−2 dB) and increased values of PSD (>2 dB) were detected in 7/19 (36.84%) and in 11 (57.89%) ODD eyes, respectively. Reduced MD values were observed in 6/19 (31.58%) ODD-S eyes and in 1 (5.26%) ODD-D eye, whereas increased PSD values were found in 8/19 (42.11%) ODD-S eyes and in 3 (15.79%) ODD-D eyes.

On average, significantly ($p < 0.01$) reduced MD and increased PSD mean values were found in the ODD Group with respect to those found in the Control Group. As shown in Figure 2A,B, in the ODD-S eyes, the reduction in MD and the increase in PSD were significantly ($p < 0.01$) correlated with the ODD visible height.

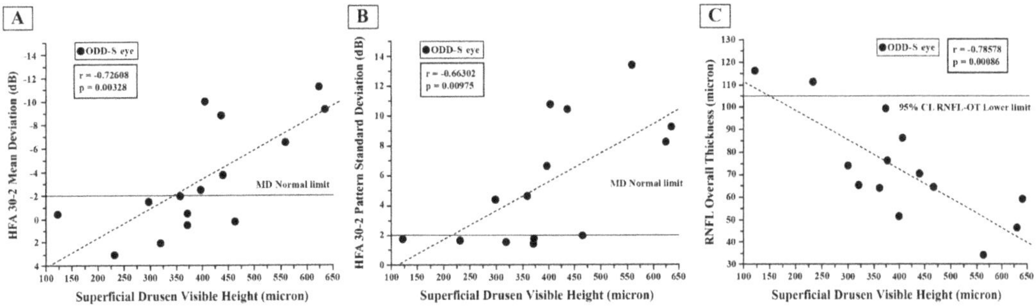

Figure 2. Individual values of superficial optic disc drusen (ODD-S) visible height plotted as a function of the corresponding values of Humphrey 30-2 automated visual field test (HFA) mean deviation (**A**), of pattern standard deviation (**B**) and of retinal nerve fiber layer (RNFL) Overall Thickness (**C**). The solid line indicates the normal limit in (**A**,**B**) and the 95% lower normal limit in (**C**). The dashed line indicates the regression analysis and correlations for which Pearson's test was used.

3.5. Retinal Ganglion Cells' Functional Changes: PERG Data

Reduced values of 60′ and 15′ PERG As were observed in 14/19 (73.68%) and in 16/19 (84.21%) ODD eyes, respectively. The 60′ PERG A was reduced in 11 (57.89%) ODD-S eyes and in 3 (15.79%) ODD-D eyes; similarly, 15′ PERG A was abnormal in 13 (68.42%) ODD-S eyes and in 3 (15.79%) ODD-D eyes. On average, significantly ($p < 0.01$) reduced mean values of 60′ and 15′ PERG As were detected in the ODD Group with respect to those detected in the Control Group.

As shown in Figures 2A and 3A, in the ODD-S eyes, both 60′ and 15′ reduced PERG As were significantly ($p < 0.01$) linearly correlated with the increase in the ODD visible height. It is worth noting that a greater percentage of reduced PERG A was detected in eyes with an ODD visible height greater than 300 microns.

3.6. Neural Conduction along the Visual Pathways' Changes: VEP Data

An increase in the 60′ and 15′ VEP IT values were found in 12 (63.16%) and in 10 (52.63%) ODD eyes, respectively. We found that 60′ VEP ITs were abnormal in 11 (57.89%) ODD-S eyes and only in 1 (5.26%) ODD-D eye; similarly, 15′ VEP ITs were found to be abnormal in 8 (42.11%) ODD-S eyes and in 2 (10.53%) ODD-D eyes. On average, the mean values of 60′ and 15′ VEP ITs were significantly ($p < 0.01$) increased in the ODD Group compared with those in the Control Group. Reduced VEP As were recorded in 11 (57.89%) ODD eyes for both 60′ and 15′ stimuli. Abnormal values were recorded in 8 (42.11%) ODD-S eyes and in 3 (15.79%) ODD-D eyes for 60′ VEP, whereas for 15′ VEP A values,

9 (47.37%) ODD-S and 3 (15.79%) ODD-D eyes were found to be abnormal. On average, the 60′ and 15′ VEP A mean values of the ODD Group were significantly ($p < 0.01$) reduced when compared to those of the Control Group.

In the ODD-S eyes, as presented in Figures 3B and 4B, both 60′ and 15′ VEP ITs were significantly ($p < 0.01$) linearly correlated with the ODD visible height, and it is worth noting that a greater percentage of increased VEP ITs was detected in ODD eyes with a visible height greater than 300 microns.

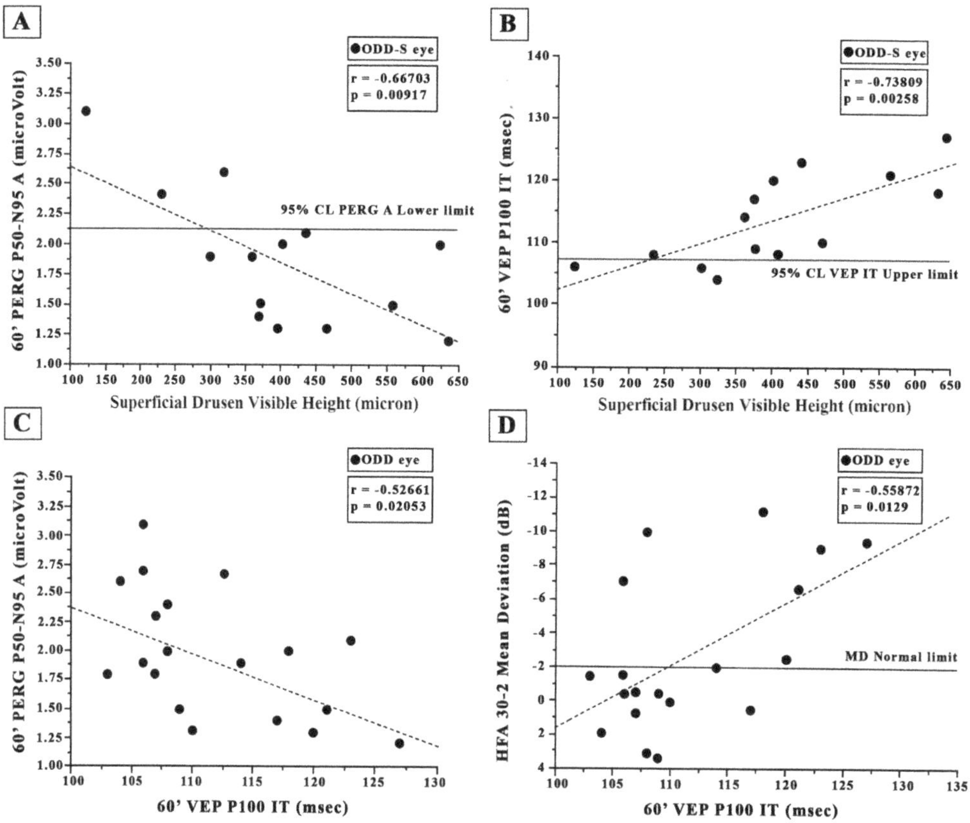

Figure 3. Individual values of superficial optic disc drusen (ODD-S) visible height plotted as a function of (**A**) the corresponding values of 60′ Pattern Electroretinogram (PERG) P50-N95 amplitude (**A**,**B**) and of 60′ Visual Evoked Potential (VEP) P100 implicit time (IT). The solid line indicates the 95% lower normal limit in (**A**) and the 95% upper normal limit in (**B**). Individual values of 60′ Visual Evoked Potential (VEP) P100 implicit time (IT) detected in all eyes with optic disc drusen (ODD) plotted as a function of the corresponding values of 60′ PERG P50-N95 A (**C**) and Humphrey 30-2 automated visual field test (HFA) mean deviation (**D**). The dashed line indicates the regression analysis and the correlations obtained with Pearson's test. 60′ refers to the visual stimuli checks subtending 60 min of visual arc.

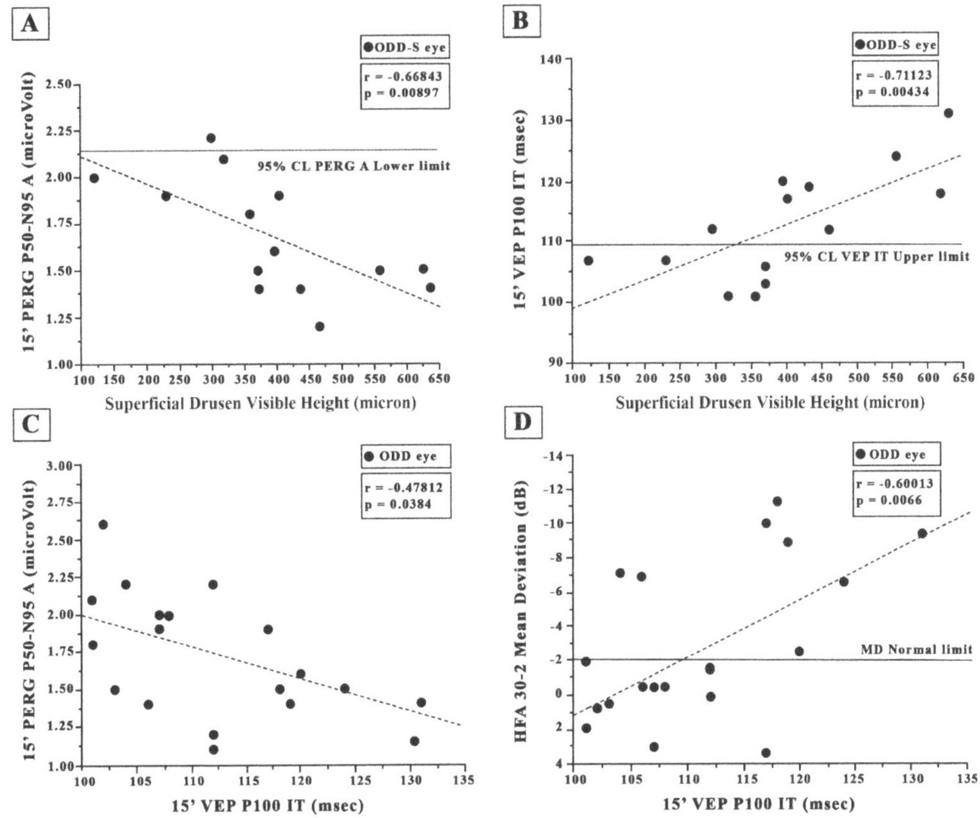

Figure 4. Individual values of superficial optic disc drusen (ODD-S) visible height plotted as a function of (**A**) the corresponding values of 15′ Pattern Electroretinogram (PERG) P50-N95 amplitude (**A**,**B**) and of 15′ Visual Evoked Potential (VEP) P100 implicit time (IT). The solid line indicates the 95% lower normal limit in (**A**) and the 95% upper normal limit in (**B**). Individual values of 15′ Visual Evoked Potential (VEP) P100 implicit time (IT) detected in all eyes with optic disc drusen (ODD) plotted as a function of the corresponding values of 15′ PERG P50-N95 A (**C**) and Humphrey 30-2 automated visual field test (HFA) mean deviation (**D**). The dashed line indicates the regression analysis and the correlations obtained with Pearson's test. 15′ refers to the visual stimuli checks subtending 15 min of visual arc.

Considering all 19 ODD eyes, the 60′ and 15′ VEP ITs values were not significantly (p textgreater 0.01) correlated with the 60′ and 15′ PERG A values (see Figures 3C and 4C). As shown in Figures 3D and 4D, the 60′ VEP IT values were associated but not significantly correlated ($p > 0.01$) with the MD values, whereas a significant ($p > 0.01$) correlation between 15′ VEP ITs and the MD values was found; both the 60′ and 15′ VEP IT values were significantly correlated with the PSD values (r = −0.645, r = 0.002 and r = 0.6854, p = 0.0012).

3.7. Retinal Nerve Fiber Layer and Ganglion Cell Thicknesses: OCT Data

A reduced RNFL thickness was found in the ODD eyes: RNFL-TT was reduced in 16 eyes (84.21%), RNFL-ST was reduced in 14 eyes (73.68%), RNFL-IT was reduced in all 19 eyes (100%), RNFL-NT was reduced in 5 eyes (26.31%), and RNFL-OT was reduced in 16 eyes (94.74%). Regarding the involvement of each sector, abnormal thickness values were found in 9 (47.37%) ODD-S eyes and in 3 (15.79%) ODD-D eyes for RNFL-TT; in 11

(67.89%) ODD-S eyes and in 3 (15.79%) ODD-D eyes for RNFL-ST; in 14 (73.68%) ODD-S eyes and 5 (26.32%) ODD-D eyes for RNFL-IT; in 5 (26.32%) ODD-S eyes and in 1 (5.26%) ODD-D eye for RNFL-NT; and in 12 (63.16%) ODD-S eyes and in 4 (21.05%) ODD-D eyes for RNFL-OT. GC-T was found to be reduced in 13 ODD eyes (73.68%), more specifically, in 10 (52.63%) ODD-S and in 3 (15.79%) ODD-D eyes, respectively. On average, in the ODD Group, the mean RNFL thickness values were significantly reduced ($p < 0.01$) as compared to those of the Controls in several sectors (RNFL-TT, ST, OT and IT) apart from the nasal one; for instance, RNFL-NT was not statistically different ($p = 0.986$) when compared to that in the Controls.

Considering selectively ODD-S eyes, the visible height was linearly significantly correlated with the RNFL-OT ($p < 0.01$, see Figure 2C) and RNFL-NT ($r = -0.815$, $p = 0.0003$) values. The ODD visible height was not significantly correlated with the RNFL-TT ($r = -0.477$, $p = 0.0873$), RNFL-ST ($r = -0.648$, $p = 0.0120$), RNFL-IT ($r = -0.558$, $p = 0.0377$) or GC-T ($r = -0.407$, $p = 0.1482$) values.

4. Discussion

To provide a contribution for a better understanding of the impact of ODD on the morpho-functional condition of different elements forming the visual pathways, our aim was to assess whether the presence of ODD (superficial or deep) could induce changes in BCVA and/or VF defects, morphological and functional impairments in RGCs and their fibers, and/or a dysfunction of the neural conduction along the small and large axons of the visual pathways. Nevertheless, due to the small number of observed ODD-D (n = 5) cases, not sufficient to provide an adequate sample size (see the Statistics Section), we were not able to make a statistical comparison between the ODD-S and ODD-D subgroups. In the eyes with ODD-S, the relevance of the visible height to the psychophysical, electrophysiological and morphological findings was also investigated.

Briefly, in the ODD Group, as compared to the Controls, we observed the following major findings:

(1) A normal BCVA (0.0 LogMAR) but a significantly reduced HFA MD and increased HFA PSD values, correlated with increased 15′ VEP ITs;
(2) Significantly reduced 60′ and 15′ PERG and VEP A values and significantly increased 60′ and 15′ VEP IT values;
(3) A significantly reduced RNFL-T in all sectors apart from the nasal one and a reduced GC-T.

In the ODD-S eyes, the values of perimetric changes, the reduced PERG As, the increased VEP ITs and the reduction in RNFL-OT were significantly linearly correlated with the ODD visible height. VF, PERG, VEP and RNFL-OT changes were greater for an ODD visible height > 300 microns. Surprisingly, most of our patients presented with unilateral drusen and not bilateral drusen, as expected. It is likely that Ss-OCT was not as able as EDI-OCT to detect small and deep drusen; therefore, it is possible that small or deep drusen of the contralateral eye were not detected.

4.1. ODD and Visual Field Changes: HFA Data

Even though our patients with ODD did not report any visual disturbances, VF defects were found in almost one-third (36.8%) of the studied ODD eyes (regarding the HFA MD values), and perimetric changes were mainly identified in the ODD-S eyes.

This agrees with all that reported in the literature, since ODD is almost always an incidental finding during an ophthalmological examination. VF defects have been associated with ODD in 51% of children [13], 75% of affected individuals overall [36] and up to 87% of cases [37], being more commonly observed in ODD-S eyes [36,38–41], with a trend of progression during adolescence and minimal worsening thereafter [42,43]. VF defects, most commonly enlarged blind spots, aspecific defects, bundle defects and concentric narrowing [21], have been suggested to be due to the compression of the RGCs' fibers by calcified ODD, leading to RGC death and axonal degeneration [16], the blockage of axonal transport [2,44] or, alternatively, vascular failure [13]. In any case, ODD make patients more susceptible to vision loss due to anterior ischemic optic neuropathy [37,45], central retinal artery occlusion [46], central retinal vein occlusion [47] and choroidal neovascularization [48]. However, ODD-D have been associated with preserved VF in many cases (95% of eyes examined by Katz and Pomeranz) [16].

Moreover, in the ODD-S eyes, the reduction in MD and the increase in the PSD values were significantly ($p < 0.01$) correlated with the ODD visible height, so the higher the ODD, the worse the perimetric impairment. Our results agree with those reported by Malmqvist et al., who suggested that a worse VF defect is associated with a larger volume of visible ODD, applying a model process going from EDI-OCT scans to the 3D volume of ODD [22].

Overall, it is worth noting that a large percentage (63.2%) of ODD eyes showed normal HFA MD and PSD values despite abnormal values of the PERG or VEP parameters being detected in the same eyes. This finding is similar to that observed in patients with ocular hypertension (OHT), in whom PERG and VEP abnormalities were detected despite the presence of unaltered HFA sensitivity [30,31]. The finding of a PERG A reduction in patients with OHT was explained by the data showing that a loss of at least 20% of RGCs is required to induce a reduction in retinal sensitivity evaluated using HFA [49], and, therefore, RGC dysfunction may precede the observation of RGC death, leading to HFA defects [30,31].

In addition, we found that the reduced HFA MD values were significantly ($p < 0.01$) correlated with the increased 15′ VEP IT values, thus meaning that the presence of ODD produced proportionate disturbances in both VF and the neural conduction of the small axons of the visual pathways. The correlation between the HFA values and the 60′ VEP IT values was near significance ($p = 0.0129$), and this can suggest that the neural conduction along the large axons might also contribute to the reduced HFA MD.

4.2. ODD and Retinal Ganglion Cell Function: PERG Data

In the ODD eyes, the function of RGCs and their fibers was studied using PERG recordings [15,28,33,50]. In the PERG analysis, we measured the P50-N95 amplitude, since this parameter is considered the most specific for assessing RGCs and their fibers' function [51,52]. Since it was described that PERG P50 IT might be influenced by the pre-ganglionic elements' function [27,30,51], this parameter was not taken into consideration. The notion that PERG A is a sensitive tool for monitoring RGC function under the compressive effect of ODD was also recently suggested by Pojda-Wilczek et al. [7].

A PERG A reduction was found in more than 70% of individual studied eyes. On average, with respect to the Control eyes, in the ODD Group, we observed a significant reduction in both 15′ and 60′ PERG A. Our findings are consistent with previously reported data [14] of reduced PERG A in ODD eyes.

Our detected PERG abnormalities can be ascribed to the RGC involvement secondary to a local disturbance of axoplasmic transport at the optic disc for the mechanical compression of prelaminar RNFL caused by ODD and for some retrograde distension of the RGC body [44]. This is also supported by experimental studies of optic neuropathies, in which it was suggested that abnormalities in retrograde axoplasmic transport alter the integrity of PERG A [53]. Thus, based on these concepts and previous findings [53], the PERG A reduction observed in our study suggests that ODD compression may induce an impaired function of the RGCs' fibers.

An interesting finding provided by our results was the significant correlation between the 15′ PERG A reduction and the increased ODD-S visible height, suggesting that "the greater the visible height, the worse the RGCs function". This might mean that ODD-S, localized above BMO, could determine direct compression at the level of intraretinal vasculature inducing localized ischemic damage [19] and, consequently, RGC dysfunction. Based on our data, it should be suggested that a minimum visible height of 300 microns is relevant for inducing RGC abnormalities.

4.3. ODD and Neural Conduction along the Visual Pathways: VEP Data

In our ODD eyes, the neural conduction along the large and small axons forming the visual pathways up to the visual cortex was assessed by recording VEP in response to 60′ and 15′ checks [26,27,29].

Abnormal values were detected for 60′ and 15′ VEP IT in a large percentage (63.15% and 52.63%, respectively) of individual ODD eyes. A similar condition was found when recording 60′ and 15′ VEP A. On average, with respect to the Control eyes, in the ODD Group, a significant increase in VEP ITs and a significant reduction in VEP A were found.

Our findings suggest an impairment of the neural conduction along the visual pathways, but this dysfunction was not univocally observed in previous studies, since abnormal VEP IT responses were reported in a wide range (from 0 to 83%) of studied ODD eyes [13,54–56].

Our detected VEP abnormalities, according to the study by Malmqivist [22], should be ascribed to hypothesized damage due to mechanical compression on the optic nerve fibers with the consequent involvement of anterograde axonal transport up to the visual cortex.

In our ODD eyes, we found a lack of correlation between the PERG A and VEP IT responses, thus suggesting that retrograde (impairment of RGCs) and anterograde (abnormal neural conduction along the small and large axons of the visual pathways) axoplasmic transport impairment might occur, but in an unrelated way.

In the ODD-S eyes, similarly to the HFA and PERG findings, increased 60′ and 15′ VEP ITs were significantly ($p < 0.01$) correlated with the ODD visible height. It is likely that, also in this case, "the higher the ODD, the worse the neural conduction along small and large axons of the visual pathways", with a relevant effect for ODD visible height values > 300 microns.

4.4. ODD and Retinal Nerve Fiber Layer and Ganglion Cell Thicknesses: OCT Data

With respect to the Control eyes, in the ODD Group, the RNFL thickness was significantly reduced in all sectors but the nasal one. These findings are in agreement with those in a previous report describing an RNFL-T reduction predominantly in other sectors [19], sparing the nasal one, but they are in contrast with those in some other reviews describing a predominance of ODD on the nasal side of the optic disc, with RNFL thinning in the same sector [4,10].

RNFL thinning that is associated with the number [5] or the ODD diameter [23] might indicate a process of indirect optic nerve axonal degeneration that can be due to either mechanical compression by the ODD [10] or vascular failure, as suggested by the observed reduced vessel density studied using Ss-OCT angiography in ODD eyes [19].

In the absence of a comparison in this study between the ODD-S and ODD-D subgroups, we were not able to compare our findings to those in previous reports finding a greater reduction in RNFL-OT in ODD-S eyes than in ODD-D eyes [17,38,39].

In our ODD-S eyes, as for the HFA, PERG and VEP findings, a linear significant correlation between the ODD visible height and the reduction in RNFL-OT was detected, suggesting that "the higher the ODD, the worse the RNFL integrity". Also in this case, a visible height > 300 microns might be suggested as relevant to inducing a structural impairment.

Regarding the reduced GC-T observed in our ODD Group when compared to the Control one, this finding is in agreement with that in other previous works [4,19,57]. We suppose that this morphological change may be due to all mechanisms previously suggested to explain the PERG A reduction, such as those briefly summarized as retrograde neurodegeneration after compression.

Nevertheless, since PERG represents an electrophysiological tool for the functional assessment of RGCs located in the entire retina and the CG thickness was measured from the macular area, we believed that it was not appropriate to perform a correlation between the functional (PERG A) and morphological (GC-T) findings.

Moreover, in the ODD-S eyes, unlike the RNFL thickness, the GC-T reduction was not significantly correlated with the ODD visible height.

It has been suggested that a macular GC analysis might be more useful for detecting early structural involvement with respect to RNFL thickness analyses, particularly in ODD-D eyes, because ODD-D often produce an RNFL thickening that can mask axonal damage, yielding a false negative result [57]. Regarding this, however, our study cannot provide results confirming this suggested evidence.

5. Conclusions

In conclusion, our findings suggest that the presence of ODD might induce morphological changes in RGCs and their fibers (as for the reduced RFNFL and GC-T) and a dysfunction of RGCs and their fibers (as derived by abnormal PERG responses) and an unrelated impairment of neural conduction along the large and small axons forming the visual pathways (indicated by abnormal VEP responses). All these changes either lead or do not lead to visual field defects. The observed morpho-functional impairment should be ascribed to alterations in retrograde (from the axons to the RGCs) and anterograde (from the RGCs up to the visual cortex) axoplasmic transport. In ODD-S eyes, a visible height of 300 microns represented the threshold for the abnormalities, suggesting that "the higher the ODD, the worse the impairment".

We acknowledge that this study may present some limitations. These are the reduced number of participants; the absence of a follow-up; the non-standardized method of measurement for the visible height of ODD; and the use of SS-OCT instead of EDI (enhanced depth imaging) OCT, which allows for a better visualization of ODD with less artifacts. Regarding this point, however, a recent study showed no significant difference between SS-OCT and the EDI-OCT acquisitions in detecting ODD [58].

Author Contributions: Conceptualization, G.A., L.Z., L.B. and V.P.; methodology, V.P.; software, A.D.R.; validation, G.A., L.Z. and V.P.; formal analysis, G.A. and L.B.; investigation, G.A. and L.B.; resources, L.B.; data curation, G.A.; writing—original draft preparation, G.A. and L.B.; writing—review and editing, L.Z. and V.P.; visualization, G.A.; supervision, V.P.; project administration, V.P.; funding acquisition, L.Z. and V.P. All authors have read and agreed to the published version of the manuscript.

Funding: This research received no external funding.

Institutional Review Board Statement: The study was conducted in accordance with the Declaration of Helsinki and was approved by the local Ethical Committee Institutional Review Board (Comitato Etico Centrale IRCCS Lazio, Sezione IFO/Fondazione Bietti, Rome, Italy) with the protocol code: NEU_03-2021; 125/21/F.

Informed Consent Statement: Informed consent was obtained from all subjects involved in the study.

Data Availability Statement: Available on request.

Acknowledgments: The contribution of Fondazione Bietti to this paper was supported by the Italian Ministry of Health and Fondazione Roma. The authors acknowledge Federica Petrocchi and Elisa Tronti for executing visual psychophysical assessments and Maria Luisa Alessi for providing technical assistance in electrophysiology and figure presentation.

Conflicts of Interest: The authors declare no conflict of interest. The funders had no role in the design of the study; in the collection, analyses, or interpretation of data; in the writing of the manuscript; or in the decision to publish the results.

Abbreviations

ODD	Optic disc drusen
ODD-S	Superficial optic disc drusen
ODD-D	Deep optic disc drusen
EDI-OCT	Enhanced depth imaging OCT
RGCs	Retinal ganglion cells
PERG	Pattern Electroretinogram
VEP	Visual Evoked Potential
CL	Confidence limit
ANOVA	One-way analysis of variance
RNFL	Retinal nerve fiber layer
BCVA	Best-corrected visual acuity measurement
ETDRS	Early Treatment Diabetic Retinopathy Study
LogMAR	Logarithm of the minimum angle of resolution
IOP	Intraocular pressure
HFA	Humphrey Field Analyzer
MD	Mean deviation
PSD	Pattern standard deviation
ISCEV	International Society for Clinical Electrophysiology of Vision
PERG A	Pattern Electroretinogram amplitude
VEP IT	Visual Evoked Potential implicit time
VEP A	Visual Evoked Potential amplitude
SNR	Signal-to-noise ratio
BMO	Bruch's membrane opening
SD	Standard deviation
GC	Ganglion cell
OHT	Ocular hypertension
VF	Visual field
SS-OCT	Swept-source optical coherence tomography
TT	Temporal Thickness
ST	Superior Thickness
IT	Inferior Thickness
NT	Nasal Thickness

References

1. Friedman, A.H.; Beckerman, B.; Gold, D.H.; Walsh, J.B.; Gartner, S. Drusen of the Optic Disc. *Surv. Ophthalmol.* **1977**, *21*, 373–390. [CrossRef] [PubMed]
2. Tso, M.O.M. Pathology and Pathogenesis of Drusen of the Optic Nervehead. *Ophthalmology* **1981**, *88*, 1066–1080. [CrossRef] [PubMed]
3. Auw-Haedrich, C.; Staubach, F.; Witschel, H. Optic Disk Drusen. *Surv. Ophthalmol.* **2002**, *47*, 515–532. [CrossRef] [PubMed]
4. Allegrini, D.; Pagano, L.; Ferrara, M.; Borgia, A.; Sorrentino, T.; Montesano, G.; Angi, M.; Romano, M.R. Optic Disc Drusen: A Systematic Review: Up-to-Date and Future Perspective. *Int. Ophthalmol.* **2020**, *40*, 2119–2127. [CrossRef]
5. Roh, S.; Noecker, R.J.; Schuman, J.S.; Hedges, T.R.; Weiter, J.J.; Mattox, C. Effect of Optic Nerve Head Drusen on Nerve Fiber Layer Thickness. *Ophthalmology* **1998**, *105*, 878–885. [CrossRef]
6. Malmqvist, L.; Bursztyn, L.; Costello, F.; Digre, K.; Fraser, J.A.; Fraser, C.; Katz, B.; Lawlor, M.; Petzold, A.; Sibony, P.; et al. The Optic Disc Drusen Studies Consortium Recommendations for Diagnosis of Optic Disc Drusen Using Optical Coherence Tomography. *J. Neuroophthalmol.* **2018**, *38*, 299–307. [CrossRef]
7. Pojda-Wilczek, D.; Wycisło-Gawron, P. The Effect of a Decrease in Intraocular Pressure on Optic Nerve Function in Patients with Optic Nerve Drusen. *Ophthalmic. Res.* **2019**, *61*, 153–158. [CrossRef]
8. Silverman, A.L.; Tatham, A.J.; Medeiros, F.A.; Weinreb, R.N. Assessment of Optic Nerve Head Drusen Using Enhanced Depth Imaging and Swept Source Optical Coherence Tomography. *J. Neuroophthalmol.* **2014**, *34*, 198–205. [CrossRef]
9. Morris, R.W.; Ellerbrock, J.M.; Hamp, A.M.; Joy, J.T.; Roels, P.; Davis, C.N. Advanced Visual Field Loss Secondary to Optic Nerve Head Drusen: Case Report and Literature Review. *Optometry* **2009**, *80*, 83–100. [CrossRef]
10. Hamann, S.; Malmqvist, L.; Costello, F. Optic Disc Drusen: Understanding an Old Problem from a New Perspective. *Acta Ophthalmol.* **2018**, *96*, 673–684. [CrossRef]
11. Robson, A.G.; Frishman, L.J.; Grigg, J.; Hamilton, R.; Jeffrey, B.G.; Kondo, M.; Li, S.; McCulloch, D.L. ISCEV Standard for Full-Field Clinical Electroretinography (2022 Update). *Doc. Ophthalmol.* **2022**, *144*, 165–177. [CrossRef] [PubMed]

12. Odom, J.V.; Bach, M.; Brigell, M.; Holder, G.E.; McCulloch, D.L.; Tormene, A.P.; Vaegan. ISCEV Standard for Clinical Visual Evoked Potentials (2009 Update). *Doc. Ophthalmol.* **2010**, *120*, 111–119. [CrossRef] [PubMed]
13. Chang, M.Y.; Pineles, S.L. Optic Disc Drusen in Children. *Surv. Ophthalmol.* **2016**, *61*, 745–758. [CrossRef] [PubMed]
14. Scholl, G.B.; Song, H.S.; Winkler, D.E.; Wray, S.H. The Pattern Visual Evoked Potential and Pattern Electroretinogram in Drusen-Associated Optic Neuropathy. *Arch. Ophthalmol.* **1992**, *110*, 75–81. [CrossRef] [PubMed]
15. Luo, X.; Frishman, L.J. Retinal Pathway Origins of the Pattern Electroretinogram (PERG). *Investig. Ophthalmol. Vis. Sci.* **2011**, *52*, 8571–8584. [CrossRef]
16. Katz, B.J.; Pomeranz, H.D. Visual Field Defects and Retinal Nerve Fiber Layer Defects in Eyes with Buried Optic Nerve Drusen. *Am. J. Ophthalmol.* **2006**, *141*, 248–253. [CrossRef]
17. Gili, P.; Flores-Rodríguez, P.; Martin-Ríos, M.D.; Carrasco Font, C. Anatomical and Functional Impairment of the Nerve Fiber Layer in Patients with Optic Nerve Head Drusen. *Graefe's Arch. Clin. Exp. Ophthalmol.* **2013**, *251*, 2421–2428. [CrossRef]
18. Lee, K.M.; Woo, S.J.; Hwang, J.-M. Morphologic Characteristics of Optic Nerve Head Drusen on Spectral-Domain Optical Coherence Tomography. *Am. J. Ophthalmol.* **2013**, *155*, 1139–1147.e1. [CrossRef]
19. Engelke, H.; Shajari, M.; Riedel, J.; Mohr, N.; Priglinger, S.G.; Mackert, M.J. OCT Angiography in Optic Disc Drusen: Comparison with Structural and Functional Parameters. *Br. J. Ophthalmol.* **2020**, *104*, 1109–1113. [CrossRef]
20. Tsikata, E.; Verticchio Vercellin, A.C.; Falkenstein, I.; Poon, L.Y.-C.; Brauner, S.; Khoueir, Z.; Miller, J.B.; Chen, T.C. Volumetric Measurement of Optic Nerve Head Drusen Using Swept Source Optical Coherence Tomography. *J. Glaucoma* **2017**, *26*, 798–804. [CrossRef]
21. Lee, K.M.; Woo, S.J.; Hwang, J.-M. Factors Associated with Visual Field Defects of Optic Disc Drusen. *PLoS ONE* **2018**, *13*, e0196001. [CrossRef]
22. Malmqvist, L.; Lindberg, A.-S.W.; Dahl, V.A.; Jørgensen, T.M.; Hamann, S. Quantitatively Measured Anatomic Location and Volume of Optic Disc Drusen: An Enhanced Depth Imaging Optical Coherence Tomography Study. *Investig. Ophthalmol. Vis. Sci.* **2017**, *58*, 2491–2497. [CrossRef]
23. Sato, T.; Mrejen, S.; Spaide, R.F. Multimodal Imaging of Optic Disc Drusen. *Am. J. Ophthalmol.* **2013**, *156*, 275–282.e1. [CrossRef]
24. Traber, G.L.; Weber, K.P.; Sabah, M.; Keane, P.A.; Plant, G.T. Enhanced Depth Imaging Optical Coherence Tomography of Optic Nerve Head Drusen: A Comparison of Cases with and without Visual Field Loss. *Ophthalmology* **2017**, *124*, 66–73. [CrossRef]
25. Scuderi, G.L.; Cesareo, M.; Perdicchi, A.; Recupero, S.M. Standard Automated Perimetry and Algorithms for Monitoring Glaucoma Progression. *Prog. Brain Res.* **2008**, *173*, 77–99. [CrossRef]
26. Parisi, V.; Scarale, M.E.; Balducci, N.; Fresina, M.; Campos, E.C. Electrophysiological Detection of Delayed Postretinal Neural Conduction in Human Amblyopia. *Investig. Ophthalmol. Vis. Sci.* **2010**, *51*, 5041–5048. [CrossRef]
27. Parisi, V.; Ziccardi, L.; Sadun, F.; De Negri, A.M.; La Morgia, C.; Barbano, L.; Carelli, V.; Barboni, P. Functional Changes of Retinal Ganglion Cells and Visual Pathways in Patients with Chronic Leber's Hereditary Optic Neuropathy during One Year of Follow-Up. *Ophthalmology* **2019**, *126*, 1033–1044. [CrossRef]
28. Parisi, V.; Manni, G.; Spadaro, M.; Colacino, G.; Restuccia, R.; Marchi, S.; Bucci, M.G.; Pierelli, F. Correlation between Morphological and Functional Retinal Impairment in Multiple Sclerosis Patients. *Investig. Ophthalmol. Vis. Sci.* **1999**, *40*, 2520–2527.
29. Ziccardi, L.; Sadun, F.; De Negri, A.M.; Barboni, P.; Savini, G.; Borrelli, E.; La Morgia, C.; Carelli, V.; Parisi, V. Retinal Function and Neural Conduction along the Visual Pathways in Affected and Unaffected Carriers with Leber's Hereditary Optic Neuropathy. *Investig. Ophthalmol. Vis. Sci.* **2013**, *54*, 6893–6901. [CrossRef]
30. Parisi, V.; Miglior, S.; Manni, G.; Centofanti, M.; Bucci, M.G. Clinical Ability of Pattern Electroretinograms and Visual Evoked Potentials in Detecting Visual Dysfunction in Ocular Hypertension and Glaucoma. *Ophthalmology* **2006**, *113*, 216–228. [CrossRef]
31. Parisi, V. Impaired Visual Function in Glaucoma. *Clin. Neurophysiol.* **2001**, *112*, 351–358. [CrossRef] [PubMed]
32. Harter, M.R.; White, C.T. Evoked Cortical Responses to Checkerboard Patterns: Effect of Check-Size as a Function of Visual Acuity. *Electroencephalogr. Clin. Neurophysiol.* **1970**, *28*, 48–54. [CrossRef] [PubMed]
33. Fiorentini, A.; Maffei, L.; Pirchio, M.; Spinelli, D.; Porciatti, V. The ERG in Response to Alternating Gratings in Patients with Diseases of the Peripheral Visual Pathway. *Investig. Ophthalmol. Vis. Sci.* **1981**, *21*, 490–493.
34. Klem, G.H.; Lüders, H.O.; Jasper, H.H.; Elger, C. The Ten-Twenty Electrode System of the International Federation. The International Federation of Clinical Neurophysiology. *Electroencephalogr. Clin. Neurophysiol. Suppl.* **1999**, *52*, 3–6. [PubMed]
35. Cruz-Herranz, A.; Balk, L.J.; Oberwahrenbrock, T.; Saidha, S.; Martinez-Lapiscina, E.H.; Lagreze, W.A.; Schuman, J.S.; Villoslada, P.; Calabresi, P.; Balcer, L.; et al. The APOSTEL Recommendations for Reporting Quantitative Optical Coherence Tomography Studies. *Neurology* **2016**, *86*, 2303–2309. [CrossRef]
36. Savino, P.J.; Glaser, J.S.; Rosenberg, M.A. A Clinical Analysis of Pseudopapilledema. II. Visual Field Defects. *Arch. Ophthalmol.* **1979**, *97*, 71–75. [CrossRef]
37. Lorentzen, S.E. Drusen of the Optic Disk. A Clinical and Genetic Study. *Acta Ophthalmol. Suppl.* **1966**, *90*, 1–180.
38. Mistlberger, A.; Sitte, S.; Hommer, A.; Emesz, M.; Dengg, S.; Hitzl, W.; Grabner, G. Scanning Laser Polarimetry (SLP) for Optic Nerve Head Drusen. *Int. Ophthalmol.* **2001**, *23*, 233–237. [CrossRef]
39. Malmqvist, L.; Wegener, M.; Sander, B.A.; Hamann, S. Peripapillary Retinal Nerve Fiber Layer Thickness Corresponds to Drusen Location and Extent of Visual Field Defects in Superficial and Buried Optic Disc Drusen. *J. Neuroophthalmol.* **2016**, *36*, 41–45. [CrossRef]

40. Wilkins, J.M.; Pomeranz, H.D. Visual Manifestations of Visible and Buried Optic Disc Drusen. *J. Neuroophthalmol.* **2004**, *24*, 125–129. [CrossRef]
41. Mustonen, E. Pseudopapilloedema with and without Verified Optic Disc Drusen. A Clinical Analysis II: Visual Fields. *Acta Ophthalmol.* **1983**, *61*, 1057–1066. [CrossRef]
42. Malmqvist, L.; Lund-Andersen, H.; Hamann, S. Long-Term Evolution of Superficial Optic Disc Drusen. *Acta Ophthalmol.* **2017**, *95*, 352–356. [CrossRef]
43. Frisén, L. Evolution of Drusen of the Optic Nerve Head over 23 Years. *Acta Ophthalmol.* **2008**, *86*, 111–112. [CrossRef]
44. Spencer, W.H. XXXIV Edward Jackson Memorial Lecture: Drusen of the Optic Disc and Aberrant Axoplasmic Transport. *Ophthalmology* **1978**, *85*, 21–38. [CrossRef]
45. Purvin, V.; King, R.; Kawasaki, A.; Yee, R. Anterior Ischemic Optic Neuropathy in Eyes with Optic Disc Drusen. *Arch. Ophthalmol.* **2004**, *122*, 48–53. [CrossRef]
46. Farah, S.G.; Mansour, A.M. Central Retinal Artery Occlusion and Optic Disc Drusen. *Eye* **1998**, *12 Pt 3a*, 480–482. [CrossRef]
47. Green, W.R.; Chan, C.C.; Hutchins, G.M.; Terry, J.M. Central Retinal Vein Occlusion: A Prospective Histopathologic Study of 29 Eyes in 28 Cases. *Retina* **1981**, *1*, 27–55. [CrossRef]
48. Duncan, J.E.; Freedman, S.F.; El-Dairi, M.A. The Incidence of Neovascular Membranes and Visual Field Defects from Optic Nerve Head Drusen in Children. *J. AAPOS* **2016**, *20*, 44–48. [CrossRef]
49. Quigley, H.A.; Dunkelberger, G.R.; Green, W.R. Retinal Ganglion Cell Atrophy Correlated with Automated Perimetry in Human Eyes with Glaucoma. *Am. J. Ophthalmol.* **1989**, *107*, 453–464. [CrossRef]
50. Maffei, L.; Fiorentini, A. Electroretinographic Responses to Alternating Gratings in the Cat. *Exp. Brain Res.* **1982**, *48*, 327–334. [CrossRef]
51. Viswanathan, S.; Frishman, L.J.; Robson, J.G. The Uniform Field and Pattern ERG in Macaques with Experimental Glaucoma: Removal of Spiking Activity. *Investig. Ophthalmol. Vis. Sci.* **2000**, *41*, 2797–2810.
52. Parisi, V. Correlation between Morphological and Functional Retinal Impairment in Patients Affected by Ocular Hypertension, Glaucoma, Demyelinating Optic Neuritis and Alzheimer's Disease. *Semin. Ophthalmol.* **2003**, *18*, 50–57. [CrossRef] [PubMed]
53. Chou, T.-H.; Park, K.K.; Luo, X.; Porciatti, V. Retrograde Signaling in the Optic Nerve Is Necessary for Electrical Responsiveness of Retinal Ganglion Cells. *Investig. Ophthalmol. Vis. Sci.* **2013**, *54*, 1236–1243. [CrossRef] [PubMed]
54. Brudet-Wickel, C.L.; Van Lith, G.H.; Graniewski-Wijnands, H.S. Drusen of the Optic Disc and Occipital Transient Pattern Reversal Responses. *Doc. Ophthalmol.* **1981**, *50*, 243–248. [CrossRef]
55. Mustonen, E.; Sulg, I.; Kallanranta, T. Electroretinogram (ERG) and Visual Evoked Response (VER) Studies in Patients with Optic Disc Drusen. *Acta Ophthalmol.* **1980**, *58*, 539–549. [CrossRef]
56. Bishara, S.; Feinsod, M. Visual Evoked Response as an Aid in Diagnosing Optic Nerve Head Drusen: Case Report. *J. Pediatr. Ophthalmol. Strabismus* **1980**, *17*, 396–398. [CrossRef]
57. Casado, A.; Rebolleda, G.; Guerrero, L.; Leal, M.; Contreras, I.; Oblanca, N.; Muñoz-Negrete, F.J. Measurement of Retinal Nerve Fiber Layer and Macular Ganglion Cell-Inner Plexiform Layer with Spectral-Domain Optical Coherence Tomography in Patients with Optic Nerve Head Drusen. *Graefe's Arch. Clin. Exp. Ophthalmol.* **2014**, *252*, 1653–1660. [CrossRef]
58. Rothenbuehler, S.P.; Malmqvist, L.; Belmouhand, M.; Bjerager, J.; Maloca, P.M.; Larsen, M.; Hamann, S. Comparison of Spectral-Domain OCT versus Swept-Source OCT for the Detection of Deep Optic Disc Drusen. *Diagnostics* **2022**, *12*, 2515. [CrossRef]

Journal of
Clinical Medicine

MDPI

Review

ROCK Inhibitors in Corneal Diseases and Glaucoma—A Comprehensive Review of These Emerging Drugs

Luca Pagano [1], Jason William Lee [2], Matteo Posarelli [3,4], Giuseppe Giannaccare [5,*], Stephen Kaye [3] and Alfredo Borgia [3,6]

1 Department of Biomedical Sciences, Humanitas University, 20072 Milano, Italy; luca.pagano@humanitas.it
2 Clinical Eye Research Centre, St Paul's Eye Unit, Royal Liverpool University Hospital, Liverpool L7 8YE, UK; jason.lee1@rlbuht.nhs.uk
3 Department of Corneal Diseases, St. Paul's Eye Unit, Royal Liverpool University Hospital, Liverpool L7 8YE, UK; mposarelli@gmail.com (M.P.); stephen.kaye@liverpoolft.nhs.uk (S.K.); alfredo.borgia@liverpoolft.nhs.uk (A.B.)
4 Ophthalmology Unit of the Department of Medicine, Surgery and Neuroscience, University of Siena, 53100 Siena, Italy
5 Eye Clinic, Department of Surgical Sciences, University of Cagliari, 09124 Cagliari, Italy
6 Eye Unit, Humanitas-Gradenigo Hospital, 10122 Turin, Italy
* Correspondence: giuseppe.giannaccare@unica.it; Tel.: +39-096-1364-7041

Abstract: Rho kinase (ROCK) inhibitors have gained significant attention as emerging novel treatment options in the field of ophthalmology in recent years. The evidence supporting their efficacy in glaucoma and corneal pathology includes both in vitro and clinical studies. Among the available options, ripasudil and netarsudil have emerged as the leading ROCK inhibitors, and some countries have approved these therapeutic options as treatments for glaucoma. Various dosing regimens have been studied, including monotherapy and combination therapy, especially for patients with secondary glaucoma who are already on multiple medications. Another rising application of ROCK inhibitors includes their use as an adjunct in surgical procedures such as Descemetorhexis Without Endothelial Keratoplasty (DWEK), Descemet Stripping Only (DSO) to accelerate visual recovery, glaucoma surgeries to reduce scarring process and allow better intraocular pressure (IOP) control, or after complicated anterior segment surgery to treat corneal oedema. This article provides a comprehensive overview of the existing literature in the field, offering recommendations for prescribing ROCK inhibitors and also discussing patient selection, drug efficacy, and possible adverse effects.

Keywords: rho kinase; cornea guttata; Descemet membrane; glaucoma; ripasudil; netarsudil

1. Introduction

Addressing glaucoma and corneal disease can present substantial difficulties, often necessitating medical therapy as the primary mode of treatment. Polypharmacy is prevalent among patients with glaucoma; half of patients with newly diagnosed glaucoma initially require more than one medication to control IOP, and a further 30% require add-on treatment after one year [1]. Furthermore, many of the current medications have systemic side effects and there is evidence suggesting that intensification of medical therapy has diminishing returns and increased clinical and economic burdens [2]. There is, therefore, an ongoing need for novel therapies, and one promising emerging therapy is Rho kinase (ROCK) inhibitors, which have gained significant attention in the last ten years. The Rho kinase (ROCK) signaling cascade is ubiquitously present in all tissues of the human body, and it regulates different cellular processes such as replication, proliferation, and apoptosis [3]. In the eye, it regulates the physiological properties of the trabecular meshwork and corneal endothelium. Thus, the ROCK signaling cascade was hypothesized to be a potential therapeutic target. In addition to opening new therapeutic options in glaucoma,

ROCK inhibitors have shown promise in the treatment of corneal endothelial diseases by promoting corneal endothelial cell regeneration and both functional and morphological recovery [4]. Laboratory studies have suggested that ROCK inhibitors improve cellular attachment and proliferation of cultured endothelial cells in vitro and improve wound healing on ex vivo corneas [5]. They facilitate cell cycle progression from the G1 to S phase and prevent actinomyosin contraction by inhibiting the Rho kinase signaling cascade [6]. Therefore, ROCK inhibitors serve a niche in either in current routinely performed anterior segment surgery to minimize complications or to enhance novel techniques such as Descemetorhexis Without Endothelial Keratoplasty (DWEK) [7]. However, there are variable levels of acceptance among healthcare professionals worldwide, and these drugs are still far from being routinely used in routine ophthalmology practice.

Three commercially available ROCK inhibitors currently exist: ripasudil (Glanatec®), netarsudil (Rhopressa®), and fasudil. Ripasudil has been used in the treatment of ocular hypertension and glaucoma in Japan since September 2014 and has been recently approved for commercial use in the United Kingdom. Netarsudil has been used for glaucoma treatment in the United States since late 2017 and more recently has been approved in Europe in November 2021. Fasudil was originally approved in Japan in 1995 for the treatment of cerebral vasospasms caused by subarachnoid hemorrhage [8], and it is used in ophthalmology for the treatment of diabetic macular edema (DME) [9]. Finally, two ROCK inhibitors have not been approved yet: SNJ-1656, currently in phase II trial for controlling intraocular pressure (IOP) [10], and Y-27632, still in a pre-clinical phase for use in corneal endothelial diseases [5].

As the utilization of ROCK inhibitors are increasing among ophthalmologists globally, it is crucial to better understand the potential benefits and safety of these pharmaceutical products for both approved and off-label use. In this regard, we present a comprehensive review covering the current level of knowledge in the existing literature, aiming to provide evidence-based recommendations for prescribing ROCK inhibitors. This review will also discuss patient selection, efficacy, and adverse effects of these drugs with a particular focus on the two FDA-approved molecules ripasudil and netarsudil.

2. The Rho Kinase Pathway

There are two isoforms of ROCK, ROCK1 (ROKβ) and ROCK2 (ROKα), which may have slightly different effects depending on the isoform [11,12]. The activation of RhoA is regulated by guanine nucleotide exchange factors (GEFs), GTPase activating proteins (GAPs), and guanine nucleotide dissociation inhibitors (GDIs) [11,12]. Once activated, RhoA proteins trigger the activation of ROCKs, which phosphorylate various target proteins involved in actin-related processes such as actomyosin contraction, cell adhesion, cell morphology and stiffness, and cell migration [11]. These general processes play a key role in modulating various eye mechanisms (Figure 1), such as aqueous humor outflow regulation [11,13], corneal tissue regeneration [10], or optic nerve vessel vasodilation [13].

In glaucoma, endothelin-1 (ET-1)-induced ROCK signaling plays a role in regulating retinal blood flow and vasomotor tone, resulting in the promotion of vasoconstriction [14]. Administration of ROCK inhibitors has been shown to enhance ocular blood flow in both normal and disease rabbit models, as well as in normal rat models. This was demonstrated by increased blood flow in the optic nerve head when assessed using LASER speckle flowgraphy [8,15]. ROCK inhibitors administration induces the relaxation of vascular smooth muscle cells, leading to the dilation of ONH blood vessels.

Additionally, ROCK inhibitors can alter the trabecular meshwork cell shapes improving the control of intraocular pressure (IOP). In the cornea, ROCK inhibition has been shown to induce metabolic changes in endothelial cells, such as increased mitochondrial metabolic activity and upregulation of oxidative phosphorylation through the AMPK pathway [16], which would support the change in cellular function described above. Furthermore, the ROCK pathway has also been implicated in retinal diseases such as diabetic retinopathy [17] and diabetic macular oedema [18].

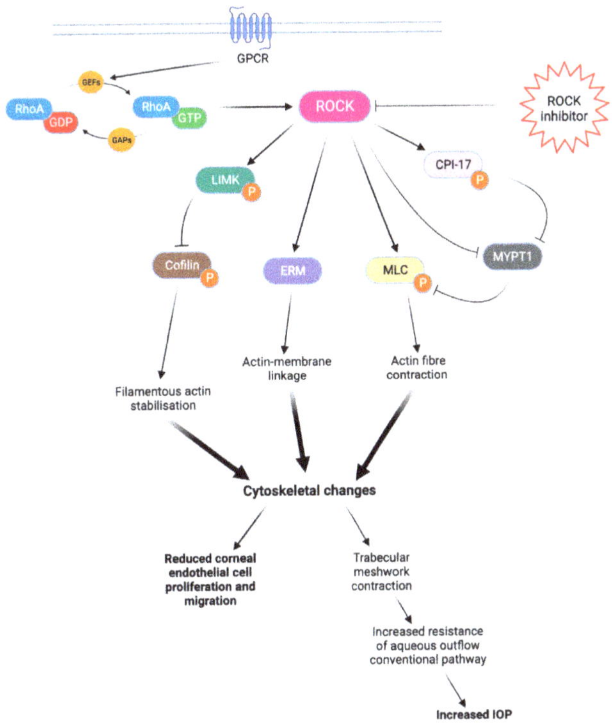

Figure 1. Rho kinase cascade of activation. When coupled with GTP, RhoA protein can phosphorylate various target proteins and ultimately lead to cytoskeletal changes. These cytoskeletal modifications limit endothelial cell proliferation and migration, as well as aqueous outflow through the conventional pathway. By blocking this cascade, ROCK inhibitors can improve corneal endothelial cell migration and reduce the IOP. ROCK: Rho kinase. LIMK: LIM kinase. ERM: ezrin-radixin-moesin. MLC: myosin light chain. CPI-17: C-kinase-potentiated protein phosphatase 1 inhibitor of 17 kDa. MYPT1: Myosin phosphatase target subunit 1. IOP: intraocular pressure.

3. Evidence for Clinical Efficacy and Safety of Ripasudil

3.1. Ripasudil in Glaucoma

In Phase 1 and Phase 2 trials, ripasudil has demonstrated a significant reduction in IOP when used as monotherapy in patients with open-angle glaucoma (POAG) or ocular hypertension (OHT) [19,20]. In particular, a dose-dependent reduction in the IOP was observed with ripasudil 0.1–0.4% twice daily versus placebo over 8 weeks. Further, Tanihara et al. investigated the use of 0.4% ripasudil as a single therapy, or in addition to either latanoprost or timolol, in POAG and OHT [21]. In these trials, ripasudil demonstrated a significantly greater IOP reduction over 8 weeks at trough and peak levels when combined with prostaglandins or beta-blockers as compared to placebo. Furthermore, the authors confirmed these results in a multicentric, prospective 52-week study that enrolled 388 patients with POAG, OHT, and exfoliation glaucoma [22]. In this study, authors divided the patients into four cohorts: cohort 1, treated with 0.4% ripasudil as monotherapy; and cohorts 2 to 4, treated with ripasudil and prostaglandins, beta-blockers, and fixed-association prostaglandins-beta-blockers, respectively. Ripasudil showed significant IOP reduction when utilized in monotherapy and additive therapy. Interestingly, 94.1% of subjects experienced adverse events, in particular conjunctiva hyperemia (75%), blepharitis (21%), allergic conjunctivitis (17%), eye irritation (10%), conjunctivitis (7%), and eyelids pruritus (4.5%). In most of the patients the conjunctival hyperemia was mild and resolved spontaneously, whereas 22% of subjects required further treatment. Interestingly, the brush cytology did not show a correlation between the presence of eosinophils and an allergic reaction. Finally, they also evaluated the effectiveness of ripasudil in a larger post-marketing observational study over 3 months, with a sample size of over 3000 participants [23]. All groups, including ripasudil as newly initiated monotherapy, combination therapy, or switched therapy, showed a significant reduction in mean IOP over the study period in multiple glaucoma subtypes including exfoliation and uveitic glaucoma. In terms of safety, only 8% of patients experience adverse drug reactions (ADRs), with the most common side effects represented by conjunctival and ocular hyperemia. The overall IOP mean reduction was -2.6 ± 4.1 mmHg compared to the baseline, with the highest reduction observed in subjects with NTG (-3.9 ± 5.3 mmHg). Within patients with secondary glaucoma, good efficacy was observed in cases of exfoliation glaucoma (-3.0 ± 5.5 mmHg), uveitis-associated glaucoma (-4.7 ± 7.2 mmHg), and steroid glaucoma (-5.5 ± 6.0 mmHg), whereas a non-significant IOP reduction was found in subjects with neovascular glaucoma (-2.8 ± 12.1 mmHg, $p = 0.669$).

Additionally, various case series and observational studies [24–27] have shown the effectiveness of ripasudil as an adjunct or monotherapy in specific subtypes of glaucoma such as exfoliation and uveitic glaucoma, and in patients where maximum medical therapy failed to control IOP adequately. In a study with 30 participants, the combination of ripasudil and prostaglandin analogs showed a significant additional reduction in intraocular pressure compared to prostaglandin analog monotherapy in patients with normal tension glaucoma [28]. The combination treatment resulted in significant IOP lowering at 1 month and 3 months. Jethva et al. conducted a small prospective study in patients with inadequately controlled IOP on two or more treatments [29]; ripasudil was added to patients' ongoing glaucoma therapy, and the authors observed a significant reduction in IOP at 3 months. Furthermore, Tanihara et al. found that ripasudil–brimonidine fixed-dose combination therapy was more effective than monotherapy of either drug and just as effective as administering ripasudil shortly followed by brimonidine, but with the added benefit of potentially improving patients' compliance [9].

Ripasudil has also been studied as an adjunct to surgical glaucoma procedures such as trabeculectomy [30]. Mimura et al. investigated the potential application of ripasudil in lowering IOP after trabeculectomy for patients with uveitic glaucoma, who often have poorer outcomes post-surgery. They found that ripasudil could reduce the need for bleb needling or revision, and all participants in the ripasudil treatment group had a significant reduction in IOP compared to the control group at 3 months post-operatively. Further trials are currently investigating the use of ripasudil drops after bleb needling without antimetabolite agents [31]. In selected cases, ripasudil treatment after bleb needle revision could suppress the fibrotic processes and improve the bleb filtration, reducing the need for antimetabolite injections.

To date, no studies have compared ripasudil as a monotherapy to first-line glaucoma drugs such as prostaglandins and beta-blockers. However, ripasudil is demonstrating promising results in reducing the IOP when used as a monotherapy or in combination with other agents or procedures. More extensive studies are needed to establish its efficacy as a standalone treatment and further explore its potential in different types of glaucoma.

3.2. Ripasudil in Corneal Diseases

Descemet's membrane removal in procedures like Descemetorhexis Without Endothelial Keratoplasty (DWEK) or Descemet's Stripping Only (DSO) for Fuchs Endothelial Corneal Dystrophy (FECD) has been shown to improve corneal clarity and vision and to concurrently reduced the need for corneal graft procedures [7]. In this scenario, the use of ripasudil as an adjunct therapy to these procedures has shown promising results [32,33]. Multiple studies have highlighted the potential of ripasudil in achieving corneal clearance and improving visual outcomes in DWEK/DSO procedures. A recent meta-analysis of 68 patients undergoing DWEK found that faster corneal clearance was achieved in patients treated with a ROCK inhibitor as compared to non-treated subjects (4.9 weeks vs. 10.1 weeks, respectively, $p < 0.001$) [34]. A follow-up study in 2021 further supported the use of ripasudil, with corneal clearance observed in the majority of the cases [35]. Macsai et al. compared DWEK combined with ripasudil to standalone DWEK [36]. Eighteen subjects were included; nine were assigned to the observation group (DWEK only) and nine to the treatment group (DWEK plus netarsudil). In the ripasudil group, patients experienced a faster visual recovery (4.6 vs. 6.5 weeks, $p < 0.01$) and a higher average at 3 months (859 vs. 552, $p < 0.01$), 6 months (934 vs. 672, $p < 0.01$), and 12 months (1086, vs. 736, $p < 0.01$) as compared to the DWEK-only group. Further, peripheral ECD did not significantly change from baseline to 12 months post-operatively (1239 vs. 1233 cells/mm^2, $p < 0.1$) in subjects treated with netarsudil, whereas the observation group had a statistically significant reduction in ECD (1257 vs. 1142 cells/mm^2, $p < 0.01$). Overall, studies have shown patients treated with DWEK/DSO require a longer time to achieve a visual outcome similar to those treated with Descemet's Membrane Endothelial Keratoplasty (DMEK) [33]. Therefore, the delay in visual recovery may give ripasudil a valuable role, considering that DWEK/DSO procedures do not require donor corneal tissue and could help overcome the problem of limited availability of corneal tissues [37]. Due to its healing effect on corneal endothelium, other applications of ripasudil have been studied. Cataract or anterior segment surgeries are known to be associated with a risk of postoperative corneal oedema due to endothelial cell damage. Studies have shown that administering ripasudil in the post-operative period has a protective effect on endothelial cell density [38], and may improve visual recovery after complicated procedures [39,40]. In both Descemet's Stripping Automated Endothelial Keratoplasty (DSAEK) and penetrating keratoplasty corneal grafts that failed to clear with conservative management, vision can be rescued with ripasudil therapy [41]. Ripasudil also shows promise in other pathology which can result in oedema such as acute hydrops in keratoconus [42]. Eslami et al. presented the case of a 32-year-old male diagnosed with corneal hydrops. The patient was started on topical netarsudil 0.4% twice a day. At 3 weeks of follow-up, VA was slightly better and corneal oedema had resolved completely. The patient underwent corneal lamellar transplant successfully, and at 14 months the BCVA was 0.18 logMAR. In this case, the use of netarsudil allowed the treatment of corneal oedema and improved the view during the corneal transplant.

3.3. *Safety Profile of Ripasudil*

The adverse effects of ripasudil have been well studied (Table 1). The most significant adverse drug reactions (ADR) reported at one year by Tanihara et al. were conjunctival hyperemia (74.6%) and blepharitis (20.6%) [22]. However, the majority of hyperemia cases were only classed as 'mild' in severity and usually resolved within 2 h [43]. The main reasons for discontinuing ripasudil were usually blepharitis and symptoms such as pruritis and eyelid redness, rather than conjunctival hyperemia [44]. There have been some case reports of a further adverse effect of honeycomb/reticular epithelial oedema [35,45,46] not reported in previously discussed larger clinical trials. This effect is usually transient, but in one case the patient required a repeat corneal graft procedure to improve visual function [45].

Tanihara et al. later followed up POAG and OHT patients over 12 months and then 24 months [47,48] and demonstrated an acceptable safety profile of twice daily ripasudil. Out of 3374 participants, the rate of adverse events was 25.3%, of which 8.6% was accountable for blepharitis (the most common adverse effect). This was only slightly elevated compared to the results at 1 year, and 87% of participants recovered from the adverse events. No serious adverse events were reported at 24 months. Ripasudil-associated blepharitis was significantly correlated with a past medical history of atopy or drug allergy. However, ripasudil is still considered safe to be used in those with a sulfonamide antibiotic allergy, as there is no evidence of cross-reactivity in the current literature [49].

Table 1. List of similarities and difference between ripasudil and netarsudil.

Similarities	Differences
Overall safety profiles acceptable for clinical use.	The adverse drug reaction (ADR) rate for netarsudil was 3.3% (RCT) versus 18.7% for ripasudil (post-marketing surveillance).
Conjunctival hyperemia is the most frequent adverse event.	Blepharitis is the most common reason for discontinuation of ripasudil treatment but is not a prominent side effect of netarsudil.
	The incidence of severe conjunctival hyperemia is greater in ripasudil compared to netarsudil.
	Netarsudil is associated with cornea verticillata as an adverse drug reaction, whereas this has not been observed with ripasudil.
Reticular honeycomb epithelial edema has been observed with both drugs.	Reticular honeycomb epithelial oedema seems to be more frequent with netarsudil, and it has not been observed in the randomized controlled trials for ripasudil.

4. Evidence for Clinical Efficacy and Safety of Netarsudil

4.1. Netarsudil in Glaucoma

Netarsudil has been shown to lower the IOP by improving the outflow facility and reducing the episcleral venous pressure (EVP) [50]. In this multicenter, randomized, placebo (vehicle)-controlled, double-masked Phase 2 study, authors included 20 patients, and eyes were randomized to be treated with placebo or netarsudil. For each subject, one eye received one drop of netarsudil 0.02%, and the fellow eye received one drop of vehicle once a day in the morning for 7 days. The primary endpoint was the change in mean diurnal trabecular outflow facility compared to baseline, and the secondary objectives were the differences in IOP and episcleral vein pressure changes between drug and placebo, as well as ocular and systemic safety. At day 8, a significant difference in diurnal outflow facility was observed in the netarsudil group as compared to the placebo (0.039 ± 0.040 µL/min/mmHg vs. 0.007 ± 0.028, $p < 0.01$). Further, IOP changes from baseline were significantly higher in the eye treated with netarsudil compared to the fellow eye (-4.52 ± 1.58 mm Hg vs. -0.98 ± 1.60 mm Hg, $p < 0.01$). Interestingly, the EVP decreased in the drug group compared to baseline (-9.5%, $p < 0.01$) and increased in the vehicle group (3.1%, $p = 0.81$), with a between-treatment difference of -12.6% ($p < 0.001$ vs. vehicle). These results suggest that netarsudil could influence the distal portion of the conventional outflow pathway beyond Schlemm's canal.

One of the first clinical studies by Bacharach et al. compared netarsudil to latanoprost in patients with POAG or OHT. In this double-masked, parallel comparison study, patients were randomized to receive netarsudil 0.01%, netarsudil 0.02%, or latanoprost 0.005% for 28 days. Subjects with POAG or OHT were included. At days 14 and 28 of treatment, all three groups showed a reduction in IOP as compared to unmedicated baseline ($p < 0.01$). Although netarsudil did not meet the criterion for noninferiority to latanoprost, authors observed that netarsudil 0.02% had similar efficacy in patients with a baseline IOP ≤ 26 mmHg [51].

The main clinical trials that support the use of netarsudil for glaucoma consist of the ROCKET and MERCURY studies. MERCURY-1 and MERCURY-2 trials demonstrated a significantly higher decrease in IOP with the netarsudil/latanoprost fixed-dose combination compared to either of the therapies individually [52,53]. In MERCURY-3, authors conducted a 6-month prospective, double-masked, randomized, multicenter, active-controlled, parallel-group, non-inferiority study [54]. They included 430 patients from 58 clinical sites of 11 European countries, and subjects were randomized to receive netarsudil/latanoprost 0.02%/0.005% (NET/LAT) or bimatoprost 0.03%/timolol maleate 0.5% (BIM/TIM). For the primary endpoint, NET/LAT FDC demonstrated non-inferiority to BIM/TIM, with a between treatment difference in IOP of ≤ 1.5 mmHg achieved at all time points and ≤ 1.0 mmHg at the majority of time points from week 2 through week 12. Interestingly, two time points showed a statistically significant difference in mean IOP: 08:00 at week 6 and week 12 in favor of BIM/TIM. These results are consistent with previous works comparing netarsudil with timolol [55]. The ROCKET trials compared netarsudil to timolol as standalone therapy for reducing IOP. The ROCKET-1 and ROCKET-2 trials showed that netarsudil was as effective as timolol in reducing the IOP in patients with a baseline IOP of <25 mmHg [56]. However, it is important to note that netarsudil use was associated with a greater incidence of adverse events such as conjunctival hyperemia that caused discontinuations of the drug (Figure 2). The ROCKET-4 study [55,57], which had broader inclusion criteria, demonstrated non-inferiority of netarsudil once daily to timolol twice daily in patients with baseline IOP < 30 mmHg. Mathur et al. conducted a real-world, open-label observational study and deemed netarsudil monotherapy to be effective yet safe [58].

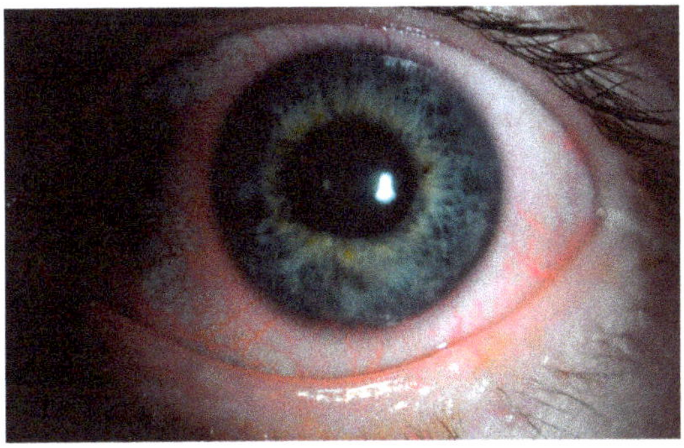

Figure 2. Unilateral mild conjunctival hyperemia (left eye) in a patient treated with latanoprost/netarsudil combination for glaucoma. The patient reported that the redness in the eye typically resolved within two hours following the application of the drops.

The effectiveness of netarsudil in specific clinical sub-cohorts, such as secondary glaucoma and patients on maximal tolerated medical therapy, is still being explored. Preliminary evidence suggests that netarsudil can provide additional IOP-lowering effects in patients with uveitic glaucoma on maximal tolerated medical therapy [59]. Netarsudil has also been shown to be effective in a cohort of patients with Sturge-Weber Syndrome on maximal medical therapy by reducing EVP [60], and it demonstrated similar efficacy to latanoprostene bunod when used as adjunct therapy in patients on maximal therapy for POAG [61]. The efficacy of netarsudil has also been compared to ripasudil in the J-ROCKET study and demonstrated a stronger IOP-lowering effect [62]. Like ripasudil, netarsudil has also been studied in the context of glaucoma surgery. Xu et al. investigated the effect of netarsudil on patients who had undergone Kahook blade goniotomy [63], and they observed a greater decrease in IOP as compared to goniotomy-naïve patients. This was thought to be due to netarsudil's effect on lowering the EVP.

4.2. Netarsudil in Corneal Diseases

A recent randomized study investigated the use of netarsudil in patients with symptomatic Fuchs Endothelial Corneal Dystrophy (FECD) [64]. The study included 29 subjects who were either given netarsudil 0.02% once daily or a placebo for three months. The results showed that netarsudil monotherapy led to a significant reduction in central corneal thickness and improvement in best-corrected visual acuity compared to the placebo. Another study by Lindstrom et al. demonstrated significant improvement in central corneal thickness as well as visual acuity and patient-reported FECD-associated symptoms when once-daily dosing was used [65].

Netarsudil has not been extensively studied as an adjunct therapy in DWEK/DSO, with only three case reports available. However, these studies showed improved endothelial cell density and resolution of corneal edema in patients treated with netarsudil [66–68]. The advantage of netarsudil is its once-daily dosing, which provides a practical benefit over ripasudil and may improve patients' compliance. Prospective trials are needed to further explore the potential application of netarsudil in corneal endothelial diseases.

4.3. Safety Profile of Netarsudil

The ROCKET [55] and MERCURY [69] trials evaluated the safety profile of netarsudil 0.02% once daily as monotherapy or as a fixed-dose combination with latanoprost 0.005%. In a pooled analysis of safety from the ROCKET trials, no serious ocular adverse events were reported when netarsudil was used as a standalone treatment, and the overall rate of serious ADRs (including non-ocular) was 3.3% for netarsudil-treated patients, similar to the rate of 3.2% in timolol-treated patients [55]. The non-ocular serious events reported for the netarsudil group included coronary artery disease, myocardial infarction, atrial fibrillation, and prostate cancer. The MERCURY-2 trial demonstrated that the most common adverse effect was conjunctival hyperemia, which occurred in 55% of patients using netarsudil as a standalone treatment. This was higher than that observed in standalone treatment with latanoprost (22.3%) and timolol (10.4%), but no patients on netarsudil discontinued the treatment. The majority of the conjunctival hyperemia cases were classified as 'mild'. The other most common adverse effects included cornea verticillata, which was reported between 9% and 15% of patients with an onset of 2–13 weeks. The corneal appearance was similar to that seen with the use of some systemic medications, most notably amiodarone. It is believed that ROCK inhibitors penetrate the lysosomes within the basal epithelial layer of the cornea; within these lysosomes, they bind to cellular lipids. These complexes of medication and lipids are resistant to enzymatic breakdown and build up as deposits in the cornea [70]. This might have notable implications for individuals with glaucoma experiencing reduced contrast sensitivity due to their underlying optic neuropathy. However, none of these adverse effects had any influence on visual acuity, and they resolved once netarsudil was discontinued.

MERCURY-2 demonstrated that the rate of serious adverse events in the fixed-dose combination group was lower than in either netarsudil or latanoprost monotherapy; none of which were considered to be treatment-related. It is interesting to note that blepharitis is not a common adverse effect of netarsudil in contrast to ripasudil, and the reasons for this remain unclear. As with ripasudil, various studies reported the incidence of honeycomb corneal oedema caused by netarsudil [46,71,72]. However, this adverse effect was not found in any participant in the MERCURY-2 study [53]. The nature of corneal oedema seems to vary between netarsudil and ripasudil, with the onset being faster in netarsudil. Patients that develop corneal oedema are likely to have risk factors such as reduced endothelial cell count, epithelial defects, or a history of penetrating keratoplasty [46,71]. Netarsudil-associated cornea oedema has been reported to occur in children [73]; one case of corneal flattening was also reported in a child [74].

5. Future Directions

ROCK inhibitors are showing promising results, but their clinical use is still limited. In future, there is the possibility that more specific molecules will be introduced to selectively target the trabecular meshwork, the corneal endothelium, and the optic nerve. More selective ROCK inhibitors could potentially increase their clinical efficacy and reduce the side effects. Further, new studies are focusing on direct genetic modulation of ROCK signaling to clarify the mechanism of aqueous outflow, as well as to find novel glaucoma gene therapies [75].

In cornea, new less-invasive surgical techniques such as DSAEK and DMEK have allowed the treatment of endothelial diseases with better clinical outcomes as compared to PK. These new procedures have the advantage over PK to offer a faster visual recovery, a better refractive outcome, and a lower rejection risk. However, they still require a learning curve, especially for DMEK surgeries, and they are associated with graft rejection risk. In this scenario, the use of ROCK inhibitors has been proposed for tissue engineering therapies [76]. In particular, the injection of corneal endothelial cells could be enhanced using ROCK inhibitors to improve cell adhesion and replications [76]. Further clinical studies are needed to confirm the safety and efficacy of these new engineering therapies as compared to conventional corneal grafts. Initiating ROCK inhibitors in the early stages of glaucoma can be advantageous as they have the potential to reduce intraocular pressure (IOP) while the trabecular meshwork is functioning properly. This approach is particularly beneficial for patients with steroid-induced ocular hypertension or uveitic glaucoma. However, a comprehensive understanding of the full benefits of ROCK inhibitor therapy in early-stage glaucoma necessitates further investigation.

Although ROCK inhibitors represent an innovative category of topical medications for lowering IOP, it is crucial to conduct more clinical trials and post-marketing studies to establish optimal treatment protocols for glaucoma patients.

Lastly, ROCK inhibitors could also serve in modulating wound healing response following glaucoma filtration surgery. The wound healing process depends on various mechanisms such as cell proliferation and migration, necessitating constant and active changes in the cell's cytoskeleton.

In vitro studies revealed the role of Rho-ROCK expression in Tenon fibroblasts (TF), which are central to ocular wound healing. Specifically, they have demonstrated that the use of ROCK inhibitors suppresses wound healing activities of TF in vitro. Exposure to ROCK inhibitors, significantly inhibits fibroblast proliferation, adhesion, and contraction [77,78]. Honjo et al. also demonstrated that topical treatment with a ROCK inhibitor effectively reduces subconjunctival scarring at day 7 after experimental glaucoma surgery in rabbits [77]. While long-term experiments on the effect of ROCK inhibition on collagen deposition and bleb survival after glaucoma filtration surgery are still lacking, some data in rabbit models and small groups have shown the inhibition of the proliferation of human TF and the differentiation of fibroblasts into myofibroblasts [79]. As a result, a postoperative topical treatment with a ROCK inhibitor (AMA0526) significantly improved the outcome of glaucoma filtration surgery. Compared to eyes treated with a vehicle, AMA0526 resulted in increased bleb area and prolonged survival. Histological evaluation revealed that blebs treated with the ROCK inhibitor exhibited reduced inflammation, angiogenesis, and collagen deposition at the filtration surgery site [79]. Additionally, experimental evidence suggests that, aside from being a regulator of the cytoskeleton, ROCK also plays a significant role in the inflammatory process [80], with potential benefits of ROCK inhibition in treating conditions like rheumatoid arthritis [81] and Crohn's disease [82], where it inhibits NF-kb activation and reduces the production of inflammatory cytokines. ROCK inhibitors have demonstrated anti-inflammatory, antiangiogenic, and antifibrotic effects in various animal models, including those for ocular conditions like corneal wound healing and age-related macular degeneration. Consequently, targeting the Rho-ROCK pathway offers promise for modulating the wound healing response following glaucoma surgery.

6. Conclusions

ROCK inhibitors such as ripasudil and netarsudil have shown promise as safe, emerging treatment options across different sub-specialties of ophthalmology. In glaucoma, they have shown efficacy as monotherapy and open new avenues for treatment for patients who have inadequately controlled IOP on maximum medical therapy. By acting on the dysfunctional trabecular meshwork, these agents address the underlying cause of glaucoma, as opposed to other agents like beta-blockers that only reduce aqueous humor secretion. In both glaucoma and corneas, ROCK inhibitors have also proven to be an effective adjunct to surgery, such as trabeculectomy or Descemetorhexis Without Endothelial Keratoplasty. Combination with other pre-existing medications such as brimonidine has shown to have further additive effects compared to monotherapy. For now, it remains unclear whether ripasudil or netarsudil is superior. Only one study so far (J-ROCKET) has compared ripasudil versus netarsudil and concluded that netarsudil had superior IOP-lowering effects with fewer side effects; however, further studies would be needed to confirm this observation as the number of cases of reticular epithelial oedema appears to be higher with netarsudil use.

Author Contributions: Conceptualization, L.P., G.G. and A.B.; methodology, L.P., J.W.L., M.P., G.G., S.K. and A.B.; writing—original draft preparation, L.P., J.W.L., M.P., G.G., S.K. and A.B.; writing—review and editing, L.P., J.W.L., M.P., G.G., S.K. and A.B. All authors have read and agreed to the published version of the manuscript.

Funding: This research received no external funding.

Institutional Review Board Statement: Not applicable.

Informed Consent Statement: Not applicable.

Data Availability Statement: Not applicable.

Conflicts of Interest: The authors declare no conflict of interest.

References

1. Singh, K.; Singh, A. Rho-kinase Inhibitors in Ocular Diseases: A Translational Research Journey. *J. Curr. Glaucoma Pract.* **2023**, *17*, 44–48. [CrossRef]
2. Patel, A.R.; Schwartz, G.F.; Campbell, J.H.; Chen, C.C.; McGuiness, C.B.; Multani, J.K.; Shih, V.; Smith, O.U. Economic and Clinical Burden Associated With Intensification of Glaucoma Topical Therapy: A US Claims-based Analysis. *J. Glaucoma* **2021**, *30*, 242–250. [CrossRef]
3. Rikitake, Y.; Liao, J.K. Rho GTPases, statins, and nitric oxide. *Circ. Res.* **2005**, *97*, 1232–1235. [CrossRef]
4. Okumura, N.; Koizumi, N.; Kay, E.P.; Ueno, M.; Sakamoto, Y.; Nakamura, S.; Hamuro, J.; Kinoshita, S. The ROCK inhibitor eye drop accelerates corneal endothelium wound healing. *Invest. Ophthalmol. Vis. Sci.* **2013**, *54*, 2493–2502. [CrossRef]
5. Peh, G.S.L.; Bandeira, F.; Neo, D.; Adnan, K.; Hartono, Y.; Ong, H.S.; Naso, S.; Venkatraman, A.; Gomes, J.A.P.; Kocaba, V.; et al. Effects of Rho-Associated Kinase (Rock) Inhibitors (Alternative to Y-27632) on Primary Human Corneal Endothelial Cells. *Cells* **2023**, *12*, 1307. [CrossRef]
6. Okumura, N.; Nakano, S.; Kay, E.P.; Numata, R.; Ota, A.; Sowa, Y.; Sakai, T.; Ueno, M.; Kinoshita, S.; Koizumi, N. Involvement of cyclin D and p27 in cell proliferation mediated by ROCK inhibitors Y-27632 and Y-39983 during corneal endothelium wound healing. *Invest. Ophthalmol. Vis. Sci.* **2014**, *55*, 318–329. [CrossRef]
7. Franceschino, A.; Dutheil, F.; Pereira, B.; Watson, S.L.; Chiambaretta, F.; Navel, V. Descemetorhexis Without Endothelial Keratoplasty in Fuchs Endothelial Corneal Dystrophy: A Systematic Review and Meta-Analysis. *Cornea* **2022**, *41*, 815–825. [CrossRef]
8. Sugiyama, T.; Shibata, M.; Kajiura, S.; Okuno, T.; Tonari, M.; Oku, H.; Ikeda, T. Effects of fasudil, a Rho-associated protein kinase inhibitor, on optic nerve head blood flow in rabbits. *Invest. Ophthalmol. Vis. Sci.* **2011**, *52*, 64–69. [CrossRef]
9. Tanihara, H.; Yamamoto, T.; Aihara, M.; Kawakita, K.; Kojima, S.; Kanazawa, M.; Nojima, T.; Suganami, H. Ripasudil-Brimonidine Fixed-Dose Combination vs. Ripasudil or Brimonidine: Two Phase 3 Randomized Clinical Trials. *Am. J. Ophthalmol.* **2023**, *248*, 35–44. [CrossRef]
10. Inoue, T.; Tanihara, H.; Tokushige, H.; Araie, M. Efficacy and safety of SNJ-1656 in primary open-angle glaucoma or ocular hypertension. *Acta Ophthalmol.* **2015**, *93*, e393–e395. [CrossRef]
11. Rao, P.V.; Pattabiraman, P.P.; Kopczynski, C. Role of the Rho GTPase/Rho kinase signaling pathway in pathogenesis and treatment of glaucoma: Bench to bedside research. *Exp. Eye Res.* **2017**, *158*, 23–32. [PubMed]
12. Moshirfar, M.; Parker, L.; Birdsong, O.C.; Ronquillo, Y.C.; Hofstedt, D.; Shah, T.J.; Gomez, A.T.; Hoopes, P.C.S. Use of Rho kinase Inhibitors in Ophthalmology: A Review of the Literature. *Med. Hypothesis Discov. Innov. Ophthalmol.* **2018**, *7*, 101–111. [PubMed]
13. Moura-Coelho, N.; Tavares Ferreira, J.; Bruxelas, C.P.; Dutra-Medeiros, M.; Cunha, J.P.; Pinto Proenca, R. Rho kinase inhibitors-a review on the physiology and clinical use in Ophthalmology. *Graefes Arch. Clin. Exp. Ophthalmol.* **2019**, *257*, 1101–1117.
14. Hein, T.W.; Rosa, R.H., Jr.; Yuan, Z.; Roberts, E.; Kuo, L. Divergent roles of nitric oxide and rho kinase in vasomotor regulation of human retinal arterioles. *Invest. Ophthalmol. Vis. Sci.* **2010**, *51*, 1583–1590. [CrossRef] [PubMed]
15. Wada, Y.; Higashide, T.; Nagata, A.; Sugiyama, K. Effects of ripasudil, a rho kinase inhibitor, on blood flow in the optic nerve head of normal rats. *Graefes Arch. Clin. Exp. Ophthalmol.* **2019**, *257*, 303–311. [CrossRef] [PubMed]
16. Ho, W.T.; Chang, J.S.; Chen, T.C.; Wang, J.K.; Chang, S.W.; Yang, M.H.; Jou, T.; Wang, I. Inhibition of Rho-associated protein kinase activity enhances oxidative phosphorylation to support corneal endothelial cell migration. *FASEB J.* **2022**, *36*, e22397. [CrossRef]
17. Arita, R.; Hata, Y.; Ishibashi, T. ROCK as a Therapeutic Target of Diabetic Retinopathy. *J. Ophthalmol.* **2010**, *2010*, 175163. [CrossRef]
18. Mateos-Olivares, M.; Garcia-Onrubia, L.; Valentin-Bravo, F.J.; Gonzalez-Sarmiento, R.; Lopez-Galvez, M.; Pastor, J.C.; Usategui-Martín, R.; Pastor-Idoate, S. Rho-Kinase Inhibitors for the Treatment of Refractory Diabetic Macular Oedema. *Cells* **2021**, *10*, 1683. [CrossRef]

19. Tanihara, H.; Inoue, T.; Yamamoto, T.; Kuwayama, Y.; Abe, H.; Araie, M.; K-115 Clinical Study Group. Phase 1 clinical trials of a selective Rho kinase inhibitor, K-115. *JAMA Ophthalmol.* **2013**, *131*, 1288–1295. [CrossRef]
20. Tanihara, H.; Inoue, T.; Yamamoto, T.; Kuwayama, Y.; Abe, H.; Araie, M.; K-115 Clinical Study Group. Phase 2 randomized clinical study of a Rho kinase inhibitor, K-115, in primary open-angle glaucoma and ocular hypertension. *Am. J. Ophthalmol.* **2013**, *156*, 731–736. [CrossRef]
21. Tanihara, H.; Inoue, T.; Yamamoto, T.; Kuwayama, Y.; Abe, H.; Suganami, H.; Araie, M.; K-115 Clinical Study Group. Additive Intraocular Pressure-Lowering Effects of the Rho Kinase Inhibitor Ripasudil (K-115) Combined With Timolol or Latanoprost: A Report of 2 Randomized Clinical Trials. *JAMA Ophthalmol.* **2015**, *133*, 755–761. [CrossRef] [PubMed]
22. Tanihara, H.; Inoue, T.; Yamamoto, T.; Kuwayama, Y.; Abe, H.; Fukushima, A.; Suganami, H.; Araie, M.; K-115 Clinical Study Group. One-year clinical evaluation of 0.4% ripasudil (K-115) in patients with open-angle glaucoma and ocular hypertension. *Acta Ophthalmol.* **2016**, *94*, e26–e34. [PubMed]
23. Tanihara, H.; Kakuda, T.; Sano, T.; Kanno, T.; Imada, R.; Shingaki, W.; Gunji, R. Safety and Efficacy of Ripasudil in Japanese Patients with Glaucoma or Ocular Hypertension: 3-month Interim Analysis of ROCK-J, a Post-Marketing Surveillance Study. *Adv. Ther.* **2019**, *36*, 333–343. [PubMed]
24. Matsumura, R.; Inoue, T.; Matsumura, A.; Tanihara, H. Efficacy of Ripasudil as a Second-line Medication in Addition to a Prostaglandin Analog in Patients with Exfoliation Glaucoma: A Pilot Study. *Clin. Drug Investig.* **2017**, *37*, 535–539.
25. Kusuhara, S.; Katsuyama, A.; Matsumiya, W.; Nakamura, M. Efficacy and safety of ripasudil, a Rho-associated kinase inhibitor, in eyes with uveitic glaucoma. *Graefes Arch. Clin. Exp. Ophthalmol.* **2018**, *256*, 809–814.
26. Futakuchi, A.; Morimoto, T.; Ikeda, Y.; Tanihara, H.; Inoue, T.; Collaborators R-Ssg. Intraocular pressure-lowering effects of ripasudil in uveitic glaucoma, exfoliation glaucoma, and steroid-induced glaucoma patients: ROCK-S, a multicentre historical cohort study. *Sci. Rep.* **2020**, *10*, 10308.
27. Inazaki, H.; Kobayashi, S.; Anzai, Y.; Satoh, H.; Sato, S.; Inoue, M.; Yamane, S.; Kadonosono, K. Efficacy of the Additional Use of Ripasudil, a Rho-Kinase Inhibitor, in Patients With Glaucoma Inadequately Controlled Under Maximum Medical Therapy. *J. Glaucoma* **2017**, *26*, 96–100.
28. Sakata, R.; Fujishiro, T.; Saito, H.; Honjo, M.; Shirato, S.; Aihara, M. The Additive Effect of ROCK Inhibitor on Prostaglandin-Treated Japanese Patients with Glaucoma Indicating 15 mmHg and Under: ROCK U-15. *Adv Ther.* **2021**, *38*, 3760–3770.
29. Jethva, J.; Bhagat, P.; Prajapati, K.; Tank, G. Safety, efficacy, and patient selection of ripasudil in patients with uncontrolled glaucoma with maximum conventional medical therapy. *Indian J. Ophthalmol.* **2022**, *70*, 2020–2023.
30. Mimura, T.; Noma, H.; Inoue, Y.; Kawashima, M.; Kitsu, K.; Mizota, A. Early Postoperative Effect of Ripasudil Hydrochloride After Trabeculectomy on Secondary Glaucoma: A Randomized Controlled Trial. *Open Ophthalmol. J.* **2022**, *16*. [CrossRef]
31. Mizuno, Y.; Komatsu, K.; Tokumo, K.; Okada, N.; Onoe, H.; Okumichi, H.; Hirooka, K.; Miura, Y.; Kiuchi, Y. A multicenter phase II study on the safety of rho-kinase inhibitor (ripasudil) with needling for the patients after trabeculectomy. *Contemp. Clin. Trials Commun.* **2023**, *33*, 101160. [PubMed]
32. Moloney, G.; Petsoglou, C.; Ball, M.; Kerdraon, Y.; Höllhumer, R.; Spiteri, N.; Beheregaray, S.; Hampson, J.; D'Souza, M.; Devasahayam, R.N. Descemetorhexis Without Grafting for Fuchs Endothelial Dystrophy-Supplementation With Topical Ripasudil. *Cornea* **2017**, *36*, 642–648. [PubMed]
33. Huang, M.J.; Kane, S.; Dhaliwal, D.K. Descemetorhexis Without Endothelial Keratoplasty Versus DMEK for Treatment of Fuchs Endothelial Corneal Dystrophy. *Cornea* **2018**, *37*, 1479–1483. [PubMed]
34. Din, N.; Cohen, E.; Popovic, M.; Mimouni, M.; Trinh, T.; Gouvea, L.; Alshaker, S.M.; Tone, S.M.O.; Chan, C.C.M.; Slomovic, A.R.M. Surgical Management of Fuchs Endothelial Corneal Dystrophy: A Treatment Algorithm and Individual Patient Meta-Analysis of Descemet Stripping Only. *Cornea* **2022**, *41*, 1188–1195. [PubMed]
35. Moloney, G.; Congote, D.G.; Hirnschall, N.; Arsiwalla, T.; Boso, A.L.; Toalster, N.; D'Souza, M.; Devasahayam, R.N. Descemet Stripping Only Supplemented With Topical Ripasudil for Fuchs Endothelial Dystrophy 12-Month Outcomes of the Sydney Eye Hospital Study. *Cornea* **2021**, *40*, 320–326.
36. Macsai, M.S.; Shiloach, M. Use of Topical Rho Kinase Inhibitors in the Treatment of Fuchs Dystrophy After Descemet Stripping Only. *Cornea* **2019**, *38*, 529–534.
37. Parekh, M.; Wongvisavavit, R.; Cubero Cortes, Z.M.; Wojcik, G.; Romano, V.; Tabernero, S.S.; Ferrari, S.; Ahmad, S. Alternatives to endokeratoplasty: An attempt towards reducing global demand of human donor corneas. *Regen. Med.* **2022**, *17*, 461–475.
38. Fujimoto, H.; Setoguchi, Y.; Kiryu, J. The ROCK Inhibitor Ripasudil Shows an Endothelial Protective Effect in Patients With Low Corneal Endothelial Cell Density After Cataract Surgery. *Transl. Vis. Sci. Technol.* **2021**, *10*, 18.
39. Azhari, J.; Patel, U.; Vakharia, M. Corneal endothelial wound healing after Descemet tear with a rho kinase inhibitor. *J. Cataract. Refract. Surg. Online Case Rep.* **2022**, *10*, e00075.
40. Fernandez Lopez, E.; Montolio-Marzo, S.; Ortega Perez, C.; Catalan Gomez, M.; Peris Martinez, C.; Pia Ludena, J.V.; Chan, E. Descemet stripping only and ripasudil for the treatment of traumatic Descemet's membrane ruptures. *Eur. J. Ophthalmol.* **2023**, *33*, NP13-8.
41. Tseng, M.; Feder, R. Topical Ripasudil for the Treatment of Segmental Corneal Edema: A Case Series. *Cornea* **2023**, *42*, 903–907. [CrossRef] [PubMed]
42. Eslami, M.; Arsiwalla, T.; Boso, A.L.M.; Moloney, G. Use of ripasudil for rapid resolution of acute hydrops in keratoconus. *Can. J. Ophthalmol.* **2022**, *57*, e126–e128. [CrossRef] [PubMed]

43. Sakamoto, E.; Ishida, W.; Sumi, T.; Kishimoto, T.; Tada, K.; Fukuda, K.; Yoneda, T.; Kuroiwa, H.; Terao, E.; Fujisawa, Y. Evaluation of offset of conjunctival hyperemia induced by a Rho-kinase inhibitor; 0.4% Ripasudil ophthalmic solution clinical trial. *Sci. Rep.* **2019**, *9*, 3755. [CrossRef] [PubMed]
44. Saito, H.; Kagami, S.; Mishima, K.; Mataki, N.; Fukushima, A.; Araie, M. Long-term Side Effects Including Blepharitis Leading to Discontinuation of Ripasudil. *J. Glaucoma* **2019**, *28*, 289–293. [CrossRef]
45. Jain, N.; Singh, A.; Mishra, D.K.; Murthy, S.I. Honeycomb epithelial oedema due to ripasudil: Clinical, optical coherence tomography and histopathological correlation. *BMJ Case Rep.* **2022**, *15*, e251074. [CrossRef]
46. Bhargava, M.; Sen, S.; Bhambhani, V.; Paul, R.S.; Dutta, C. Reticular epithelial corneal edema as a novel side-effect of Rho Kinase Inhibitors: An Indian scenario. *Indian. J. Ophthalmol.* **2022**, *70*, 1163–1170. [CrossRef]
47. Tanihara, H.; Kakuda, T.; Sano, T.; Kanno, T.; Gunji, R. Safety and efficacy of ripasudil in Japanese patients with glaucoma or ocular hypertension: 12-month interim analysis of ROCK-J, a post-marketing surveillance study. *BMC Ophthalmol.* **2020**, *20*, 275.
48. Tanihara, H.; Kakuda, T.; Sano, T.; Kanno, T.; Kurihara, Y. Long-Term Intraocular Pressure-Lowering Effects and Adverse Events of Ripasudil in Patients with Glaucoma or Ocular Hypertension over 24 Months. *Adv. Ther.* **2022**, *39*, 1659–1677. [CrossRef]
49. Giles, A.; Foushee, J.; Lantz, E.; Gumina, G. Sulfonamide Allergies. *Pharmacy* **2019**, *7*, 132. [CrossRef]
50. Sit, A.J.; Gupta, D.; Kazemi, A.; McKee, H.; Challa, P.; Liu, K.C.; Lopez, J.; Kopczynski, C.; Heah, T. Netarsudil Improves Trabecular Outflow Facility in Patients with Primary Open Angle Glaucoma or Ocular Hypertension: A Phase 2 Study. *Am. J. Ophthalmol.* **2021**, *226*, 262–269. [CrossRef]
51. Bacharach, J.; Dubiner, H.B.; Levy, B.; Kopczynski, C.C.; Novack, G.D.; AR-13324-CS202 Study Group. Double-masked, randomized, dose-response study of AR-13324 versus latanoprost in patients with elevated intraocular pressure. *Ophthalmology* **2015**, *122*, 302–307. [CrossRef]
52. Asrani, S.; Robin, A.L.; Serle, J.B.; Lewis, R.A.; Usner, D.W.; Kopczynski, C.C.; Heah, T.; Ackerman, S.L.; Alpern, L.M.; Bashford, K.; et al. Netarsudil/Latanoprost Fixed-Dose Combination for Elevated Intraocular Pressure: Three-Month Data from a Randomized Phase 3 Trial. *Am. J. Ophthalmol.* **2019**, *207*, 248–257. [CrossRef]
53. Walters, T.R.; Ahmed, I.I.K.; Lewis, R.A.; Usner, D.W.; Lopez, J.; Kopczynski, C.C.; Heah, T. Once-Daily Netarsudil/Latanoprost Fixed-Dose Combination for Elevated Intraocular Pressure in the Randomized Phase 3 MERCURY-2 Study. *Ophthalmol. Glaucoma* **2019**, *2*, 280–289. [CrossRef]
54. Stalmans, I.; Lim, K.S.; Oddone, F.; Fichtl, M.; Belda, J.I.; Hommer, A.; Laganovska, G.; Schweitzer, C.; Voykov, B.; Zarnowski, T. MERCURY-3: A randomized comparison of netarsudil/latanoprost and bimatoprost/timolol in open-angle glaucoma and ocular hypertension. *Graefes Arch. Clin. Exp. Ophthalmol.* **2023**. [CrossRef] [PubMed]
55. Singh, I.P.; Fechtner, R.D.; Myers, J.S.; Kim, T.; Usner, D.W.; McKee, H.; Sheng, H.; Lewis, R.A.; Heah, T.; Kopczynski, C.C. Pooled Efficacy and Safety Profile of Netarsudil Ophthalmic Solution 0.02% in Patients With Open-angle Glaucoma or Ocular Hypertension. *J. Glaucoma* **2020**, *29*, 878–884. [CrossRef] [PubMed]
56. Serle, J.B.; Katz, L.J.; McLaurin, E.; Heah, T.; Ramirez-Davis, N.; Usner, D.W.; Novack, G.D.; Kopczynski, C.C. Two Phase 3 Clinical Trials Comparing the Safety and Efficacy of Netarsudil to Timolol in Patients With Elevated Intraocular Pressure: Rho Kinase Elevated IOP Treatment Trial 1 and 2 (ROCKET-1 and ROCKET-2). *Am. J. Ophthalmol.* **2018**, *186*, 116–127. [CrossRef] [PubMed]
57. Khouri, A.S.; Serle, J.B.; Bacharach, J.; Usner, D.W.; Lewis, R.A.; Braswell, P.; Kopczynski, C.C.; Heah, T.; Benza, R.; Boyle, J.W. Once-Daily Netarsudil Versus Twice-Daily Timolol in Patients With Elevated Intraocular Pressure: The Randomized Phase 3 ROCKET-4 Study. *Am. J. Ophthalmol.* **2019**, *204*, 97–104. [CrossRef] [PubMed]
58. Mathur, M.C.; Ratnam, P.V.; Saikumar, S.J.; John, M.; Ravishankar, S.; Dinesh, M.B.; Chandil, P.; Pahuja, K.; Cherlikar, V.; Wadhwani, S.; et al. Netarsudil monotherapy as the initial treatment for open-angle glaucoma and ocular hypertension in Indian patients: A real-world evaluation of efficacy and safety. *Indian J. Ophthalmol.* **2023**, *71*, 2500–2503. [CrossRef]
59. Oydanich, M.; Roll, E.H.; Uppuluri, S.; Khouri, A.S. Effectiveness of netarsudil 0.02% in lowering intraocular pressure in patients with secondary glaucoma. *Can. J. Ophthalmol.* **2023**. [CrossRef]
60. Kaufman, A.R.; Elhusseiny, A.M.; Edward, D.P.; Vajaranant, T.S.; Aref, A.A.; Abbasian, J. Topical netarsudil for treatment of glaucoma with elevated episcleral venous pressure: A pilot investigation in sturge-weber syndrome. *Eur. J. Ophthalmol.* **2023**, *33*, 1969–1976. [CrossRef]
61. Mehta, A.A.; Kanu, L.N.; Sood-Mendiratta, S.; Quinones, R.; Hawkins, A.; Lehrer, R.A.; Malhotra, K.; Papas, R.; Hillman, D.; Wilensky, J.T.; et al. Experience with netarsudil 0.02% and latanoprostene bunod 0.024% as adjunctive therapy for glaucoma. *Eur. J. Ophthalmol.* **2022**, *32*, 322–326.
62. Araie, M.; Sugiyama, K.; Aso, K.; Kanemoto, K.; Iwata, R.; Hollander, D.A.; Senchyna, M.; Kopczynski, C.C. Phase 3 Clinical Trial Comparing the Safety and Efficacy of Netarsudil to Ripasudil in Patients with Primary Open-Angle Glaucoma or Ocular Hypertension: Japan Rho Kinase Elevated Intraocular Pressure Treatment Trial (J-ROCKET). *Adv. Ther.* **2023**, *40*, 4639–4656. [PubMed]
63. Xu, H.; Thomas, M.T.; Lee, D.; Hirabayashi, M.T.; An, J.A. Response to netarsudil in goniotomy-treated eyes and goniotomy-naive eyes: A pilot study. *Graefes Arch. Clin. Exp. Ophthalmol.* **2022**, *260*, 3001–3007. [CrossRef] [PubMed]
64. Price, M.O.; Price, F.W., Jr. Randomized, Double-Masked, Pilot Study of Netarsudil 0.02% Ophthalmic Solution for Treatment of Corneal Edema in Fuchs Dystrophy. *Am. J. Ophthalmol.* **2021**, *227*, 100–105. [PubMed]

65. Lindstrom, R.L.; Lewis, A.E.; Holland, E.J.; Sheppard, J.D.; Hovanesian, J.A.; Senchyna, M.; Holander, D.A. Phase 2, Randomized, Open-Label Parallel-Group Study of Two Dosing Regimens of Netarsudil for the Treatment of Corneal Edema Due to Fuchs Corneal Dystrophy. *J. Ocul. Pharmacol. Ther.* **2022**, *38*, 657–663.
66. Ploysangam, P.; Patel, S.P. A Case Report Illustrating the Postoperative Course of Descemetorhexis without Endothelial Keratoplasty with Topical Netarsudil Therapy. *Case Rep. Ophthalmol. Med.* **2019**, *2019*, 6139026. [CrossRef]
67. Hirabayashi, K.E.; Mark, D.; Lau, J.; Lin, C.C. Descemet Stripping Only for a Chronic Descemet Detachment After Cataract Surgery. *Cornea* **2020**, *39*, 379–381.
68. Chen, S.L.; LoBue, S.A.; Goyal, H. Case report: The use of netarsudil to improve corneal edema after laser peripheral iridotomy and Descemet's membrane endothelial keratoplasty. *Am. J. Ophthalmol. Case Rep.* **2021**, *22*, 101087.
69. Asrani, S.; Bacharach, J.; Holland, E.; McKee, H.; Sheng, H.; Lewis, R.A.; Kopczynski, C.C.; Heah, T. Fixed-Dose Combination of Netarsudil and Latanoprost in Ocular Hypertension and Open-Angle Glaucoma: Pooled Efficacy/Safety Analysis of Phase 3 MERCURY-1 and -2. *Adv. Ther.* **2020**, *37*, 1620–1631.
70. Lyons, L.J.; Wu, K.Y.; Baratz, K.H.; Sit, A.J. Honeycomb Epithelial Edema Associated with Rho Kinase Inhibition: A Case Series and Review of the Literature. *Cornea* **2022**, *41*, 243–248.
71. Jeang, L.J.; Shah, A.S.; Hammer, J.D.; Tuli, S.S. Reticular epithelial edema after penetrating keratoplasty in a patient taking netarsudil. *Digit. J. Ophthalmol.* **2022**, *28*, 34–37. [CrossRef] [PubMed]
72. Parmar, D.P.; Bhole, P.K.; Garde, P.V. Reticular corneal epithelial edema with topical netarsudil. *Oman J. Ophthalmol.* **2023**, *16*, 94–97. [PubMed]
73. Guzman Aparicio, M.A.; Liebman, D.L.; Chodosh, J.; Freitag, S.K.; Kazlas, M.; Mai, D.D.; Marando, C.M.; Mukai, S.; Wu, A.M.; Chen, T.C. Two pediatric cases of reticular corneal epithelial edema associated with netarsudil. *Am. J. Ophthalmol. Case Rep.* **2022**, *27*, 101638. [CrossRef]
74. Ganesh, D.; Coleman, A.L.; Shibayama, V.P.; Tseng, V.L. Netarsudil-Induced Corneal Flattening in a Child with Secondary Open-Angle Glaucoma. *Case Rep. Ophthalmol.* **2022**, *13*, 330–335. [PubMed]
75. Inoue, T.; Tanihara, H. Rho-associated kinase inhibitors: A novel glaucoma therapy. *Prog. Retin. Eye Res.* **2013**, *37*, 1–12.
76. Okumura, N.; Kinoshita, S.; Koizumi, N. Application of Rho Kinase Inhibitors for the Treatment of Corneal Endothelial Diseases. *J. Ophthalmol.* **2017**, *2017*, 2646904.
77. Honjo, M.; Tanihara, H.; Kameda, T.; Kawaji, T.; Yoshimura, N.; Araie, M. Potential role of Rho-associated protein kinase inhibitor Y-27632 in glaucoma filtration surgery. *Invest. Ophthalmol. Vis. Sci.* **2007**, *48*, 5549–5557.
78. Tura, A.; Grisanti, S.; Petermeier, K.; Henke-Fahle, S. The Rho-kinase inhibitor H-1152P suppresses the wound-healing activities of human Tenon's capsule fibroblasts in vitro. *Invest. Ophthalmol. Vis. Sci.* **2007**, *48*, 2152–2161. [CrossRef]
79. Van de Velde, S.; Van Bergen, T.; Vandewalle, E.; Kindt, N.; Castermans, K.; Moons, L.; Stalmans, I. Rho kinase inhibitor AMA0526 improves surgical outcome in a rabbit model of glaucoma filtration surgery. *Prog. Brain Res.* **2015**, *220*, 283–297.
80. Doe, C.; Bentley, R.; Behm, D.J.; Lafferty, R.; Stavenger, R.; Jung, D.; Bamford, M.; Panchal, T.; Grygielko, E.; Wright, L.L.; et al. Novel Rho kinase inhibitors with anti-inflammatory and vasodilatory activities. *J. Pharmacol. Exp. Ther.* **2007**, *320*, 89–98.
81. He, Y.; Xu, H.; Liang, L.; Zhan, Z.; Yang, X.; Yu, X.; Ye, Y.; Sun, L. Antiinflammatory effect of Rho kinase blockade via inhibition of NF-kappaB activation in rheumatoid arthritis. *Arthritis Rheum.* **2008**, *58*, 3366–3376. [CrossRef] [PubMed]
82. Segain, J.P.; Raingeard de la Bletiere, D.; Sauzeau, V.; Bourreille, A.; Hilaret, G.; Cario-Toumaniantz, C.; Pacaud, P.; Galmiche, J.P.; Loirand, G. Rho kinase blockade prevents inflammation via nuclear factor kappa B inhibition: Evidence in Crohn's disease and experimental colitis. *Gastroenterology* **2003**, *124*, 1180–1187. [CrossRef] [PubMed]

Journal of
Clinical Medicine

MDPI

Article

Optic Neuritis: The Influence of Gene Polymorphisms and Serum Levels of *STAT4* (rs10181656, rs7574865, rs7601754, rs10168266)

Greta Gedvilaite [1,2,*], Monika Duseikaitė [1], Gabrielė Dubinskaite [2], Loresa Kriauciuniene [1], Reda Zemaitiene [3] and Rasa Liutkevicienė [1]

1 Laboratory of Ophthalmology, Institute of Neuroscience, Lithuanian University of Health Sciences, LT-50161 Kaunas, Lithuania; monika.duseikaite@lsmuni.lt (M.D.); loresa.kriauciuniene@lsmuni.lt (L.K.); rasa.liutkeviciene@lsmuni.lt (R.L.)

2 Medical Faculty, Lithuanian University of Health Sciences, LT-50161 Kaunas, Lithuania; gabriele.dubinskaite@stud.lsmuni.lt

3 Department of Ophthalmology, Lithuanian University of Health Sciences, LT-50161 Kaunas, Lithuania; reda.zemaitiene@lsmuni.lt

* Correspondence: greta.gedvilaite@lsmuni.lt

Abstract: The aim of the study was to evaluate the associations of *STAT4* (rs10181656, rs7574865, rs7601754, rs10168266) gene polymorphisms and STAT4 serum level in patients with optic neuritis. Eighty-one subjects with optic neuritis (ON) and 158 healthy subjects participated in the study. Genotyping was performed using real-time polymerase chain reaction to obtain data. STAT4 serum level was determined using the ELISA method. Statistical analysis revealed that *STAT4* rs7574865 allele G was statistically significantly more frequent in patients with ON and multiple sclerosis (MS) than in the control group (84.38% vs. 65.93%, $p = 0.003$). *STAT4* rs10168266 allele C was statistically significantly more frequent in the ON group with MS than in the control group (89.06% vs. 71.75%, $p = 0.003$). The haplotypes G-G-A-C and C-T-A-T of *STAT4* (rs10181656, rs7574865, rs7601754, rs10168266) were associated with an 11.5- and 19.5-fold increased odds of ON occurrence ($p = 0.003$; $p = 0.008$, respectively). In optic neuritis without MS occurrence, *STAT4* (rs10181656, rs7574865, rs7601754, rs10168266) haplotypes G-G-A-C and C-T-A-T were found to be associated with 32.6- and 9-fold increased odds of ON without MS ($p = 0.002$, $p = 0.016$, respectively). The current findings may indicate a risk role of *STAT4* (rs10181656, rs7574865, rs7601754, rs10168266) G-G-A-C and C-T-A-T haplotypes in the occurrence of optic neuritis.

Keywords: optic nerve; optic neuritis; *STAT4*; rs10181656; rs7574865; rs7601754; rs10168266; STAT4 ELISA

1. Introduction

The optic nerve, also known as cranial nerve II, is a structure of ganglion cell fibers that connects the brain with the retina and is responsible for transmission of visual information. The optic nerve, which is enveloped by three meninges (hard, soft, and arachnoid), is anatomically divided into four parts: the crystalline lens (*pars intraocularis*), the orbit (*pars intraorbitalis*), the part located in the cranial box (*pars intracranialis*), and the part of the nerve located in the bony canal (*pars intracanalicularis*) [1,2]. Due to its structure and location in the cranial cavity, the optic nerve is one of the most sensitive structures in the body and is most frequently damaged by various diseases, conditions, or injuries [3,4]. Changes in the optic nerve can also be a local sign of systemic diseases, such as idiopathic intracranial hypertension (IIH). In other cases, a para-physiological finding (optic nerve drusen) can simulate a serious pathology and mislead the clinician. For this reason, ultrasound examination of the optic nerve is of fundamental importance [5,6].

Under the influence of various environmental and genetic factors, visual impairment manifests itself in specific symptoms that may indicate possible damage to the aforementioned structure. One of the most common diseases of the optic nerve is optic neuritis (ON). This pathology usually occurs in people aged 18–45 years. The prevalence of optic neuritis is 1–5 cases per 100,000 population [3]. The best-studied and best-known causes of the disease are multiple sclerosis (MS), ischemia, infectious and autoimmune processes, so that ON can still be divided into typical and atypical forms [7,8].

Although the causes mentioned above are undoubtedly associated with optic nerve inflammation, the importance of genetic factors remains unclear. The influence of hereditary or congenital factors on the manifestation of certain diseases is increasingly recognized.

Members of the Signal Transducer and Activator of Transcription (STAT) proteins are responsible for physiological cellular processes in the body, such as proliferation, differentiation, apoptosis, angiogenesis, and the regulation of the immune system [9,10]. However, as with any other healthy part of the body system, genetic damage occurs, leading to inappropriate expression of STAT proteins. All this can be associated with pathological processes such as malignant cell transformation and metastasis [10]. The fourth member of the STAT family, STAT4, which is localized in the cytoplasm, can be phosphorylated by membrane-bound receptors, dimerized, and translocated to the nucleus, where it differentially regulates gene expression. This transcription factor transmits interleukin (IL)-12, (IL)-23, and type I interferon cytokine signals in T cells and monocytes. It leads to the differentiation of T helper type 1 and T helper type 17, the activation of monocytes, and the production of interferon, so the factor may be involved in many autoimmune diseases [11]. *STAT4* single nucleotide polymorphisms (SNPs) are known to be associated with an increased risk of autoimmune diseases, such as systemic lupus erythematosus (SLE), primary Sjogren's syndrome (pSS), rheumatoid arthritis (RA), or thyroid disease [12], so an association with other less well-studied diseases is possible. Therefore, the aim of this study is to determine the associations of *STAT4* (rs10181656, rs7574865, rs7601754, rs10168266) with the manifestation of optic neuritis.

1.1. Clinic

The initial clinical manifestations are loss of vision in one eye, pain that worsens with eye movement, and impaired color perception [3]. Patients describe seeing as if through a fog, and initial changes can occur within a few hours to days. The earliest onset of dyschromatopsia (impaired color perception) affects a broad spectrum of colors [8]. As visual acuity can vary from minimal to complete vision loss, patients may complain of "flashes" of light during eye movements, known as photocopies [13,14] When the depth perception of moving objects is altered, the disorder is referred to as Pulfrich phenomenon [15]. During the visual recovery phase, there may be a brief deterioration in vision after a hot shower or exercise (when body temperature rises)—this is known as the Unthoff symptom [16]. Central and peripheral ocular changes may occur during optic neuritis and are characteristic of 97% of patients. Central disturbances occur more frequently but recover more slowly. Almost all patients with bilateral ON have an afferent pupillary defect [14].

Based on the site of involvement, ON can be categorized as follows:

1. Retrobulbar neuritis with normal appearance of the optic disc;
2. Papillitis with a swollen optic disc;
3. Perineuritis, which affects the optic nerve sheath, while the optic disc may or may not be swollen;
4. Neuroretinitis with optic nerve oedema and macular exudates [17]. Retrobulbar neuritis and papillitis are mainly associated with MS, while perineuritis and neuroretinitis are more commonly associated with infectious or inflammatory pathologies [18].

1.2. STAT

Signal transducers and activators of transcription (STATs) are a family of proteins responsible for the essential and multifunctional regulation of physiological cellular processes, including proliferation, differentiation, apoptosis, angiogenesis, and immune regulation. As the name implies, these factors can transmit signals from the cell membrane to the cell nucleus and thereby activate gene transcription [9]. In their inactive form, STAT proteins are located in the cytoplasm. They become active through phosphorylation of tyrosine and serine amino acids. Dimers are already formed in the active state. Then they migrate to the nucleus, bind to DNA and regulate gene transcription [11,13,19]. Seven members of the STAT family have been identified in the human genome: STAT1, STAT2, STAT3, STAT4, STAT5A, STAT5B, and STAT6 [20]. Each STAT protein has its own function, and STAT3 and STAT5 are considered oncogenes [21].

1.3. STAT4 Gene

Several *STAT4* single nucleotide polymorphisms (SNPs) have previously been associated with an increased risk of autoimmune diseases such as systemic lupus erythemosus (SLE), primary Sjogren's syndrome (pSS), rheumatoid arthritis (RA) and thyroid disease [12,22,23].

The four *STAT4* polymorphisms investigated in this study (rs10181656, rs7574865, rs7601754, rs10168266) are located at different sites on the chromosome (Figure 1). SNP rs7574865 and rs10181656 are located in intron 3, while rs7601754 and rs10168266 are located in intron 4 and intron 5, respectively [12]. STAT4 is activated by interleukin (IL)-12 and IL -23, which promotes the differentiation of CD40+ T cells into Th1 and Th17 cells and the production of interferon-γ (IFN-γ) and IL-17. The Th1 signaling pathway is considered to be the most important proinflammatory part of pathogenesis in multiple sclerosis (MS). In contrast, the Th17 signaling pathway is involved in the pathogenetic mechanisms of MS. It is well known that ON is closely related to MS, and it is often difficult to distinguish the specific symptoms of these diseases [24,25], so the SNPs studied in our work could have a direct impact on the manifestation of ON.

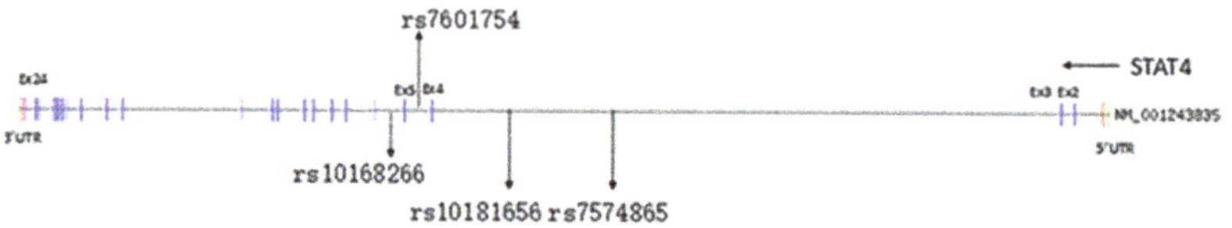

Figure 1. STAT4 SNPs location.

1.4. Optic Neuritis and Multiple Sclerosis

Multiple sclerosis is a chronic inflammatory, demyelinating disease of the central nervous system characterized by white matter damage and axonal loss. The causes of this disease are not yet fully understood, but it is often associated with viral infections or other autoimmune processes. The diagnosis is made on the basis of clinical symptoms or instrumental tests [24].

When optic neuritis and multiple sclerosis occur together, it is often difficult to distinguish the specific signs of these diseases, as ON can be part of the manifestations of multiple sclerosis [26]. In about 20% of MS patients, this disease first manifests as inflammation of the optic nerve; in about 50% of MS patients, inflammation of the optic nerve occurs during their lifetime [24,25].

2. Materials and Methods

2.1. Ethics Statement

To determine whether there was an association between *STAT4* and ON, we conducted a study involving subjects who had signed personal forms for approval by the Kaunas Regional Biomedical Research Ethics Committee (No. BE-2-102).

2.2. Subjects

Subjects with ON were included according to the inclusion/diagnostic criteria (Table 1) [27].

Table 1. Optic neuritis (ON) inclusion/diagnostic criteria [27].

Symptoms	Typical ON
Age	Young patient < 50 years
Visual acuity loss time	Acute/subacute visual acuity loss
Visual acuity loss progression	Visual acuity loss progressing for few days or few weeks
Damage	Mostly one eye
Visual acuity	↓ in 90% of cases
Visual field	Changes noticed in 97% of cases
Color vision	In acute period, blue-yellow color vision loss; in subacute period, red-green color vision loss
Visual evoked potentials (VEP)	↓ VEP latency
Optical coherence tomography (OCT)	Optic nerve disc edema (mostly in superior and nasal quadrants), noticed in 20% of patients
Pain	Acute painful visual acuity loss, especially ↑ with eye movement
Optic nerve disc	Mostly normal optic nerve disc
Vitreous	Normal
Orbit	Normal
Anamnesis	ON in anamnesis or MS in anamnesis. Patients without MS had MS-like lesions but were not followed up after ON treatment in our study, only redirected for neurological follow-up.
Neurological symptoms	Neurological symptoms, allowing to suspect MS
Treatment effect using steroids	Shortens the duration of the disease
Improvement	Spontaneous improvement in 2–3 weeks
Prognosis	Mostly good
Recurrence (5–10 years)	28%

Patients with other diseases of the optic nerve, systemic illnesses (diabetes mellitus, oncological diseases, systemic tissue disorders, chronic infectious diseases, conditions after organ or tissue transplantation), opacities of the optical system or because of poor quality of fundus photography were excluded [27,28].

The diagnosis of MS was made on the basis of consultation with the neurologist and MRI records. The neurological diagnosis of MS was established according to the revised and widely accepted McDonald criteria [29].

The control group comprised healthy individuals admitted to the Department of Ophthalmology at the Hospital of Lithuanian University of Health Sciences for routine ophthalmological examinations. Matching was performed based on the age and gender of patients diagnosed with optic neuritis (ON). Inclusion in the control group required participants to exhibit no ophthalmological eye disorders during the examination and to provide informed consent. Exclusion criteria encompassed any pre-existing eye disorders and the use of epileptic and sedative medications.

2.3. Genotyping

The analysis of *STAT4* gene polymorphisms, specifically rs10181656, rs7574865, rs7601754, and rs10168266, was conducted at the Laboratory of Ophthalmology, Neuroscience Institute, LUHS. Genotyping of *STAT4* polymorphisms was carried out using the real-time polymerase chain reaction (RT-PCR) method. The identification of all single-nucleotide polymorphisms was performed through TaqMan® Genotyping assays (Applied Biosystems, New York, NY, USA; Thermo Fisher Scientific, Inc., Waltham, MA, USA), specifically using the assays: C__30530761_10, C__29882391_10, C__11515729_20, and C__29936344_10, following the manufacturer's protocols on a StepOne Plus system (Applied Biosystems). The genotyping process utilized the "StepOnePlus" real-time PCR quantification system (Thermo Fisher Scientific, Singapore).

2.4. Serum IL-9 Levels Measurement

Serum STAT4 levels were measured in duplicate in control subjects and patients with ON. The determination was performed by enzyme-linked immunosorbent assay (ELISA) using the Signal Transducer And Activator Of Transcription 4 (STAT4) ELISA kit (Cat. No. abx156860), standard curve sensibility range: 0.312–20 ng/mL, sensitivity <0.12 ng/mL. Serum levels were analyzed according to the manufacturer's instructions using a Multiskan FC Microplate Photometer (Thermo Scientific, Waltham, MA, USA/Canada) at 450 nm.

2.5. Statistical Analysis

Statistical data analysis for genotype and allele distribution and binary logistic regression was carried out with the program "IBM SPSS Statistics 29.0", while haplotype analysis was performed with the online program "SNPStats". Qualitative data are presented in absolute numbers and percentages. The hypothesis about the distribution of the quantitative data was tested using the Shapiro–Wilk test. The median was calculated for the test characteristics that did not fulfil the criteria of normal distribution.

After evaluating the age of the subjects and if the studied groups did not meet the criterion of normal distribution, the Mann–Whitney U test was used (to assess the difference between two independent groups). Binary logistic regression calculations were also performed, evaluating the influence of genotypes on the occurrence of ON, indicating the 95% likelihood ratio (OR) and confidence interval (CI).

In our study, we applied the Bonferroni correction because of multiple comparisons. Therefore, differences are considered statistically significant if the *p*-value is <0.05/4 (<0.0125). Only statistically significant results are presented in this article.

3. Results

During the study, subjects were divided into two groups. The first group consisted of subjects with optic neuritis (ON) with or without multiple sclerosis ($n = 81$). Of these, 28 were men (34.56%), 53 were women (65.44%), and the average age of the subjects was 33 years. Of these, 24 were examined for multiple sclerosis. The control group was composed of 158 subjects: 37 males (23.41%), 121 females (76.59%), and their average age was 29.5 years. The characteristics of the subjects are shown in Table S1 of the Supplementary Materials.

The genotypes and allele distributions of *STAT4* genes rs10181656, rs7574865, rs7601754, and rs10168266 were analysed in the ON group and compared with the control group. However, no statistically significant differences were found between the groups (Supplementary Materials, Table S2). Binary logistic regression also revealed no statistically significant differences between patients with optic neuritis and the control group (Supplementary Materials, Table S3).

STAT4 rs10181656, rs7574865, rs7601754, rs10168266 genotype and allele distribution were compared by age group (≤30 and >30 years) and gender. Unfortunately, no statistically significant differences were found (Supplementary Material, Tables S4 and S5). Binary logistic regression between patients with optic neuritis and the control group also did not yield statistically significant results when divided by age groups (≤30 and >30 years) and gender (Supplementary Materials, Tables S6 and S7).

Another analysis was performed when subjects with ON were divided into two groups: with multiple sclerosis and without multiple sclerosis. Statistically significant differences were found when comparing ON with MS and the control group. The *STAT4* rs7574865 G allele was statistically significantly more frequent in the group of ON patients with MS than in the control group (84.38% vs. 65.93%, $p = 0.003$). In addition, *STAT4* rs10168266 C allele was statistically significantly more frequent in ON group of patients with MS than in control group (89.06% vs. 71.75%, $p = 0.003$). The results are shown in Table 2. However, binary logistic regression did not yield statistically significant results between patients with MS and without MS (Supplementary Materials, Table S8).

Table 2. Distribution of *STAT4* (rs10181656, rs7574865, rs7601754, rs10168266) genotypes, optic nerve inflammation groups in patients with and without multiple sclerosis.

Gene	Genotype	With MS			Without MS		
		ON Group (n = 32) n (%)	Control Group (n = 158) n (%)	p-Value	ON Group (n = 42) n (%)	Control Group (n = 158) n (%)	p-Value
STAT4 (rs10181656)	CC	20 (62.5)	90 (56.96)	0.721	26 (61.9)	90 (56.96)	0.827
	CG	11 (34.38)	58 (36.71)		14 (33.33)	58 (36.71)	
	GG	1 (3.13)	10 (6.33)		2 (4.76)	10 (6.33)	
	Allele:						
	C	51 (79.69)	238 (65.38)	0.024	66 (78.57)	238 (65.38)	0.020
	G	13 (20.31)	126 (34.62)		18 (21.43)	126 (34.62)	
STAT4 (rs7574865)	GG	23 (71.88)	91 (57.59)	0.303	25 (59.52)	91 (57.59)	0.968
	GT	8 (25)	56 (35.44)		14 (33.33)	56 (35.44)	
	TT	1 (3.13)	11 (6.96)		3 (7.14)	11 (6.96)	
	Allele:						
	G	54 (84.38)	238 (65.93)	0.003	64 (76.19)	238 (65.93)	0.070
	T	10 (15.63)	123 (34.07)		20 (23.81)	123 (34.07)	
STAT4 (rs7601754)	AA	22 (68.75)	121 (76.58)	0.631	31 (73.81)	121 (76.58)	0.927
	GA	9 (28.13)	34 (21.52)		10 (23.81)	34 (21.52)	
	GG	1 (3.13)	3 (1.9)		1 (2.38)	3 (1.9)	
	Allele:						
	A	53 (82.81)	276 (79.54)	0.547	72 (85.71)	276 (79.54)	0.198
	G	11 (17.19)	71 (20.46)		12 (14.29)	71 (20.46)	
STAT4 (rs10168266)	CC	26 (81.25)	105 (66.46)	0.213	27 (64.29)	105 (66.46)	0.873
	CT	5 (15.63)	49 (31.01)		13 (30.95)	49 (31.01)	
	TT	1 (3.13)	4 (2.53)		2 (4.76)	4 (2.53)	
	Allele:						
	C	57 (89.06)	259 (71.75)	0.003	67 (79.76)	259 (71.75)	0.135
	T	7 (10.94)	102 (28.25)		17 (20.24)	102 (28.25)	

p-value—significance level; After Bonferroni correction, differences were considered statistically significant when $p < 0.0125$.

STAT4 (rs10181656, rs7574865, rs7601754, rs10168266) haplotype analysis was performed. Pairwise linkage disequilibrium (LD) between studied polymorphisms was observed. The deviation between the predicted haplotype frequency and the observed frequency (D') was calculated, and the square of the correlation coefficient (r^2) was estimated. Data are presented in Table 3.

Table 3. Linkage disequilibrium between studied polymorphisms in patients with optical neuritis and control group.

SNPs	ON vs. Controls		
	D′	r^2	*p*-Value
rs10181656–rs7574865	0.867	0.743	<0.001
rs10181656–rs7601754	0.858	0.034	<0.001
rs10181656–rs10168266	0.707	0.348	<0.001
rs7574865–rs7601754	0.998	0.046	<0.001
rs7574865–rs10168266	0.814	0.467	<0.001
rs7601754–rs10168266	0.998	0.032	<0.001

D′: the deviation between the expected haplotype frequency and the observed frequency; r^2: the square of the haplotype frequency correlation coefficient.

Haplotype frequencies and statistical analysis on the occurrence of ON have shown that individuals carrying *STAT4* rs10181656, rs7574865, rs7601754, rs10168266 haplotypes G-G-A-C and C-T-A-T were associated with 11.5- and 19.5-fold increased odds of ON (OR = 11.51; 95% CI: 2.29–57.80; p = 0.003; OR = 19.47; 95% CI: 2.25–168.17; p = 0.008, respectively) (Table 4).

Table 4. Haplotype association with the predisposition to optical neuritis occurrence.

Haplotype	*STAT4* rs10181656	*STAT4* rs7574865	*STAT4* rs7601754	*STAT4* rs10168266	Frequency		OR (95% CI)	*p*-Value
					Control	ON		
1	C	G	A	C	59.43	58.29	1.00	–
2	G	T	A	T	14.57	11.01	0.55 (0.27–1.09)	0.087
3	C	G	G	C	11.78	14.81	1.24 (0.69–2.24)	0.470
4	G	T	A	C	9.16	4.15	0.47 (0.19–1.17)	0.100
5	C	G	A	T	2.59	0.70	0.29 (0.05–1.62)	0.160
6	G	G	A	C	0.64	5.17	11.51 (2.29–57.80)	0.003
7	C	T	A	T	0.32	4.30	19.47 (2.25–168.17)	0.008
rare	*	*	*	*	NA	NA	0.65 (0.06–7.49)	0.760

OR: odds ratio; CI: confidence interval; *p*-value: significance level (after Bonferroni correction statistically significant when $p < 0.0125$). * rare—polymorphic alleles with <1% frequency; NA—not applicable.

In addition, we performed haplotype analysis in ON with and without MS groups vs. the control group. Statistical analysis of the incidence of ON without MS has shown that individuals carrying *STAT4* rs10181656, rs7574865, rs7601754, rs10168266 haplotypes C-T-A-T and G-G-A-C were respectively associated with 32.6- and 9-fold increased odds of ON without MS occurrence (OR = 32.55; 95% CI: 3.66–289.72; p = 0.002; OR = 9.05; 95% CI: 1.53–53.35; p = 0.016, respectively) (Table 5). Unfortunately, haplotype analysis of ON with MS vs. control group did not reveal any statistically significant results (Supplementary Materials, Table S9).

Table 5. Haplotype association with the predisposition to optical neuritis without MS occurrence.

Haplotype	*STAT4* rs10181656	*STAT4* rs7574865	*STAT4* rs7601754	*STAT4* rs10168266	Frequency Control	Frequency ON	OR (95% CI)	*p*-Value
1	C	G	A	C	59.43	55.58	1.00	–
2	G	T	A	T	14.57	11.52	0.57 (0.24–1.38)	0.210
3	C	G	G	C	11.78	14.28	1.21 (0.57–2.61)	0.620
4	G	T	A	C	9.16	4.81	0.50 (0.15–1.64)	0.260
5	C	G	A	T	2.59	1.24	0.49 (0.06–4.41)	0.530
6	C	T	A	T	0.32	7.47	32.55 (3.66–289.72)	0.002
7	G	G	A	C	0.64	5.09	9.05 (1.53–53.35)	0.016

OR: odds ratio; CI: confidence interval; *p*-value: significance level (after Bonferroni correction statistically significant when $p < 0.0125$).

STAT4 serum levels in ON patients and control group subjects were evaluated. We found that STAT4 serum levels were not statistically significantly different between groups (0.290 (0.248) ng/mL vs. 0.314 (0.292) ng/mL, $p = 0.263$) (Figure 2).

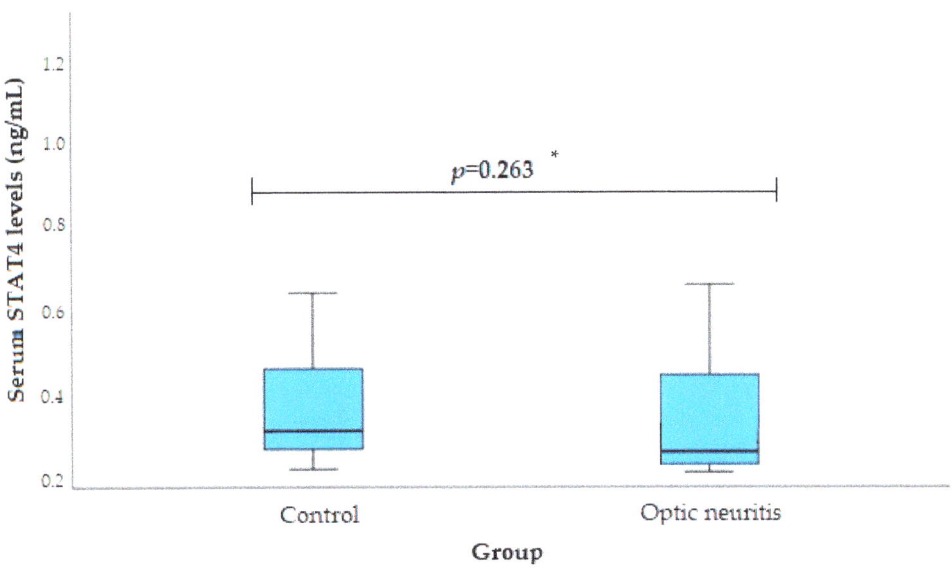

Figure 2. Serum STAT4 levels (ng/mL) in ON and control groups. * Mann–Whitney U test was used.

4. Discussion

In this study, we investigated the associations of *STAT4* gene (rs10181656, rs7574865, rs7601754, rs10168266) polymorphisms and STAT4 serum level with ON. According to the scientific literature, the rs10181656, rs7574865, rs7601754 and rs10168266 polymorphisms influence the manifestation of various diseases, including autoimmune diseases. Associations have been found with Graves' disease (GD) and Hashimoto's thyroiditis (HT) as well as an increased risk of rheumatoid arthritis, systemic lupus erythematosus and type 1 diabetes [12,30–34]. However, no study has examined the impact of the occurrence of ON.

Hye-Soon Lee and co-authors conducted a study to determine the association of rs7574865, rs8179673, rs10181656 with type 1 diabetes. Patients were categorized into early- and late-period subgroups based on the time of diagnosis. Rs7574865, rs8179673 and rs10181656 showed statistically significant associations with diabetes type 1 in the early-onset subgroup (rs7574865, OR = 1.44 (1.03–2.01), $p < 0.05$), but not in the late-onset subgroup. This provides evidence that *STAT4* is not only disease-specific but also associated with early development of type 1 diabetes [23]. Yongsoo Park and co-authors also studied *STAT4* gene expression in type 1 CD. The results show an association between *STAT4* haplotype (rs11889341, rs7574865, rs8179673, and rs10181656) and type 1 diabetes and rheumatoid arthritis. Researchers have found that *STAT4* alleles and the same haplotypes can influence cytokine signaling and thus the development of autoimmune thyroid disease (AITD) and type 1 diabetes [35].

Based on the further aims of our work, an analysis of *STAT4* polymorphisms (rs10181656, rs7574865, rs7601754, rs10168266) was performed to determine associations with ON in subjects with ON and control groups as a function of subject age. We did not obtain statistically significant data ($p < 0.0125$). Bi C and co-authors conducted a case-control study in a Han population in northeastern China. Two SNPs in the *STAT4* gene and their association with type 1 diabetes were investigated. This disease is associated with autoimmune body lesions such as ON. The results of this study showed that one of the two SNPs studied (rs7574865) was strongly associated with type 1 diabetes in a northeast Chinese population compared with healthy controls ($p < 0.05$). Another SNP (rs3024866) showed a weak association with the onset of type 1 diabetes, but when the researchers stratified patients by age of onset, the alleles of all four single nucleotide polymorphisms and the same haplotypes showed a significant association with susceptibility to type 1 diabetes in the early-onset subgroup ($p < 0.01$) and not in the late-onset subgroup [22].

STAT4 is a central mediator in the development of inflammation during protective immune responses and immune-mediated disease [36]. Rheumatoid arthritis (RA) is a chronic systemic inflammatory disease characterized by articular and extra-articular manifestations, including cardiovascular disease [37]. Both genetic and environmental factors have been reported to influence the pathogenesis of RA. STAT4 contributes to the differentiation and proliferation of Th1 and Th17 cells, which play a critical role in chronic inflammatory diseases [38]. Researchers found that increased expression of STAT4 protein in dendritic cells in the synovial membrane is associated with serum rheumatoid factor, which is a risk factor for RA [39,40]. Diabetic retinopathy (DR) is considered one of the most important microvascular complications of diabetes, usually resulting from moderate to severe vision loss [41]. One of the main reasons for this irreversible visual impairment is retinal neovascularization. DR is usually associated with dysfunction of signaling pathways and abnormal expression of functional molecules [42]. Jun Shao and co-authors conducted a case-control study in China, experimenting with certified hRECs cells. The results of this study showed that miR-223-3p plays a key role in the development of DR and that the STAT4 protein recognizes mir223-3p as a direct target and can enhance the expression of mir223-3p. This study revealed a new potential signaling pathway in the progression of DR [43].

The study's main limitation is its small sample size due to the rarity of ON. Future studies should prioritize increasing the number of subjects to enhance result accuracy. A larger sample size offers advantages such as increased trait variation, higher significance levels, and lower measurement error [44]. These improvements bolster the study's reliability and its potential to inform further exploration of ON pathology, contributing to strategies for preventing rapid disease progression. Addressing this limitation remains a priority in future research efforts, emphasizing our commitment to advancing ON understanding. The results of the research conducted can be used to further study this pathology and prevent the rapid progression of the disease. Considering the crucial roles of *STAT4* in inflammation and autoimmunity, targeting this gene may offer a novel avenue for therapeutic intervention in ON, especially in the context of MS [45]. The molecular insights provided by our study contribute to understanding the underlying mechanisms of ON and MS pathogenesis. This understanding, combined with the known efficacy of current immunosuppressive treatments in modulating these processes, opens up possibilities for developing targeted and personalized therapeutic options. Therefore, the performed scientific researches contribute to establishing a relationship between *STAT4* gene SNP (rs10181656, rs7574865, rs7601754, rs10168266) and autoimmune diseases. With a larger sample size, it is worthwhile to search for other associations of *STAT4* harboring other SNPs with ON.

5. Conclusions

In conclusion, the G-G-A-C and C-T-A-T haplotypes of the STAT4 gene, represented by rs10181656, rs7574865, rs7601754, and rs10168266, exhibit significant associations with ON occurrences. Specifically, these haplotypes are linked to an 11.5- and 19.5-fold increased odds of ON, both with *p*-values of 0.003 and 0.008, respectively. Moreover, when considering cases of optic neuritis without MS, the same STAT4 haplotypes, G-G-A-C and C-T-A-T, demonstrate notable associations with 32.6- and 9-fold increased odds, supported by *p*-values of 0.002 and 0.016, respectively. Collectively, the current evidence suggests a potential risk role of the STAT4 G-G-A-C and C-T-A-T haplotypes in the context of both ON and ON without MS.

Supplementary Materials: The following supporting information can be downloaded at: https://www.mdpi.com/article/10.3390/jcm13010010/s1, Table S1: Characteristics; Table S2: Distribution of *STAT4* rs10181656, rs7574865, rs7601754, rs10168266 genotypes in patients with optic neuritis and controls; Table S3: STAT4 (rs10181656, rs7574865, rs7601754, rs10168266) binary logistic regression analysis of genotypes; Table S4: *STAT4* (rs10181656, rs7574865, rs7601754, rs10168266) distribution of genotypes in patients with optic neuritis and controls according to the age of the subjects; Table S5: Distribution of *STAT4* (rs10181656, rs7574865, rs7601754, rs10168266) genotypes in patients with optic neuritis and controls according to gender; Table S6: Binary logistic regression analysis of *STAT4* (rs10181656, rs7574865, rs7601754, rs10168266) genotypes by age of the subjects; Table S7: Binary logistic regression analysis of *STAT4* (rs10181656, rs7574865, rs7601754, rs10168266) genotypes by gender; Table S8: Binary logistic regression analysis of STAT4 (rs10181656, rs7574865, rs7601754, rs10168266) genotypes in patients with multiple sclerosis (with MS) and without multiple sclerosis (without MS); Table S9: Haplotype association with the predisposition to optical neuritis with MS occurrence.

Author Contributions: Conceptualization, G.G., M.D. and R.L.; methodology, G.G. and M.D.; software, G.G.; validation, G.G. and M.D.; formal analysis, G.G.; investigation, G.D., G.G. and M.D.; resources, R.L., L.K. and R.Z.; data curation, G.G. and R.L.; writing—original draft preparation, G.G., M.D. and R.L.; writing—review and editing, G.G., M.D. and R.L.; visualization, G.G., M.D. and R.L.; supervision, R.L.; project administration, R.L.; funding acquisition, G.G. All authors have read and agreed to the published version of the manuscript.

Funding: This research received no external funding.

Institutional Review Board Statement: The study was conducted in accordance with the Declaration of Helsinki, and approved by the Biomedical Research, Lithuanian University of Health Sciences (No. BE-2-102, 25 November 2016).

Informed Consent Statement: Informed consent was obtained from all subjects involved in the study.

Data Availability Statement: Data is contained within the article and Supplementary Materials.

Conflicts of Interest: The authors declare no conflict of interest.

References

1. Pukenytė, R.; Šustickas, G.; Ščerbak, J.; Aukštikalnis, D.; Ašoklis, R. Regos nervo sužalojimas: Literatūros apžvalga. *Liet. Chirurgija* **2011**, *9*, 18–24. [CrossRef]

2. Dhillon, N. Anatomy. In *Current Diagnosis & Treatment Otolaryngology—Head and Neck Surgery*, 4th ed.; Lalswani, A.K., Ed.; McGraw-Hill Education: New York, NY, USA, 2020.
3. Punytė, V.; Liutkevičienė, R.; Gelžinis, A.; Žemaitienė, R. Optic neuritis. *J. Med. Sci.* **2020**, *8*, 170–175.
4. Bennett, J.L. Optic Neuritis. In *CONTINUUM Lifelong Learning in Neurology*; Lippincott Williams and Wilkins: Philadelphia, PA, USA, 2019; Volume 25, pp. 1236–1264.
5. Rosa, N.; De Bernardo, M.; Di Stasi, M.; Cione, F.; Capaldo, I. A-Scan Ultrasonographic Evaluation of Patients with Idiopathic Intracranial Hypertension: Comparison of Optic Nerves. *J. Clin. Med.* **2022**, *11*, 6153. [CrossRef] [PubMed]
6. Rosa, N.; De Bernardo, M.; Abbinante, G.; Vecchio, G.; Cione, F.; Capasso, L. Optic Nerve Drusen Evaluation: A Comparison between Ultrasound and OCT. *J. Clin. Med.* **2022**, *11*, 3715. [CrossRef] [PubMed]
7. Morrow, M.J. Ischemic Optic Neuropathy. *Continuum* **2019**, *25*, 1215–1235. [CrossRef]
8. Toosy, A.T.; Mason, D.F.; Miller, D.H. Optic neuritis. In *The Lancet Neurology*; Elsevier: Amsterdam, The Netherlands, 2014; Volume 13, pp. 83–99.
9. Verhoeven, Y.; Tilborghs, S.; Jacobs, J.; De Waele, J.; Quatannens, D.; Deben, C.; Prenen, H.; Pauwels, P.; Trinh, X.B.; Wouters, A.; et al. The Potential and Controversy of Targeting STAT Family Members in Cancer. In *Seminars in Cancer Biology*; Academic Press: Cambridge, MA, USA, 2020; Volume 60, pp. 41–56. [CrossRef]
10. Bowman, T.; Garcia, R.; Turkson, J.; Jove, R. STATs in Oncogenesis. In *Oncogene*; Nature Publishing Group: Berlin, Germany, 2000; Volume 19, pp. 2474–2488.
11. Wilhelm, H.; Schabet, M. The Diagnosis and Treatment of Optic Neuritis. *Dtsch. Arztebl. Int.* **2015**, *112*, 616–626. [CrossRef]
12. Shi, Z.; Zhang, Q.; Chen, H.; Lian, Z.; Liu, J.; Feng, H.; Miao, X.; Du, Q.; Zhou, H. STAT4 Polymorphisms are Associated with Neuromyelitis Optica Spec-trum Disorders. *NeuroMol. Med.* **2017**, *19*, 493–500. [CrossRef]
13. Newman, N.J. The Optic Neuritis Treatment Trial. *Ophthalmology* **2020**, *127*, S172–S173. [CrossRef]
14. Slavinskaitė, A.; Banevičius, M.; Kriaučiūnienė, L.; Zlatkutė, E.; Vilkevičiūtė, A.; Liutkevičienė, R. Regos nervo neurito pagrindiniai diagnostikos ir gydymo principai. *Neurol. Semin.* **2016**, *20*, 17–22.
15. Sobhanian, M.J.; Agarwal, R.; Meltzer, E.; Kildebeck, E.; Frohman, B.S.; Frohman, A.N.; Galetta, S.L.; Saidha, S.; White, O.; Villoslada, P.; et al. Identification and treatment of the visual processing asymmetry in MS patients with optic neuritis: The Pulfrich phenomenon. *J. Neurol. Sci.* **2018**, *387*, 60–69. [CrossRef]
16. Jain, A.; Rosso, M.; Santoro, J.D. Wilhelm Uhthoff and Uhthoff's phenomenon. *Mult. Scler. J.* **2020**, *26*, 1790–1796. [CrossRef] [PubMed]
17. Hoorbakht, H.; Bagherkashi, F. Optic neuritis, its differential diagnosis and management. *Open Ophthalmol. J.* **2012**, *6*, 65–72. [CrossRef] [PubMed]
18. Pau, D.; Al Zubidi, N.; Yalamanchili, S.; Plant, G.T.; Lee, A.G. Optic neuritis. *Eye* **2011**, *25*, 833–842. [CrossRef] [PubMed]
19. Mehrpouya-Bahrami, P.; Moriarty, A.K.; De Melo, P.; Keeter, W.C.; Alakhras, N.S.; Nelson, A.S.; Hoover, M.; Barrios, M.S.; Nadler, J.L.; Serezani, C.H.; et al. STAT4 is expressed in neutrophils and promotes antimicrobial immunity. *J. Clin. Investig.* **2021**, *6*, e141326. [CrossRef] [PubMed]
20. Ihle, J.N. The Stat Family in Cytokine Signaling. In *Current Opinion in Cell Biology*; Elsevier Ltd.: Amsterdam, The Netherlands, 2001; Volume 13, pp. 211–217. [CrossRef]
21. Calò, V.; Migliavacca, M.; Bazan, V.; Macaluso, M.; Buscemi, M.; Gebbia, N.; Russo, A. STAT proteins: From normal control of cellular events to tumorigenesis. *J. Cell. Physiol.* **2003**, *197*, 157–168. [CrossRef]
22. Bi, C.; Li, B.; Cheng, Z.; Hu, Y.; Fang, Z.; Zhai, A. Association study of STAT4 polymorphisms and type 1 diabetes in Northeastern Chinese Han population. *Tissue Antigens* **2013**, *81*, 137–140. [CrossRef]
23. Lee, H.-S.; Park, H.; Yang, S.; Kim, D.; Park, Y. STAT4 Polymorphism Is Associated with Early-Onset Type 1 Diabetes, but not with Late-Onset Type 1 Diabetes. In *Annals of the New York Academy of Sciences*; Blackwell Publishing Inc.: Oxford, UK, 2008; Volume 1150, pp. 93–98. [CrossRef]
24. Hauser, S.L.; Cree, B.A. Treatment of Multiple Sclerosis: A Review. *Am. J. Med.* **2020**, *133*, 1380–1390.e2. [CrossRef]
25. Zafeiropoulos, P.; Katsanos, A.; Kitsos, G.; Stefaniotou, M.; Asproudis, I. The contribution of multifocal visual evoked potentials in patients with optic neuritis and multiple sclerosis. A review. *Doc. Ophthalmol.* **2021**, *142*, 283–292. [CrossRef]
26. Guier, C.P.; Stokkermans, T.J. Optic Neuritis. In *StatPearls*; StatPearls Publishing: Treasure Island, FL, USA, 2022.
27. Liutkeviciene, R.; Vilkeviciute, A.; Banevicus, M.; Miezyte, R.; Kriauciuniene, L. Association of MMP-2 (-1306 C/T) gene polymor-phism with predisposition of optic neuritis together with multiple sclerosis. *Medicina* **2018**, *54*, 29. [CrossRef]
28. Gedvilaite, G.; Vilkeviciute, A.; Kriauciuniene, L.; Asmoniene, V.; Liutkeviciene, R. Does CETP rs5882, rs708272, SIRT1 rs12778366, FGFR2 rs2981582, STAT3 rs744166, VEGFA rs833068, IL6 rs1800795 polymorphisms play a role in optic neuritis development? *Ophthalmic Genet.* **2019**, *40*, 219–226. [CrossRef]
29. Swanton, J.K.; Rovira, A.; Tintore, M.; Altmann, D.R.; Barkhof, F.; Filippi, M.; Huerga, E.; A Miszkiel, K.; Plant, G.T.; Polman, C.; et al. MRI criteria for multiple sclerosis in patients presenting with clinically isolated syndromes: A multicentre retrospective study. *Lancet Neurol.* **2007**, *6*, 677–686. [CrossRef] [PubMed]
30. Remmers, E.F.; Plenge, R.M.; Lee, A.T.; Graham, R.R.; Hom, G.; Behrens, T.W.; de Bakker, P.I.; Le, J.M.; Lee, H.-S.; Batliwalla, F.; et al. STAT4 and the Risk of Rheumatoid Arthritis and Systemic Lupus Erythematosus. *N. Engl. J. Med.* **2007**, *357*, 977–986. [CrossRef] [PubMed]

31. Ghanavati, F.; Nezhad, S.R.K.; Hajjari, M.R.; Akhoond, M.R. Association of Signal Transducer and Activator of Transcription 4 rs10181656 Polymorphism with Rheumatoid Arthritis and Systemic Sclerosis in Khuzestan Province in Southwestern Iran. *Arch. Rheumatol.* **2019**, *34*, 434–442. [CrossRef] [PubMed]
32. Wang, J.M.; Xu, W.D.; Huang, A.F. Association of STAT4 Gene Rs7574865, Rs10168266 Polymorphisms and Systemic Lupus Er-ythematosus Susceptibility: A Meta-analysis. *Immunol. Investig.* **2021**, *50*, 282–294. [CrossRef] [PubMed]
33. Zhong, X.; Luo, M.; Wu, Y.; Zhou, X.; Yu, X.; Liu, L.; Chen, S. Genetic variants in STAT4 and their interactions with environmental factors for the incidence of hepatocellular carcinoma. *Cancer Biomark.* **2021**, *32*, 3–9. [CrossRef]
34. Gao, W.; Dong, X.; Yang, Z.; Mao, G.; Xing, W. Association between rs7574865 polymorphism in STAT4 gene and rheumatoid arthritis: An updated meta-analysis. *Eur. J. Intern. Med.* **2020**, *71*, 101–103. [CrossRef] [PubMed]
35. Park, Y.; Lee, H.-S.; Park, Y.; Min, D.; Yang, S.; Kim, D.; Cho, B. Evidence for the role of STAT4 as a general autoimmunity locus in the Korean population. *Diabetes/Metab. Res. Rev.* **2011**, *27*, 867–871. [CrossRef] [PubMed]
36. Kaplan, M.H. STAT4: A Critical Regulator of Inflammation In Vivo. *Immunol. Res.* **2005**, *31*, 231–242. [CrossRef]
37. Totoson, P.; Maguin-Gaté, K.; Prati, C.; Wendling, D.; Demougeot, C. Mechanisms of endothelial dysfunction in rheumatoid arthritis: Lessons from animal studies. *Arthritis Res. Ther.* **2014**, *16*, 202. [CrossRef]
38. Yang, C.; Mai, H.; Peng, J.; Zhou, B.; Hou, J.; Jiang, D. STAT4: An immunoregulator contributing to diverse human diseases. *Int. J. Biol. Sci.* **2020**, *16*, 1575–1585. [CrossRef]
39. Walker, J.G.; Ahern, M.J.; Coleman, M.; Weedon, H.; Papangelis, V.; Beroukas, D.; Roberts-Thomson, P.J.; Smith, M.D. Characterisation of a dendritic cell subset in synovial tissue which strongly expresses Jak/STAT transcription factors from patients with rheumatoid arthritis. *Ann. Rheum. Dis.* **2007**, *66*, 992–999. [CrossRef] [PubMed]
40. Gu, E.; Lu, J.; Xing, D.; Chen, X.; Xie, H.; Liang, J.; Li, L. Rs7574865 polymorphism in signal transducers and activators of transcription 4 gene and rheumatoid arthritis: An updated meta-analysis of 28 case-control comparisons. *Int. J. Rheum. Dis.* **2015**, *18*, 3–16. [CrossRef] [PubMed]
41. Hendric, A.M.; Gibson, M.V.; Kulshreshtha, A. Diabetic Retinopathy. In *Primary Care: Clinics in Office Practice*; Elsevier: Amsterdam, The Netherlands, 2015; Volume 42, pp. 451–464. ISBN 9780323395793. ISSN 0095-4543. [CrossRef]
42. Campochiaro, P.A.; Peters, K.G. Targeting Tie2 for Treatment of Diabetic Retinopathy and Diabetic Macular Edema. *Curr. Diabetes Rep.* **2016**, *16*, 126. [CrossRef] [PubMed]
43. Shao, J.; Fan, G.; Yin, X.; Gu, Y.; Wang, X.; Xin, Y.; Yao, Y. A novel transthyretin/STAT4/miR-223-3p/FBXW7 signaling pathway affects neovascularization in diabetic retinopathy. *Mol. Cell. Endocrinol.* **2019**, *498*, 110541. [CrossRef]
44. Cione, F.; Gioia, M.; Pagliarulo, S. Bias That Should Be Avoided to Obtain a Reliable Study of IOL Power Calculation After Myopic Refractive Surgery. *J. Refract. Surg.* **2023**, *39*, 68. [CrossRef]
45. Liang, Y.; Pan, H.-F.; Ye, D.-Q. Therapeutic potential of STAT4 in autoimmunity. *Expert Opin. Ther. Targets* **2014**, *18*, 945–960. [CrossRef]

Journal of
Clinical Medicine

MDPI

Article

The Effect of Esophagogastroduodenoscopy on Intraocular Pressure

Maddalena De Bernardo [1], Antonella Santonicola [2,*], Marco Gioia [1], Livio Vitiello [1], Ferdinando Cione [1], Sergio Pagliarulo [1], Paola Iovino [2] and Nicola Rosa [1]

1 Eye Unit, Department of Medicine, Surgery and Dentistry "Scuola Medica Salernitana", University of Salerno, Baronissi, 84081 Salerno, Italy; mdebernardo@unisa.it (M.D.B.); mgioia@unisa.it (M.G.); livio.vitiello@gmail.com (L.V.); fcione@unisa.it (F.C.); sergiopagliarulo88@gmail.com (S.P.); nrosa@unisa.it (N.R.)

2 Gastroenterology Unit, Department of Medicine, Surgery and Dentistry "Scuola Medica Salernitana", University of Salerno, Baronissi, 84081 Salerno, Italy; piovino@unisa.it

* Correspondence: antonellasantonicola83@gmail.com

Abstract: Background: Esophagogastroduodenoscopy (EGD) is an endoscopic examination of the upper gastrointestinal tract that requires insufflation with gas, leading to intra-abdominal hypertension (IAH). There is evidence suggesting that IAH positively correlates with intracranial pressure (ICP) and possibly with intraocular pressure (IOP). The aim of this study was to examine the effect of a routine screening EGD on the IOP. Methods: In this observational study, 25 patients were recruited; 15 males with a mean age of 50 ± 18 years and 10 females with a mean age of 45 ± 14 years. EGD was conducted under sedation in 21 subjects. Both eyes' IOP measurements were performed using Tonopen Avia in the sitting and left lateral decubitus positions before sedation and the start of EGD, and subsequently in the left lateral decubitus position when the endoscope reached the duodenum (D2) and at the end of the procedure. The final measurement was performed in the sitting position 10 min after the end of the procedure. Results: The mean IOP in the sitting position was 15.16 ± 2.27 mmHg, and in the left lateral decubitus position, 15.68 ± 2.82 mmHg. When the gastroscope entered the D2, it was 21.84 ± 6.55 mmHg, at the end of the procedure, 15.80 ± 3.25 mmHg, and 10 min later, 13.12 ± 3.63 mmHg. There was a statistically significant IOP increase when the gastroscope entered the duodenum ($p < 0.01$). At the end of the gastroscopy, the IOP significantly decreased compared to the one registered when the gastroscope entered the D2 ($p < 0.001$) and it became similar to the values measured before the EGD, in the same left lateral decubitus position ($p > 0.05$). Conclusion: Significant changes in IOP were observed during the EGD. IOP fluctuations during EGD should be taken into account, especially in patients that need repeated EGDs during their life or in patients with glaucoma. Further studies are needed to better understand the short-effect and long-effect influence of an IOP increase in these patients.

Keywords: intraocular pressure; esophagogastroduodenoscopy; supine position; lateral decubitus position; sedation; intra-abdominal insufflation

1. Introduction

Intraocular pressure (IOP) is still a key parameter in the evaluation and management of glaucomatous patients, as well as the only adjustable risk factor linked to glaucoma progression. IOP could be affected by several factors. Among the factors, body position, diurnal variations, heart rate, and medications seem to play a role [1].

Endoscopic procedures continue to play a pivotal role in the diagnosis and treatment of upper and lower gastrointestinal (GI) disorders. Recently, Kent et al. observed a statistically significant IOP decrease at the end of colonoscopy [2]. In fact, the endoscopic examination of the colon requires air insufflation to adequately visualize the colonic mucosal and detect any lesions. The air insufflation of the colon is associated with the increased intra-abdominal pressure that could influence both the intracranial pressure and the IOP [3–9]. Esophagogastroduodenoscopy (EGD) is a high-frequently performed endoscopic procedure that examines the esophagus, stomach, and the first part of the small bowel (duodenum). The procedure is often performed under sedation with a fiber optic camera on a flexible tube and it is used to investigate, diagnose, and treat several diseases [10]. In recent years, a standard protocol for EGD has been highly recommended to ensure a good-quality endoscopy, with the detection of all the precancerous lesions and early cancers in the upper GI tract [11,12]. In particular, the importance of a complete mucosal inspection, achieved by a combination of adequate air insufflation, aspiration, and the use of mucosal cleansing techniques has been underlined. In addition, a high-quality EGD requires time; the whole procedure should take on average 7 min, but the duration can be prolonged in the case of high-risk and surveillance procedures such as Barrett's esophagus or gastric atrophy surveillance [11].

The air insufflation for the luminal distension during EGD might lead to the increase in intra-abdominal pressure that possibly influences the IOP. However, to date, there are no studies investigating this topic.

The aim of the present study is to verify if IOP changes occur during routine EGD.

2. Materials and Methods

This is an observational prospective study. The study protocol was approved by the institutional ethics committee (Cometico Campania Sud prot. Number 16544). A written informed consent was obtained from each subject, after the nature and the intent of the study had been fully explained. Recruitment was performed at a single investigational site between February and July 2021. The study included subjects scheduled to undergo EGD for the diagnosis, screening, and follow-up of main gastrointestinal diseases, performed either under conscious sedation or without it. Inclusion criteria were subjects aged 18 years or older, with no history of glaucoma, no significant ocular or orbital pathologies, no specific abnormalities that may affect the IOP measurements' performance or reliability, no history of severe ocular trauma or surgery, including ocular laser procedures [13], and no chronic ophthalmic medication use.

IOP was measured using Tonopen AVIA® (TPA) (Reichert Ophthalmic Instruments, Depew, NY, USA), previously administering lidocaine 40 mg/mL eye drops. The IOP measurement was performed by an ophthalmologist who was familiar with the procedure. To measure the IOP, TPA utilizes the same GAT physical principle, on a smaller applanated area. In fact, the transducer tip, protected by a single-use latex tip cover before each measurement, has a 1.0 mm diameter. The mean IOP readings were automatically averaged by the instrument, when ten valid readings were obtained, by lightly touching the central cornea. The measurement was shown on the liquid crystal display, which is situated on the side of the device, and together it displayed the "statistical confidence indicator", indicating that the standard deviation of the valid measurements is 5% or less of the number shown. The higher the value, the more reliable the measurement is. Only values higher than 90 were accepted. IOP measurements were performed in both eyes in the sitting and left lateral decubitus positions before sedation and the start of EGD, and subsequently in the left lateral decubitus position when the endoscope reached the duodenum (D2) and at the end of the procedure. The final measurement was performed in the sitting position 10 min after the end of the procedure. All measurements were made with precision so that the average of the 10 measurements made by the tonometer achieved 95% reliability. The mean IOP of both eyes for each time point of the procedure was computed and compared.

Conscious sedation with intravenous midazolam (5 mg) and eventually fentanyl (0.05 mg) was proposed to all participants, in order to avoid the discomfort of the procedure, even if maintaining autonomous respiratory function.

Statistical Analysis

The sample size was calculated as follows: α error was set at 0.05, 1-β error was set at 0.80, and effect size was set at 0.8, and a non-central parameter λ of 16, critical F of 2.87, numerator df 4, denominator df 20, total simple size 25, and power of 0.82 were obtained.

Kolmogorov–Smirnov test was performed to evaluate the normal distribution of data and ANOVA post-hoc test with Bonferroni correction and Friedman test were used to compare the IOP measurements within the 4 time points during the examination; $p < 0.05$ was considered significant.

All data were analyzed with SPSS Software (IBM SPSS Statistics version 25).

3. Results

Fifteen males (60%) with a mean age of 50 ± 18 years (range 24–78) and ten females (40%) with a mean age of 45 ± 14 years (range 21–67) and mean weight of 73.76 ± 14.43 kg (range 50–117) were evaluated. Intravenous midazolam (5 mg) for conscious sedation during the EGD was performed in 13 patients, whereas 8 patients were sedated with midazolam (5 mg) and fentanyl (0.05 mg) by an experienced gastroenterologist. Four subjects refused sedation.

In all patients, the mean IOP in the sitting position was 15.16 ± 2.27 mmHg, and in the left lateral decubitus position, 15.68 ± 2.82 mmHg; when the gastroscope reached the second part of the duodenum (D2), the IOP was 21.84 ± 6.55 mmHg and, immediately after the gastroscope was removed (end of the procedure left lateral decubitus position), the IOP was 15.80 ± 3.25 mmHg (Table 1). The IOP in the sitting position, 10 min after the EGD, was 13.12 ± 3.63 mmHg. When the gastroscope entered the D2, a statistically significant IOP increase ($p < 0.01$) was observed. The IOP values at the end of the gastroscopy significantly decreased ($p < 0.001$), becoming similar to those measured before the EGD, in the same left lateral decubitus position. A further decrease was observed in the IOP values 10 min after the EGD, which became similar to those measured before the EGD, in the same sitting position (Table 2).

Table 1. Intraocular pressure evaluation (in mmHg) during different procedure times with Tonopen Avia.

	Sitting Position Pre-EGD	Left Lateral Decubitus Position Pre-EGD	Second Part of Duodenum in Left Lateral Decubitus Position	End of Procedure in Left Lateral Decubitus Position	Sitting Position 10 min after EGD
Mean	15.18	15.68	21.58	16.40	13.34
SD	2.40	2.45	6.13	3.42	3.16
Median	15.00	15.50	21.50	16.50	13.50
Min	8.50	11.00	11.50	10.50	7.50
Max	20.50	22.00	36.50	25.00	21.00

In the 21 patients under sedation, the mean IOP in the sitting position was 14.81 ± 2.25 mmHg, and in the left lateral decubitus position, 15.57 ± 2.60 mmHg; when the gastroscope reached the second part of the duodenum (D2), it was 21.88 ± 6.60 mmHg, and immediately after the gastroscope was removed (end of the procedure in left lateral decubitus position), the IOP was 16.40 ± 3.72 mmHg, while 10 min later, it was 12.98 ± 3.05 mmHg. When the gastroscope entered the duodenum (D2), a statistically significant IOP increase ($p < 0.01$) was observed.

Sedated patients were further divided into two groups, one sedated with midazolam alone, the other with a mixture of midazolam and fentanyl, to detect the eventual influence of different sedations on the IOP. A similar tendency in IOP variations was observed, without statistically significant differences among the two groups in all the examined positions ($p > 0.05$).

Table 2. ANOVA post-hoc test with Bonferroni correction between intraocular pressure evaluations (in mmHg) during different procedure times. The mean difference is significant at level <0.05.

				95% Confidence Interval	
		Mean Difference	p	Lower Limit	Upper Limit
Sitting position	Left lateral decubitus position	−0.50	1.000	−3.5487	2.5487
	D2	−6.40	**0.000**	−9.4487	−3.3513
	End of procedure	−1.22	1.000	−4.2687	1.8287
	10 min later	1.84	0.869	−1.2087	4.8887
Left lateral decubitus position	Sitting position	0.50	1.000	−2.5487	3.5487
	D2	−5.90	**0.000**	−8.9487	−2.8513
	End of procedure	−0.72	1.000	−3.7687	2.3287
	10 min later	2.34	0.301	−0.7087	5.3887
D2	Sitting position	6.40	**0.000**	3.3513	9.4487
	Left lateral decubitus position	5.90	**0.000**	2.8513	8.9487
	End of procedure	5.18	**0.000**	2.1313	8.2287
	10 min later	8.24	**0.000**	5.1913	11.2887
End of procedure	Sitting position	1.22	1.000	−1.8287	4.2687
	Left lateral decubitus position	0.72	1.000	−2.3287	3.7687
	D2	−5.18	**0.000**	−8.2287	−2.1313
	10 min later	3.06	0.048	0.0113	6.1087
10 min later	Sitting position	−1.84	0.869	−4.8887	1.2087
	Left lateral decubitus position	−2.34	0.301	−5.3887	0.7087
	D2	−8.24	**0.000**	−11.2887	−5.1913
	End of procedure	−3.06	0.048	−6.1087	−0.0113

In the four patients that refused sedation, the mean IOP was 17.12 ± 2.49 mmHg, and in the left lateral decubitus position, 16.25 ± 1.55 mmHg; when the gastroscope reached the second part of the duodenum (D2), it was 20.00 ± 2.48 mmHg, and immediately after the gastroscope was removed (end of the procedure in left lateral decubitus position), the IOP was 16.37 ± 1.03 mmHg, while 10 min later, it was 15.25 ± 3.48 mmHg. In this group, a similar trend in IOP variations was observed, but it did not reach a statistical significance ($p = 0.358$).

4. Discussion

The IOP increase is considered the main cause of optic nerve damage as well as the only modifiable known risk factor in glaucoma patients. An acute IOP increase does not cause chronic glaucoma, but a strict IOP control is imperative for patients with a known diagnosis of glaucoma, where a transient IOP change can also be a determinant.

Previous studies showed a relation between intra-abdominal pressure, intracranial pressure, and IOP, and some authors evaluated the IOP changes after laparoscopy [6] and colonoscopy [2].

Grosso et al. [6] revealed a mean IOP increase of 4 mmHg after pneumoperitoneum induction, with 58.6% of the patients showing an IOP increase of 5 mmHg or more. Moreover, the Trendelenburg position during surgery exhibited both an IOP increase and a great percentage of cases with an IOP increase of 5 mmHg or more.

Ackerman et al. [6] reviewed the literature concerning the impact of a steep Trendelenburg position during robot-assisted laparoscopic radical prostatectomy on intraocular pressure.

Other studies [14–18] showed a direct association between a steep Trendelenburg position and increased IOP.

Yoo et al. showed low intra-abdominal pressure resulting in the significant attenuation of the IOP increase in 67 patients undergoing robotic-assisted laparoscopic radical prostatectomy, divided into a moderate neuromuscular blockade group and deep neuromuscular blockade [14].

Hoshikawa et al. demonstrated that the IOP increased in a time-dependent fashion in 31 anesthetized patients undergoing robotic-assisted radical prostatectomy in a steep Trendelenburg position [15].

Mondzelewski et al. reported a significant elevation in IOP in 18 patients during robotic-assisted laparoscopy in a steep Trendelenburg position [16].

Both Kim et al. and Raz et al. found an IOP increase in patients during robotic-assisted radical prostatectomy in a steep Trendelenburg position, which was attenuated by the continuous infusion of dexmedetomidine or a modified Trendelenburg position [17,18].

Ece et al. [4] showed that 12 mmHg or more pressure after pneumoperitoneum induction led to a significant IOP rise, with an average of 8.5 ± 3.4 mmHg. Moreover, they postulated a correlation between the IOP elevation and the intracranial pressure increase, caused by the intra-abdominal pressure elevation.

Kent et al. [2] measured the right eye IOP in a left decubitus position in 23 healthy adults undergoing routine colonoscopy. The authors demonstrated that the IOP did not increase during colonoscopy, although patients were in the left decubitus position. On the contrary, they revealed that the IOP progressively decreased during the progression of the endoscope with a maximal decrease when it reached the cecum.

However, to the best of our knowledge, no previous studies have investigated IOP changes during EGD. We found that the IOP increased when the endoscope passed through the pylorus and entered the duodenum. The suggested mechanism underlying these results is unknown. However, an increase in intra-abdominal pressure during EGD has been detected in an animal study [3]. When intra-abdominal pressure increases, an impaired venous drainage of the lumbar venous plexus is detected, eventually leading to the increase in intracranial pressure [19]. Moreover, the intracranial pressure elevation has been suggested to be related to the IOP increase. Specifically, the IOP rise could be due to the elevation in ophthalmic venous pressure, which would be directly transmitted to the ocular fluid [7,9,20].

In this study, the EGD was performed in 21/25 subjects under conscious sedation. Previous papers showed that midazolam does not modify IOP, whereas fentanyl induces an IOP decrease during its administration [21,22]. Therefore, we hypothesize that the IOP increase during the EGD was not related to drug administration. Moreover, our results highlighted an IOP increase mainly in the group of patients that underwent sedation, without significant differences between patients who received midazolam and those who received midazolam and fentanyl. A similar trend in IOP variations was also observed in the small group of patients who did not undergo any conscious sedation, but it did not reach a statistical significance, possibly due to the small number of patients. Further studies in a larger group of patients without sedation are needed to better clarify the role of anesthesia in the IOP changes.

The left lateral decubitus position could also contribute to explaining our findings. In fact, previous studies demonstrated that the right or left lateral decubitus position might be associated with a small IOP increase in the lower side, compared to the sitting position [23]. However, in our study, we found a significant IOP elevation in both eyes, when the gastroscope reached the second part of the duodenum (D2). So, we can speculate that other factors, other than the body position, might play a role.

The elevation in IOP is considered the major risk factor for glaucoma; in addition, it has been related to an increased risk of several ophthalmic conditions such as retinal vein occlusion and anterior ischemic optic neuropathy. Moreover, the failure to achieve the target IOP has been associated with a more rapid visual field worsening in patients with glaucoma [24].

In the last few decades, endoscopic procedures have grown up worldwide, becoming an important diagnostic and therapeutic tool in daily clinical practice. The introduction of image-enhanced endoscopy and magnifying endoscopy has improved the possibility to also detect pre-neoplastic and neoplastic lesions of the upper GI tract during gastroscopy [25]. Moreover, in recent years, scientific societies have highly stressed the importance of "quality gastroscopy", performed according to a standardized protocol in order to maximize the detection of all the precancerous lesions and early cancers in the upper GI tract [11]. A high-quality EGD requires adequate air insufflation to better visualize the GI lumen and implies the use of several pieces of technical equipment to obtain the meticulous inspection of the mucosa and eventually the acquisition of histological samples [11].

Despite these undoubted advantages, we might take into account that the IOP increases during these endoscopic procedures and it could be a potential risk factor for optic nerve damage in glaucoma patients. It is important to underline that a transient IOP elevation during diagnostic procedures does not necessarily induce glaucoma, but care should be taken in patients with a previous glaucoma diagnosis.

One of the main limitations of this study was the use of TPA instead of GAT. In fact, GAT is based on the so-called Imbert–Fick law and is the gold standard for IOP measurement [26]. However, several factors, such as the central corneal thickness (CCT), curvature (Km), and structure, can influence its accuracy. In addition, taking into account the changes in the body position of the patients during the present study, GAT was unable to be properly managed. Furthermore, TPA has been used in similar studies where a handheld tonometer was required [27], showing comparable results.

Another limitation is the different sedating procedure among the patients, as a small group refused any kind of sedation, whereas most of the participants received midazolam alone or in combination with fentanyl. Although a similar trend in IOP variations was observed, further studies on a larger population could better clarify the role of sedation on IOP.

5. Conclusions

In conclusion, the IOP increase is considered the main cause of optic nerve damage in glaucoma patients, and IOP fluctuations during endoscopic procedures should be taken into account, especially, in patients that need repeated gastroscope procedures during their life or in patients with glaucoma. This is particularly important if glaucoma is in an advanced state where IOP spikes could induce severe damage.

In this paper, we detected significant changes in IOP changes during routine EGD. However, further studies are needed to better understand the short-effect and long-effect influence of the IOP increase in these patients and to suggest in future a possible preventive therapy.

Author Contributions: N.R., M.D.B. and P.I. conceived the study. M.D.B. wrote the original draft. M.G., F.C., S.P., A.S. and L.V. performed data acquisition and analysis. M.D.B. and P.I. interpreted the data. All authors reviewed and approved the manuscript. All authors have read and agreed to the published version of the manuscript.

Funding: This research received no external funding.

Institutional Review Board Statement: The study was conducted in accordance with the Declaration of Helsinki, and approved by the Cometico Campania Sud, (CECS) with prot. No. 16544.

Informed Consent Statement: Informed consent was obtained from all subjects involved in the study.

Data Availability Statement: The datasets generated and analyzed during the current study are available from the corresponding author on reasonable request.

Conflicts of Interest: The authors declare no conflicts of interest.

References

1. De Bernardo, M.; Borrelli, M.; Cembalo, G.; Rosa, N. Intraocular Pressure Measurements in Standing Position with a Rebound Tonometer. *Medicina* **2019**, *55*, 701. [CrossRef] [PubMed]
2. Kent, I.; Geffen, N.; Stein, A.; Rudnicki, Y.; Friehmann, A.; Avital, S. The effect of colonoscopy on intraocular pressure: An observational prospective study. *Graefes Arch. Clin. Exp. Ophthalmol.* **2020**, *258*, 607–611. [CrossRef] [PubMed]

3. Von Delius, S.; Karagianni, A.; Henke, J.; Preissel, A.; Meining, A.; Frimberger, E.; Schmid, R.M.; Huber, W. Changes in intra-abdominal pressure, hemodynamics, and peak inspiratory pressure during gastroscopy in a porcine model. *Endoscopy* **2007**, *39*, 962–968. [CrossRef]
4. Ece, I.; Vatansev, C.; Kucukkartallar, T.; Tekin, A.; Kartal, A.; Okka, M. The increase of intra-abdominal pressure can affect intraocular pressure. *Biomed. Res. Int.* **2015**, *2015*, 986895. [CrossRef] [PubMed]
5. Palamar, M.; Dag, M.Y.; Yagci, A. The effects of Valsalva maneuver on Ocular Response Analyzer measurements. *Clin. Exp. Optom.* **2015**, *98*, 447–450. [CrossRef]
6. Ackerman, R.S.; Cohen, J.B.; Getting, R.E.G.; Patel, S.Y. Are you seeing this: The impact of steep Trendelenburg position during robot-assisted laparoscopic radical prostatectomy on intraocular pressure: A brief review of the literature. *J. Robot. Surg.* **2019**, *13*, 35–40. [CrossRef]
7. Sajjadi, S.A.; Harirchian, M.H.; Sheikhbahaei, N.; Mohebbi, M.R.; Malekmadani, M.H.; Saberi, H. The relation between intracranial and intraocular pressures: Study of 50 patients. *Ann. Neurol.* **2006**, *59*, 867–870. [CrossRef]
8. Ren, R.; Zhang, X.; Wang, N.; Li, B.; Tian, G.; Jonas, J.B. Cerebrospinal fluid pressure in ocular hypertension. *Acta Ophthalmol.* **2011**, *89*, 142–148. [CrossRef]
9. Yavin, D.; Luu, J.; James, M.T.; Roberts, D.J.; Sutherland, G.R.; Jette, N.; Wiebe, S. Diagnostic accuracy of intraocular pressure measurement for the detection of raised intracranial pressure: Meta-analysis: A systematic review. *J. Neurosurg.* **2014**, *121*, 680–687. [CrossRef]
10. Coleman, W.H. Gastroscopy: A primary diagnostic procedure. *Prim Care* **1988**, *15*, 1–11. [CrossRef]
11. Beg, S.; Ragunath, K.; Wyman, A.; Banks, M.; Trudgill, N.; Pritchard, D.M.; Riley, S.; Anderson, J.; Griffiths, H.; Bhandari, P.; et al. Quality standards in upper gastrointestinal endoscopy: A position statement of the British Society of Gastroenterology (BSG) and Association of Upper Gastrointestinal Surgeons of Great Britain and Ireland (AUGIS). *Gut* **2017**, *66*, 1886–1899. [CrossRef] [PubMed]
12. Kim, S.Y.; Park, J.M. Quality indicators in esophagogastroduodenoscopy. *Clin. Endosc.* **2022**, *55*, 319–331. [CrossRef] [PubMed]
13. De Bernardo, M.; Capasso, L.; Caliendo, L.; Vosa, Y.; Rosa, N. Intraocular Pressure Evaluation after Myopic Refractive Surgery: A Comparison of Methods in 121 Eyes. *Semin. Ophthalmol.* **2016**, *31*, 233–242. [CrossRef] [PubMed]
14. Yoo, Y.C.; Kim, N.Y.; Shin, S.; Choi, Y.D.; Hong, J.H.; Kim, C.Y.; Park, H.; Bai, S.J. The Intraocular Pressure under Deep versus Moderate Neuromuscular Blockade during Low-Pressure Robot Assisted Laparoscopic Radical Prostatectomy in a Randomized Trial. *PLoS ONE* **2015**, *10*, e0135412. [CrossRef] [PubMed]
15. Hoshikawa, Y.; Tsutsumi, N.; Ohkoshi, K.; Serizawa, S.; Hamada, M.; Inagaki, K.; Tsuzuki, K.; Koshimizu, J.; Echizen, N.; Fujitani, S.; et al. The effect of steep Trendelenburg positioning on intraocular pressure and visual function during robotic-assisted radical prostatectomy. *Br. J. Ophthalmol.* **2014**, *98*, 305–308. [CrossRef] [PubMed]
16. Mondzelewski, T.J.; Schmitz, J.W.; Christman, M.S.; Davis, K.D.; Lujan, E.; L'Esperance, J.O.; Auge, B.K. Intraocular Pressure During Robotic-assisted Laparoscopic Procedures Utilizing Steep Trendelenburg Positioning. *J. Glaucoma* **2015**, *24*, 399–404. [CrossRef] [PubMed]
17. Kim, N.Y.; Yoo, Y.C.; Park, H.; Choi, Y.D.; Kim, C.Y.; Bai, S.J. The effect of dexmedetomidine on intraocular pressure increase in patients during robot-assisted laparoscopic radical prostatectomy in the steep Trendelenburg position. *J. Endourol.* **2015**, *29*, 310–316. [CrossRef]
18. Raz, O.; Boesel, T.W.; Arianayagam, M.; Lau, H.; Vass, J.; Huynh, C.C.; Graham, S.L.; Varol, C. The effect of the modified Z trendelenburg position on intraocular pressure during robotic assisted laparoscopic radical prostatectomy: A randomized, controlled study. *J. Urol.* **2015**, *193*, 1213–1219. [CrossRef]
19. Avital, S.; Brasesco, O.; Basu, A.; Szomstein, S.; Sands, L.; Wexner, S.D.; Rosenthal, R. Effects of colonoscopy on intracranial pressure: Observation in a large animal model. *Endoscopy* **2004**, *36*, 997–1000. [CrossRef]
20. De Bernardo, M.; Vitiello, L.; Rosa, N. Optic nerve ultrasonography for evaluating increased intracranial pressure in severe preeclampsia. *Int J Obstet Anesth.* **2019**, *38*, 147. [CrossRef] [PubMed]
21. Oberacher-Velten, I.; Prasser, C.; Rochon, J.; Ittner, K.P.; Helbig, H.; Lorenz, B. The effects of midazolam on intraocular pressure in children during examination under sedation. *Br. J. Ophthalmol.* **2011**, *95*, 1102–1105. [CrossRef]
22. Sator-Katzenschlager, S.M.; Oehmke, M.J.; Deusch, E.; Dolezal, S.; Heinze, G.; Wedrich, A. Effects of remifentanil and fentanyl on intraocular pressure during the maintenance and recovery of anaesthesia in patients undergoing non-ophthalmic surgery. *Eur. J. Anaesthesiol.* **2004**, *21*, 95–100. [CrossRef]
23. Malihi, M.; Sit, A.J. Effect of head and body position on intraocular pressure. *Ophthalmology* **2012**, *119*, 987–991. [CrossRef]
24. Villasana, G.A.; Bradley, C.; Ramulu, P.; Unberath, M.; Yohannan, J. The Effect of Achieving Target Intraocular Pressure on Visual Field Worsening. *Ophthalmology* **2022**, *129*, 35–44. [CrossRef]
25. The, J.L.; Shabbir, A.; Yuen, S.; So, J.B. Recent advances in diagnostic upper endoscopy. *World J Gastroenterol.* **2020**, *26*, 433–447.

26. De Bernardo, M.; Casaburi, C.; De Pascale, I.; Capasso, L.; Cione, F.; Rosa, N. Comparison between dynamic contour tonometry and Goldmann applanation tonometry correcting equations. *Sci. Rep.* **2022**, *12*, 20190. [CrossRef]
27. De Bernardo, M.; Abbinante, G.; Borrelli, M.; Di Stasi, M.; Cione, F.; Rosa, N. Intraocular Pressure Measurements in Standing, Sitting, and Supine Position: Comparison between Tono-Pen Avia and Icare Pro Tonometers. *J. Clin. Med.* **2022**, *11*, 6234. [CrossRef]

Journal of
Clinical Medicine

MDPI

Article

Short Wavelength Automated Perimetry, Standard Automated Perimetry, and Optical Coherence Tomography in Dominant Optic Atrophy

Marco Lombardo [1,*], Andrea Cusumano [1], Raffaele Mancino [1], Francesco Aiello [1], Roberto Pietro Sorge [2], Carlo Nucci [1] and Massimo Cesareo [1]

[1] Ophthalmology Unit, Department of Experimental Medicine, University of Rome Tor Vergata, 00133 Rome, Italy

[2] Laboratory of Biometry, Department of Systems Medicine, University of Rome Tor Vergata, 00133 Rome, Italy

* Correspondence: lombardom301@gmail.com; Tel.:+39-062-090-2972; Fax:+39-062-090-2973

Abstract: Background: Blue-yellow axis dyschromatopsia is well-known in Autosomal Dominant Optic Atrophy (ADOA) patients, but there were no data on the correlation between retinal structure and short-wavelength automated perimetry (SWAP) values in this pathology. **Methods:** In this cross-sectional case-control study, we assessed the correlation between best corrected visual acuity (BCVA), standard automated perimetry (SAP), SWAP, and optical coherence tomography (OCT) parameters of 9 ADOA patients compared with healthy controls. Correlation analysis was performed between BCVA, mean deviation, pattern standard deviation (PSD), and fovea sensitivity (FS) values and the OCT thickness of each retinal layer and the peripapillary retinal nerve fiber layer (pRNFL). **Results:** The following significant and strong correlations were found: between BCVA and ganglion cell layer (GCL) and the global (G) pRNFL thicknesses; between SAP FS and GCL and the G-pRNFL thicknesses; between SWAP PSD and total retina, GCL, inner plexiform layer, inner nuclear layer, inner retinal layer and the temporal pRNFL thicknesses. We found a constant shorter duration of the SITA-SWAP compared with the SITA-STANDARD strategy. **Conclusions:** SWAP, SAP, and BCVA values provided relevant clinical information about retinal involvement in our ADOA patients. The perimetric functional parameters that seemed to correlate better with structure involvement were FS on SAP and PSD on SWAP.

Keywords: optic neuropathies; ADOA; autosomal dominant optic atrophy; SWAP; short wavelength automated perimetry; OCT; optical coherence tomography

1. Introduction

Autosomal dominant optic atrophy (ADOA) is the most common hereditary optic neuropathy with a prevalence of 1/10,000 to 1/30,000 in the world [1].

Mutations in the *OPA1* gene cause 57 to 89% of ADOA cases. This gene encodes the mitochondrial dynamin-related GTPases in the inner mitochondrial membrane and is involved in many mitochondrial activities. In particular, the *OPA1* protein plays a crucial role in regulating mitochondrial fusion and apoptosis by modulating the inner mitochondrial membrane [1]. To date, more than 400 *OPA1* mutations have been reported. Of the reported pathogenic *OPA1* variants, 28% are missense variants, 24% are classified to induce aberrant splicing, 22% are frameshift variants, 15% are nonsense variants, and 7% are structural variants [2].

The resulting mitochondrial dysfunction mostly affects retinal ganglion cells, probably due to some peculiar characteristics of this type of cell [3].

The first clinical manifestations begin gradually from infancy and include a variable reduction of visual acuity, sometimes asymmetrically; temporal or diffuse pallor or excavation of the optic disc, and centro-cecal or central scotoma in visual field testing. Since there is a remarkable phenotypic heterogeneity even within the same family, the final visual acuity can vary from a slight decrease to legal blindness [4–7].

Another peculiar feature of the disease is an altered color perception, particularly dyschromatopsia on the blue-yellow axis, demonstrated by color perception tests: tritanopia is the typical defect found at the Farnsworth-Munsell (FM) 100-hue test and seems to be one of the most sensitive indicators of ADOA along with optic disc pallor [5,8].

Visual field tests have long been used in clinical ophthalmology and medical practice in general to determine the differential light sensitivity corresponding to the visual field examined. Testing of multiple retinal locations allows the detection and classification of visual abnormalities ranging from a general depression of sensitivity to the identification of specific regions of sensitivity loss [9]. Its ability to provide this important clinical information has allowed the diffusion of the method and its subsequent validation as an ophthalmic diagnostic tool to evaluate, not only the function of the retina and the optic nerve, but of the entire visual pathway.

White-on-white or standard automated perimetry (SAP) has become a common test for diagnosing and monitoring all types of optic neuropathies [10].

Short-wavelength automated perimetry (SWAP) presents a blue stimulus to selectively stimulate the blue cones. It also uses a high-luminance yellow background to saturate the red and green cones and the rods [11].

It was designed to find a method to diagnose early initial damage of ganglion cells, particularly in glaucoma, but this type of perimetry has been shown to have problems that have limited the diffusion of this method. It has a greater variability associated with the estimation of the threshold, absorption of the stimulus by ocular media, increase in the duration of the exam, and an additional learning effect [11]; the latter two were largely resolved with the advent of the Swedish interactive thresholding algorithm (SITA) strategy [12].

In 2006 Walters et al. published a case study on 5 patients affected by ADOA in which they found a clear difference between the mean values of mean deviation (MD) at SAP versus SWAP. MD values at SWAP were on average 11.46 decibels (dB) lower than at SAP. The authors suggested that this difference may help diagnose ADOA both in the early and advanced phases [13].

Optical coherence tomography (OCT) is a non-invasive diagnostic imaging technique. It allows for microscopic visualization and analysis of retinal structures by tomographic sections of the retina. It is based on the interference between the signal of an object under investigation and a local reference signal. OCT can produce a cross-sectional image of the object in real time, i.e., a two-dimensional image in space using confocal optics. In this way, both lateral and axial resolution are determined by the numerical aperture of the microscope objective. In OCT, the axial resolution is mainly determined by the optical source and therefore the retina of the human eye can be acquired with a very high axial resolution [14]. This technology has had extensive development not only in the medical field but also in the industrial and agricultural fields [15]. It has become part of clinical practice in ophthalmology thanks to its ease and speed of execution and its application has spread not only to retinal diseases, but also to those of the optic nerve and neurological or systemic diseases.

Numerous works have studied ADOA using spectral-domain OCT, showing a reduction in the thickness of the inner retina of patients, due to the ganglion cell layer involvement at the posterior pole and the reduction of the peripapillary retinal nerve fiber layer (pRNFL) thickness, especially in the temporal sector [16,17].

On the contrary, there are few works about the correlation between the structural parameters measured by OCT and the parameters expressing the function of the visual system; some of the functional parameters tested were visual acuity, electro-functional neurophysiological exams, and differential light sensitivity data measured at microperimetry [18–22].

This study aims to assess the correlation between SAP, SWAP and OCT parameters of patients with ADOA genetically confirmed by the presence of the *OPA1* gene mutation. Given the typical dyschromatopsia on the blue-yellow axis and the preliminary results of the case series by Walters et al. [13], the hypothesis was that SWAP can also provide important information on retinal structural involvement in patients affected by ADOA.

2. Materials and Methods

This cross-sectional, case-control, observational study included 9 patients (5 males and 4 females) from 3 unrelated families with a genetically established diagnosis of ADOA caused by the *OPA1* gene mutation. They were enrolled and examined at the Regional Reference Center for Low Vision and Visual Rehabilitation at the University of Rome Tor Vergata between April 2021 and April 2022 and were compared with 9 healthy controls (HCs), age and sex-matched, randomly enrolled in our general clinic.

Informed consent was obtained from all participants in accordance with the Declaration of Helsinki. The study was approved by the internal review board of the University of Tor Vergata in Rome (ethics approval ID: 265.21).

Genetic counseling was offered to all patients and their families. 7 patients had exon 29 mutation with the nucleotide change c.2873_2876del and the amino acid change p.(Val958Glyfs*3). One patient had a mutation at exon 8 with c.815T>C and p.L272P amino acid change and one patient at exon 19 with C.1870 of G nucleotide change (splicing defect). All these mutations were registered in the *OPA1* mutations database [23].

All patients and HCs underwent a comprehensive ophthalmologic examination including best corrected visual acuity (BCVA) measurement with standardized ETDRS tables; FM 100 Hue test; SAP with SITA-Standard program 24-2 and SWAP with SITA-SWAP program 24-2 of a Humphrey Field Analyzer in randomized order (Figure 1); Goldmann applanation tonometry; slit-lamp biomicroscopy with dilated fundus examination with assessment of lens opacity by *Lens Opacities Classification System III* (LOCS III) grading. All participants underwent the "Posterior Pole" scanning protocol of SD-OCT (Spectralis; Heidelberg Engineering, Heidelberg, Germany) to obtain the following automatic layer segmentation: total retinal (RETINA); retinal nerve fiber layer (RNFL); ganglion cell layer (GCL); inner plexiform layer (IPL); inner nuclear layer (INL); outer plexiform layer (OPL); outer nuclear layer (ONL); retinal pigment epithelium (RPE); inner retinal layers (IRL) and outer retinal layers (ORL). Within the "Posterior Pole" scan, macular ETDRS grid data were acquired for each retinal layer in the following sectors: center (C); inner-temporal (ITEM); inner-superior (ISUP); inner-nasal (INAS); inner-inferior (IINF); outer-temporal (OTEM); outer-superior (OSUP); outer-nasal (ONAS); outer-inferior (OINF). The average values of the aforementioned sectors were also calculated. Peripapillary RNFL thickness (pRNFL) was also measured in all subjects using the peripapillary RNFL scanning protocol (3.5 mm diameter). The following thickness values were obtained: global (G); temporal (T); temporal-superior (TS); nasal-superior (NS); nasal (N); nasal-inferior (NI); temporal-inferior (TI); papillo-macular bundle (PMB); N/T. All SD-OCT scans were acquired by the same experienced operator after pharmacologic mydriasis. Only scans with signal quality > 25 were included, while scans with altered segmentation, insufficient illumination or the presence of artifacts were excluded. No manual segmentation correction was required. Exclusion criteria were the presence of retinal and/or optic nerve pathology excluding ADOA, previous intraocular surgery except for uncomplicated phacoemulsification with intraocular lens implantation, current use of any drug therapy known to be toxic to the retina and/or optic nerve, cylindrical refractive errors greater than 2 diopters, spherical refractive errors greater ± 3 diopters; patients with lens opacity that could alter blue-yellow visual field results were also excluded. Regarding the perimetry tests, they were almost all found to be reliable (false positive or negative errors < 15%; fixation losses < 3) probably because all patients were familiar with performing these tests routinely every year. Only one eye of a patient was excluded due to poor fixation ability. Global indices, including the mean deviation (MD) and pattern standard deviation (PSD) of each perimetry, were registered. Foveal sensitivity (FS) values were also registered. Inclusion criteria for the control group were: BCVA of at least 0.0 logMAR, spherical or cylindrical refractive errors lower than 3 and 2 diopters, respectively, normal intraocular pressure (<21 mmHg), normal optic disc appearance, no significant ocular diseases, and no family history of glaucoma or systemic disease with possible ocular involvement. The evaluation methods were comparable between cases and HCs since both groups, who were homogeneous in terms of sex and age, underwent the same tests without requiring any manual corrections by the operators.

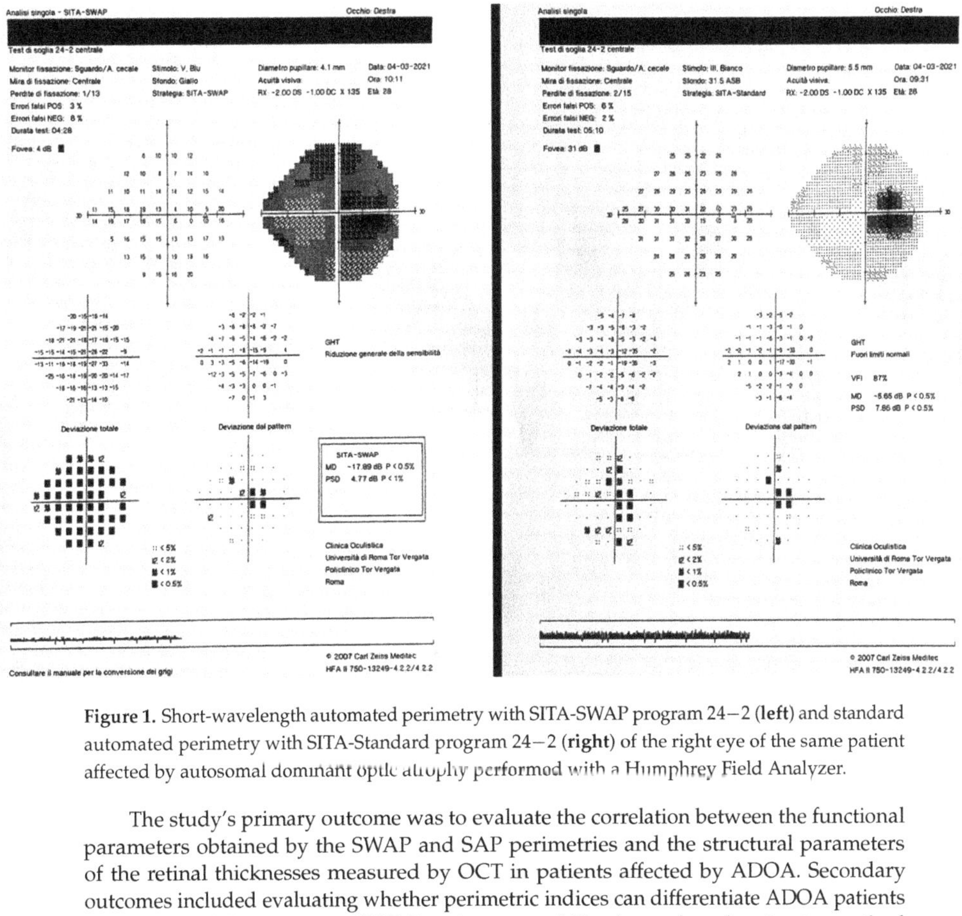

Figure 1. Short-wavelength automated perimetry with SITA-SWAP program 24−2 (**left**) and standard automated perimetry with SITA-Standard program 24−2 (**right**) of the right eye of the same patient affected by autosomal dominant optic atrophy performed with a Humphrey Field Analyzer.

The study's primary outcome was to evaluate the correlation between the functional parameters obtained by the SWAP and SAP perimetries and the structural parameters of the retinal thicknesses measured by OCT in patients affected by ADOA. Secondary outcomes included evaluating whether perimetric indices can differentiate ADOA patients from HCs and determining if SWAP perimetry could be the preferred perimetry method for this population.

Statistical Analysis

All data were initially entered into an Excel spreadsheet (Microsoft, Redmond, MA, USA) and analysis was performed using the statistical package for the social sciences Windows, version 15.0 (SPSS, Chicago, IL, USA). Descriptive statistics consisted of mean ± standard deviation for the parameters with normal distributions (after confirmation with histograms and Kolgomorov-Smirnov test), median and range (minimum and maximum) for variables with non-normal distributions. Comparison of normal variables between groups (ADOA vs. HCs) was performed with Anova one-way test while the proportions of occurrences were tested by the chi-square test. AUROC (area under receiver operating characteristics) curve analysis was used to identify the indices of the two perimetry exams with the best ability to discriminate between ADOA patients and HCs. ROC curve analysis provided cut-off values for all parameters. The possible linear correlation between the structural parameters (provided by the SD-OCT) and the functional parameters (MD, PSD, FS of each perimetry test and BCVA), was calculated using Pearson's linear correlation coefficient (r). The p-value < 0.05 was considered as the threshold for statistical significance.

3. Results

All patients and HCs who met the inclusion and exclusion criteria were confirmed eligible for the present study. A total of 17 eyes of 9 patients (average age 42.55 $\pm$ 15.94 years, range: 28–72 years) with a diagnosis of ADOA genetically confirmed by mutation of the *OPA1* gene were analyzed. They were compared with 17 eyes of 9 HCs (average age 43.11 $\pm$ 16.75 years, range: 27–74 years). The characteristics of patients, including lens opacity evaluations by LOCS III classification, are summarized in Table 1.

Table 1. Demographic and clinical characteristics of autosomal dominant optic atrophy patients enrolled in the present study.

Case Number	Sex	Age Range (Years)	Eye	BCVA (logMAR)	LOCS III
1	M	25–30	R	0.5	N = 1; C = 1; P = 1
			L	0.4	N = 1; C = 1; P = 1
2	M	25–30	R	0.5	N = 1; C = 1; P = 1
			L	0.5	N = 1; C = 1; P = 1
3	M	30–35	R	0.1	N = 1; C = 1; P = 1
			L	0.0	N = 1; C = 1; P = 1
4	M	30–35	R	0.5	N = 1; C = 1; P = 1
			L	0.5	N = 1; C = 1; P = 1
5	M	55–60	R	1.0	N = 2; C = 1; P = 1
			L	0.7	N = 2; C = 1; P = 1
6	F	25–30	R	0.5	N = 1; C = 1; P = 1
			L	0.5	N = 1; C = 1; P = 1
7	F	50–55	R	0.1	N = 2; C = 1; P = 1
			L	0.1	N = 2; C = 1; P = 1
8	F	50–55	R	1.3	N = 2; C = 1; P = 1
9	F	70–75	R	0.0	pseudophakia
			L	0.2	pseudophakia

M: male; F: female; R: right; L: left; BCVA: best corrected visual acuity; LOCS III: lens opacities classification system III.

One patient and one HC were pseudophakic with clear lens implantation in both eyes. Regarding ADOA patients, the average BCVA was 0.44 $\pm$ 0.35 logMAR (range: 0.0–1.3). The mean duration of the SAP was 6 min and 20 s while it was 4 min and 52 s for the SWAP with all the latter examinations taking less time than the SAP exams ($p < 0.001$). HCs also took less time in performing perimetry with the SITA-SWAP than with the SITA-Standard strategy. Absolute MD values were on average higher at SWAP (-15.32 dB) than at SAP (-5.63 dB), while PSD values were on average higher at SAP (5.62) than at SWAP (4.58). FS values were on average more markedly reduced at SWAP (10.94 dB) compared to SAP (29.47 dB). The distribution of all values investigated was normal, allowing the possible linear correlation between the parameters to be calculated using Pearson's coefficient.

The following significant ($p \leq 0.001$) correlations were found:

A strong negative correlation between BCVA values (measured in logMAR unit) and average GCL thickness (r = -0.784) on the ETDRS grid;

A strong negative correlation between BCVA values and the G-pRNFL thickness (r = −0.740);
A strong positive correlation between SAP FS and average GCL thickness (r = 0.749) on the ETDRS grid;
A strong positive correlation between SAP FS and the G-pRNFL thickness (r = 0.707);
Strong negative correlations between SWAP PSD and RETINA (r = −0.726), GCL (r = −0.702), IPL (r = −0.705), INL (r = −0.766), IRL (r = −0.700) average thicknesses on the ETDRS grid;
A strong negative correlation between SWAP PSD and the T-pRNFL thickness (r = −0.736).

All correlations between the functional parameters and the mentioned retinal layers and their significance levels are reported in Table 2.

Table 2. Pearson's correlation coefficients and their significance levels between optical coherence tomography thicknesses and functional parameters in our cohort of autosomal dominant optic atrophy patients. Significant correlations are highlighted in bold type.

		MD SAP	**MD SWAP**	**PSD SAP**	**PSD SWAP**	**FS SAP**	**FS SWAP**	**BCVA**
G-pRNFL	r	0.00232	0.10835	−0.40134	**−0.55558**	**0.70773**	−0.06758	**−0.74007**
	p	0.99296	0.67891	0.11033	**0.02059**	**0.00148**	0.79664	**0.00068**
T-pRNFL	r	−0.00967	−0.31899	**−0.53518**	**−0.73675**	0.45797	−0.34587	**−0.53818**
	p	0.97062	0.21205	**0.02684**	**0.00074**	0.06451	0.17388	**0.02584**
Average RETINA	r	−0.11448	−0.21884	−0.35899	**−0.72688**	**0.56497**	−0.21187	**−0.62560**
	p	0.66174	0.39874	0.15703	**0.00095**	**0.01812**	0.41429	**0.00723**
Average GCL	r	−0.04230	−0.08871	−0.39781	**−0.70236**	**0.74976**	0.15548	**−0.78435**
	p	0.87194	0.73494	0.11379	**0.00167**	**0.00053**	0.55126	**0.00019**
Average IPL	r	−0.15004	0.03093	−0.46004	**−0.70537**	**0.54795**	−0.07439	**−0.66833**
	p	0.56544	0.90618	0.06316	**0.00156**	**0.02278**	0.77661	**0.00336**
Average INL	r	−0.05794	−0.22725	−0.45809	**−0.76630**	**0.59467**	0.00954	**−0.60471**
	p	0.82519	0.38039	0.06443	**0.00033**	**0.01181**	0.97101	**0.01013**
Average IRLs	r	−0.21088	0.00596	−0.24905	**−0.70039**	0.29028	0.06938	**−0.61769**
	p	0.41654	0.98188	0.33507	**0.00174**	0.25837	0.79134	**0.00824**

MD: mean deviation; PSD: pattern standard deviation; FS: fovea sensitivity; SAP: standard automated perimetry; SWAP: short-wavelength automated perimetry; BCVA: best corrected visual acuity; G-pRNFL: global peripapillary retinal nerve fiber layer; T-pRNFL: temporal peripapillary retinal nerve fiber layer; GCL: ganglion cell layer; IPL: inner plexiform layer; INL: inner nuclear layer; IRLs: inner retinal layers; r: Pearson's correlation coefficient; *p*: significance level.

The use of ROC curves using OCT parameters has already been shown to be useful in this type of patient in previous works [22,24]. We decided to use this type of analysis also for the values obtained from the two functional tests.

The analysis of the ROC curves revealed that the parameters of both perimetry tests could well distinguish ADOA patients from HCs. SAP MD and FS along with SWAP MD and PSD showed an area under the curve of 1.000. SAP PSD and SAP FS showed an area under the curve of 0.986 and 0.939, respectively. ROC curves are shown in Figure 2.

SAP MD

AREA	*p*	
1.000	<0.000	
cut-off	**Sensitivity**	**Specificity**
−5.44	1	0.588235
−4.96	1	0.647059
−4.55	1	0.705882
−4.32	1	0.764706
−4.12	1	0.823529
−3.86	1	0.882353
−3.13	1	0.941176
−2.29	1	1
−2.01	0.941176	1
−1.23	0.882353	1
−0.43	0.823529	1
−0.36	0.764706	1
−0.34	0.705882	1

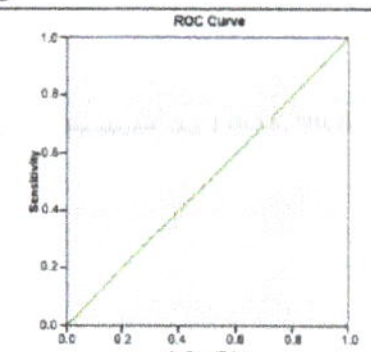

SWAP MD

AREA	*p*	
1.000	<0.000	
cut-off	**Sensitivity**	**Specificity**
14.07	1	0.647059
−14.04	1	0.705882
−12.54	1	0.764706
−10.81	1	0.823529
−9.98	1	0.882353
−9.78	1	0.941176
−7.05	1	1
−4.35	0.941176	1
−3.92	0.882353	1
−3.40	0.823529	1
−3.13	0.764706	1
−2.83	0.705882	1
−2.56	0.647059	1

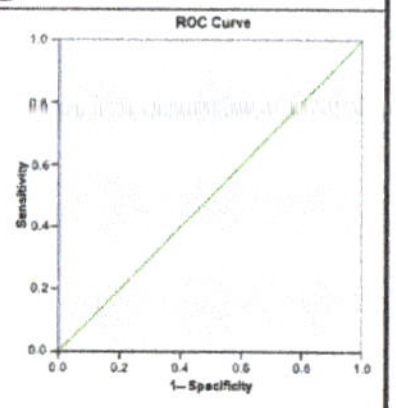

SAP PSD

AREA	*p*	
0.986	<0.000	
cut-off	**Sensitivity**	**Specificity**
1.56	1	0.647059
1.80	1	0.705882
2.05	1	0.764706
2.12	1	0.823529
2.19	1	0.882353
2.24	0.941176	0.882353
2.27	0.882353	0.882353
2.37	0.882353	0.941176
2.59	0.882353	1
2.76	0.823529	1
2.85	0.764706	1
3.36	0.705882	1
4.39	0.647059	1

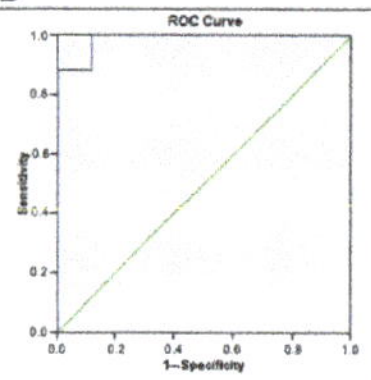

SWAP PSD

AREA	*p*	
1.000	<0.000	
cut-off	**Sensitivity**	**Specificity**
2.31	1	0.470588
2.35	1	0.529412
2.39	1	0.588235
2.44	1	0.647059
2.51	1	0.705882
2.60	1	0.764706
2.68	1	0.882353
2.79	1	0.941176
2.90	1	1
3.07	0.941176	1
3.21	0.882353	1
3.24	0.823529	1
3.37	0.764706	1

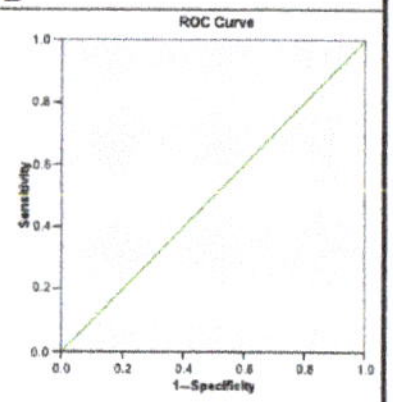

SAP FS

AREA	*p*	
1.000	<0.000	
cut-off	**Sensitivity**	**Specificity**
18.0	1	0
20.0	1	0.058824
22.5	1	0.117647
24.5	1	0.176471
26.0	1	0.235294
27.5	1	0.294118
29.0	1	0.352941
30.5	1	0.411765
31.5	1	0.647059
32.5	1	0.705882
34.0	1	0.823529
35.5	1	1
36.5	0.588235	1
37.5	0.235294	1
39.0	0	1

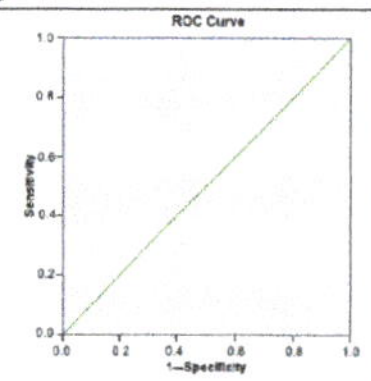

SWAP FS

AREA	*p*	
0.939	<0.000	
cut-off	**Sensitivity**	**Specificity**
0.0	1	0
2.5	1	0.058824
4.5	1	0.235294
5.5	1	0.294118
6.5	1	0.411765
9.0	1	0.470588
13.0	1	0.647059
15.5	1	0.705882
16.5	0.941176	0.705882
17.5	0.941176	0.823529
19.0	0.882353	0.823529
20.5	0.882353	0.882353
21.5	0.823529	0.882353
22.5	0.705882	0.941176
23.5	0.647059	0.941176

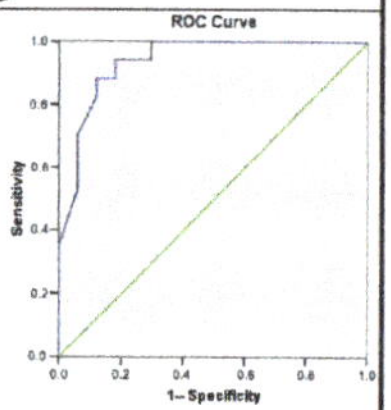

Figure 2. ROC curves of the mean deviation (MD), pattern standard deviation (PSD), and foveal sensitivity (FS) of standard automated perimetry (SAP) and short-wavelength automated perimetry (SWAP); *p*: level of significance (*p*-value).

4. Discussion

The study of the visual field in ADOA patients has always been clinically relevant since the earliest definitions of the pathology [25]. Another fundamental feature of this disease was the temporal involvement of the optic nerve; later studies with OCT revealed that not only the PMB is involved, but all the peripapillary nerve fibers and the ganglion cell population at the posterior pole [22,26]. These features, together with a typical dyschromatopsia in the blue-yellow axis, make SAP, SWAP, microperimetry, and OCT ideal for the morphological and functional assessment of this pathology. In addition, the generalized reduction in retinal sensitivity due to cataracts that typically influences perimetry results, in particular SWAP, is less relevant in this type of patient given the young age at diagnosis [27].

Only one work to date has evaluated both types of perimetry in the same ADOA patients, demonstrating the usefulness of SWAP in this disease [13]. In agreement with this study, despite the different threshold strategies, we found a 9.69 dB separation between the mean MD data of the two perimetries, with the SWAP MD consistently reduced more than that of SAP in each patient ($p < 0.001$) (Figure 3). This finding could strengthen the hypothesis that this difference may be an indicator of ADOA.

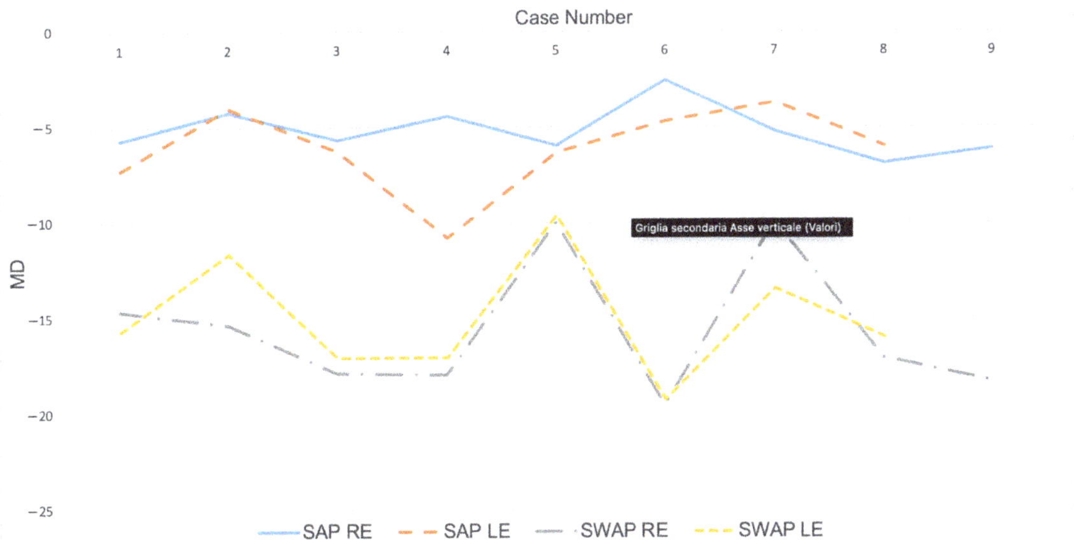

Figure 3. Graphical representation of mean deviation (MD) of each autosomal dominant optic atrophy patient measured at standard automated perimetry (SAP) and short-wavelength automated perimetry (SWAP) showing the difference between the two tests. RE: right eye; LE: left eye.

To date, no study tried to correlate SWAP values with structural data measured with OCT. We found significant correlations between the MD, PSD and FS values of both perimetry exams and the thickness values measured by OCT. Each type of perimetry was found to correlate better with specific morphological values on OCT, suggesting that both examinations are useful to investigate different aspects of the same pathology.

One of the strongest and most significant correlations found was between the PSD at the SWAP and the T value of the pRNFL thickness. The correlation proved to be negative, meaning that an increase in PSD corresponds to a decrease in OCT values. Since the reduction in differential light sensitivity in these patients was shown to be greater at the level of the papillomacular bundle (centrocecal scotoma) than at other points, we can assume that the PSD value increases in relation to the greater involvement of this bundle than the surrounding retina. The PSD value at the SWAP also showed a strong negative correlation with the thicknesses of RETINA, GCL, IPL, INL, and IRL of the ETDRS grid. The thickness of the inner retinal layers is typically reduced in this disease, not only at the level of the papillomacular bundle, but in all the posterior pole, especially in more advanced stages. This appears to be caused by a primary involvement of the more damage-sensitive small fibers of the parvocellular and koniocellular nuclei and by the subsequent damage of the residual larger ganglion cells [17]. Only moderate and not significant (except for the T-pRNFL value) correlations were found between the PSD at the SAP and the same OCT values mentioned above both in the ETDRS grid and in the peripapillary zone. A possible explanation for the better correlation of SWAP compared to SAP may result from the more selective stimulus-response of the blue cones and thus the corresponding koniocellular ganglion cells, which seem to be more sensitive to damage along with parvocellular cells [2]. In the case of the standard stimulus, cones and rods are stimulated, and therefore every type of ganglion cell.

A strong positive correlation was found between the FS value at the SAP and the thickness of the GCL layer of the ETDRS grid. The same strong correlation was also found with the G-pRNFL thickness. This may be due to the higher concentration of photoreceptors at the foveal level, which transduces the signal to the same conspicuous number of ganglion cells whose axons go to form the pRNFL. Primary damage to these ganglion cells can progressively lead to a reduction in nerve fibers and a consequent decrease in the sensitivity of the corresponding photoreceptors at the foveal level.

A slightly higher correlation coefficient also emerged between BCVA values and the aforementioned OCT thicknesses; this is because, as expected, SAP FS correlates strongly in turn with BCVA (r = −0.740; $p < 0.001$). A possible explanation for the absence of correlation between FS at the SWAP and OCT values may be due to the almost complete absence of blue cones at the level of the fovea [28,29].

No correlations were found between the parameters of the two perimetries and the RNFL value on the ETDRS grid. We can therefore conclude that regarding RNFL thickness, the peripapillary zone has a better functional correlation than the posterior pole because pRNFL thickness includes all the retinal ganglion cell fibers instead of those from only the posterior pole.

Regarding the ability of SAP and SWAP to distinguish between ADOA patients and HCs, all perimeter indices considered showed excellent sensitivity and specificity. MD values of both perimetry tests showed an AUROC equal to 1, indicating that these patients, both for SAP and, as previously mentioned, even more so for SWAP, have a diffuse light sensitivity defect very different from HCs. PSD value showed a greater area under the ROC curve for SWAP, while the area of FS was greater in SAP. This finding could precisely reflect the greater structural correlation of these parameters.

Performing two types of perimetry in ADOA patients can be difficult in routine clinical practice; since the BCVA assessment is a simpler, standardized and faster procedure than a perimetry exam, and provides better correlations with structural parameters than SAP, we suggest, for the assessment of functional response to structural involvement, the possibility of performing only SWAP in ADOA patients without significant lens opacity, along with visual acuity measurement, which remains a routine practice in ophthalmologic examinations. Another evidence in favor of this possibility is that, in our cohort of patients and HCs, the test durations with the SITA-SWAP strategy were consistently shorter than that with the SITA-SAP strategy. To the best of our knowledge, this is the first study to emphasize the fact that, with the SITA strategy, the duration of the SWAP perimetry is shorter than that of the SAP. This data could partially solve the problem of the "fatigue effect". This perimetry also showed a more depressed MD than at SAP in ADOA patients. The problem of variability in threshold estimation described for SWAP, in our cohort of patients, did not affect distinguishing them from controls. On the other hand, the influence of long-term fluctuation could not be assessed in this study, as this will require repeated examination in the future. Even the low MD values at SWAP may limit the ability to detect changes in time.

5. Conclusions

Both SAP and SWAP could provide relevant clinical information on retinal involvement in our cohort of ADOA patients. The most important functional parameters that seemed to correlate better with structure involvement were FS on SAP and PSD on SWAP. The main limitations of this study were the retrospective nature, the limited number of patients and the comparison of two perimetry tests, which, even if performed correctly by the same patient, still have different dynamic ranges, normative values and variability characteristics. Further studies with larger numbers of patients with ADOA will be needed to corroborate these findings and define which functional examination may be the most suitable, not only for studying current structural involvement, but also for monitoring disease progression.

Author Contributions: Conceptualization, M.L. and M.C.; Data curation, M.L., R.P.S. and M.C.; Formal analysis, R.P.S.; Investigation, M.L. and A.C.; Methodology, M.L. and M.C.; Project administration, R.M., C.N. and M.C.; Resources, C.N.; Supervision, R.M., C.N. and M.C.; Validation, A.C. and F.A.; Visualization, M.L., A.C. and F.A.; Writing—original draft, M.L. and M.C. All authors have read and agreed to the published version of the manuscript.

Funding: This research received no external funding.

Institutional Review Board Statement: The study was conducted according to the guidelines of the Declaration of Helsinki, and approved by the Institutional Review Board of the University of Tor Vergata (protocol code 265.21).

Informed Consent Statement: Informed consent was obtained from all subjects involved in the study.

Data Availability Statement: The datasets generated during the current study are available from the corresponding author on reasonable request.

Conflicts of Interest: The authors declare no conflict of interest.

References

1. Han, J.; Li, Y.; You, Y.; Fan, K.; Lei, B. Autosomal dominant optic atrophy caused by six novel pathogenic *OPA1* variants and genotype–phenotype correlation analysis. *BMC Ophthalmol.* **2022**, *22*, 322. [CrossRef]
2. Lenaers, G.; Neutzner, A.; Le Dantec, Y.; Jüschke, C.; Xiao, T.; Decembrini, S.; Swirski, S.; Kieninger, S.; Agca, C.; Kim, U.S.; et al. Dominant optic atrophy: Culprit mitochondria in the optic nerve. *Prog. Retin. Eye Res.* **2021**, *83*, 100935. [CrossRef] [PubMed]
3. Lenaers, G.; Hamel, C.P.; Delettre, C.; Amati-Bonneau, P.; Procaccio, V.; Bonneau, D.; Reynier, P.; Milea, D. Dominant optic atrophy. *Orphanet J. Rare Dis.* **2012**, *7*, 46. [CrossRef] [PubMed]
4. Eliott, D.; Traboulsi, E.I.; Maumenee, I.H. Visual Prognosis in Autosomal Dominant Optic Atrophy (Kjer Type). *Am. J. Ophthalmol.* **1993**, *115*, 360–367. [CrossRef] [PubMed]
5. Votruba, M. Clinical Features in Affected Individuals From 21 Pedigrees with Dominant Optic Atrophy. *Arch. Ophthalmol.* **1998**, *116*, 351. [CrossRef]
6. Johnston, R.L.; Seller, M.J.; Behnam, J.T.; Burdon, M.A.; Spalton, D.J. Dominant optic atrophy. *Ophthalmology* **1999**, *106*, 123–128. [CrossRef] [PubMed]
7. Cohn, A.C.; Toomes, C.; Potter, C.; Towns, K.V.; Hewitt, A.W.; Inglehearn, C.F.; Craig, J.E.; Mackey, D.A. Autosomal Dominant Optic Atrophy: Penetrance and Expressivity in Patients with *OPA1* Mutations. *Am. J. Ophthalmol.* **2007**, *143*, 656–662.e1. [CrossRef] [PubMed]
8. Puomila, A.; Huoponen, K.; Mäntyjärvi, M.; Hämäläinen, P.; Paananen, R.; Sankila, E.-M.; Savontaus, M.-L.; Somer, M.; Nikoskelainen, E. Dominant optic atrophy: Correlation between clinical and molecular genetic studies: Acta Ophthalmologica Scandinavica 2005. *Acta Ophthalmol. Scand.* **2005**, *83*, 337–346. [CrossRef] [PubMed]
9. Bosworth, C.F.; Sample, P.A.; Johnson, C.A.; Weinreb, R.N. Current Practice with Standard Automated Perimetry. *Semin. Ophthalmol.* **2000**, *15*, 172–181. [CrossRef]
10. Hepworth, L.R.; Rowe, F.J. Programme choice for perimetry in neurological conditions (PoPiN): A systematic review of perimetry options and patterns of visual field loss. *BMC Ophthalmol.* **2018**, *18*, 241. [CrossRef]
11. Wild, J.M. Short wavelength automated perimetry. *Acta Ophthalmol. Scand.* **2001**, *79*, 546–559. [CrossRef] [PubMed]
12. Bengtsson, B. A New Rapid Threshold Algorithm for Short-Wavelength Automated Perimetry. *Investig. Ophthalmol. Vis. Sci.* **2003**, *44*, 1388. [CrossRef] [PubMed]
13. Walters, J.W. Short wavelength-automated perimetry compared with standard achromatic perimetry in autosomal dominant optic atrophy. *Br. J. Ophthalmol.* **2006**, *90*, 1267–1270. [CrossRef] [PubMed]
14. Podoleanu, A.G. Optical coherence tomography. *J. Microsc.* **2012**, *247*, 209–219. [CrossRef] [PubMed]
15. Wijesinghe, R.E.; Lee, S.-Y.; Ravichandran, N.K.; Han, S.; Jeong, H.; Han, Y.; Jung, H.-Y.; Kim, P.; Jeon, M.; Kim, J. Optical coherence tomography-integrated, wearable (backpack-type), compact diagnostic imaging modality for in situ leaf quality assessment. *Appl. Opt.* **2017**, *56*, D108. [CrossRef] [PubMed]
16. Yu-Wai-Man, P.; Bailie, M.; Atawan, A.; Chinnery, P.F.; Griffiths, P.G. Pattern of retinal ganglion cell loss in dominant optic atrophy due to *OPA1* mutations. *Eye* **2011**, *25*, 596–602. [CrossRef] [PubMed]
17. Barboni, P.; Savini, G.; Cascavilla, M.L.; Caporali, L.; Milesi, J.; Borrelli, E.; La Morgia, C.; Valentino, M.L.; Triolo, G.; Lembo, A.; et al. Early Macular Retinal Ganglion Cell Loss in Dominant Optic Atrophy: Genotype-Phenotype Correlation. *Am. J. Ophthalmol.* **2014**, *158*, 628–636.e3. [CrossRef]
18. Russo, A.; Delcassi, L.; Marchina, E.; Semeraro, F. Correlation between visual acuity and OCT-measured retinal nerve fiber layer thickness in a family with ADOA and an *OPA1* mutation. *Ophthalmic Genet.* **2013**, *34*, 69–74. [CrossRef]
19. Rönnbäck, C.; Milea, D.; Larsen, M. Imaging of the Macula Indicates Early Completion of Structural Deficit in Autosomal-Dominant Optic Atrophy. *Ophthalmology* **2013**, *120*, 2672–2677. [CrossRef]
20. Park, S.W.; Hwang, J.-M. Optical coherence tomography shows early loss of the inferior temporal quadrant retinal nerve fiber layer in autosomal dominant optic atrophy. *Graefe's Arch. Clin. Exp. Ophthalmol.* **2015**, *253*, 135–141. [CrossRef]
21. Reis, A.; Mateus, C.; Viegas, T.; Florijn, R.; Bergen, A.; Silva, E.; Castelo-Branco, M. Physiological evidence for impairment in autosomal dominant optic atrophy at the pre-ganglion level. *Graefe's Arch Clin Exp. Ophthalmol.* **2013**, *251*, 221–234. [CrossRef]
22. Cesareo, M.; Ciuffoletti, E.; Martucci, A.; Sebastiani, J.; Sorge, R.P.; Lamantea, E.; Garavaglia, B.; Ricci, F.; Cusumano, A.; Nucci, C.; et al. Assessment of the retinal posterior pole in dominant optic atrophy by spectral-domain optical coherence tomography and microperimetry. *PLoS ONE* **2017**, *12*, e0174560. [CrossRef]

23. Bibliome Variant Database. Available online: https://bibliome.ai/ (accessed on 20 June 2023).
24. Cesareo, M.; Giannini, C.; Di Marino, M.; Aloe, G.; Martucci, A.; Aiello, F.; Cusumano, A.; Mancino, R.; Ricci, F.; Sorge, R.P.; et al. Optical coherence tomography angiography in the multimodal assessment of the retinal posterior pole in autosomal dominant optic atrophy. *Acta Ophthalmol.* **2022**, *100*, E798–E806. [CrossRef] [PubMed]
25. Kjer, P. Hereditary Infantile Optic Atrophy with Dominant Transmission. *Hum. Hered.* **1957**, *7*, 290–291. [CrossRef] [PubMed]
26. Ito, Y.; Nakamura, M.; Yamakoshi, T.; Lin, J.; Yatsuya, H.; Terasaki, H. Reduction of Inner Retinal Thickness in Patients with Autosomal Dominant Optic Atrophy Associated with *OPA1* Mutations. *Investig. Ophthalmol. Vis. Sci.* **2007**, *48*, 4079. [CrossRef]
27. Moss, I.D.; Wild, J.M.; Whitaker, D.J. The Influence of Age-Related Cataract on Blue-on-Yellow Perimetry. *Investig. Ophthalmol.* **1995**, *36*, 764–773.
28. Williams, D.R.; MacLeod, D.I.A.; Hayhoe, M.M. Punctate sensitivity of the blue-sensitive mechanism. *Vis. Res.* **1981**, *21*, 1357–1375. [CrossRef]
29. Calkins, D.J. Seeing with S cones. *Prog. Retin. Eye Res.* **2001**, *20*, 255–287. [CrossRef]

Journal of
Clinical Medicine

MDPI

Review

Optic Nerve Neuroprotection in Glaucoma: A Narrative Review

Angela D'Angelo [1], Livio Vitiello [2,*], Filippo Lixi [3], Giulia Abbinante [2], Alessia Coppola [2], Vincenzo Gagliardi [2], Alfonso Pellegrino [2] and Giuseppe Giannaccare [3]

1 Department of Medicine and Surgery, University of Naples "Federico II", 80138 Naples, NA, Italy; dangeloangela99@gmail.com
2 Eye Unit, "Luigi Curto" Hospital, Azienda Sanitaria Locale Salerno, 84035 Polla, SA, Italy; giulia.abbinante@gmail.com (G.A.); alessiacoppola330@gmail.com (A.C.); v.gagliardi@aslsalerno.it (V.G.); al.pellegrino@aslsalerno.it (A.P.)
3 Eye Clinic, Department of Surgical Sciences, University of Cagliari, 09124 Cagliari, CA, Italy; f.lixi0106@gmail.com (F.L.); giuseppe.giannaccare@gmail.com (G.G.)
* Correspondence: livio.vitiello@gmail.com

Abstract: In recent years, researchers have been interested in neuroprotective therapies as a cutting-edge therapeutic strategy to treat neurodegenerative disorders by shielding the brain system from harmful events. Millions of individuals worldwide suffer from glaucoma, an ocular neurodegenerative disease characterized by gradual excavation of the optic nerve head, retinal axonal damage, and consequent visual loss. The pathology's molecular cause is still mostly unknown, and the current treatments are not able to alter the disease's natural progression. Thus, the modern approach to treating glaucoma consists of prescribing medications with neuroprotective properties, in line with the treatment strategy suggested for other neurodegenerative diseases. For this reason, several naturally derived compounds, including nicotinamide and citicoline, have been studied throughout time to try to improve glaucoma management by exploiting their neuroprotective properties. The purpose of this review is to examine the naturally derived compounds that are currently utilized in clinical practice for neuroprotection in glaucomatous patients based on scientific data, emphasizing these compounds' pivotal mechanism of action as well as their proven therapeutic and neuroprotective benefits.

Keywords: glaucoma; neurodegenerative diseases; neuroprotection; optic nerve

1. Introduction

Neurodegeneration is characterized by a gradual loss of neurons and associated processes (axons, dendrites, and synapses), together with a concurrent impairment of neuronal function [1]. Nowadays, glaucoma is recognized as a chronic neurodegenerative disease, affecting the entire visual pathway from the eye to the visual cortex. It is one of the leading causes of low vision in the elderly globally, and its effects, as a social health issue, are only going to get worse with time. Indeed, by 2040, it is predicted to have an impact on over 112 million individuals all over the world [2]. Considering its neurodegenerative nature, pharmacological approaches used in different degenerative brain disorders could also be beneficial in treating glaucoma and other optic neuropathies [3]. In particular, the death of retinal ganglion cells (RGCs) is one of the pivotal pathophysiological events in glaucoma [4]. For this reason, in recent years, neuroprotection has drawn increasing attention as a novel approach to stop or slow the development of morphological and functional glaucomatous impairments, particularly focusing on delaying the RGC degeneration. In fact, neuroprotection aims to preserve the structure and function of the neurons, trying to lower the rate of neuronal loss over the time [5].

For this reason, several molecules, including citicoline, have been tested over the years to try to improve the management of glaucoma by exploiting their neuroprotective properties [3]. However, the intricacy of the visual system's anatomy and tissues, the timing of patient enrollment in clinical trials, the lack of valid endpoints, and the incomplete understanding of the main molecular basis of neurodegenerative diseases, including glaucoma, are some of the major factors that make it difficult to design effective neuroprotective strategies [6].

The aim of this review is to analyze the main naturally derived molecules currently used in clinical practice according to scientific evidence for neuroprotection in glaucomatous patients, focusing on their main mechanisms of action and their demonstrated therapeutic and neuroprotective effects, to provide some useful information to clinicians involved in the clinical management of this ocular neurodegenerative disease.

2. Main Naturally Derived Compounds with Neuroprotective Properties

2.1. Citicoline

Citicoline, also known as cytidine-5′-diphosphocholine or CDP-choline, is a mononucleotide composed of ribose, pyrophosphate, and cytosine [3]. It is a naturally occurring endogenous substance that acts as an intermediary in the synthesis of phosphatidylcholine, a crucial phospholipid in neuronal membranes. This occurs through the activation of biosynthesis pathways leading to the formation of structural phospholipids in neuronal membranes [4]. Citicoline increases the metabolism of cerebral structures, preventing phospholipid degradation and promoting an elevation in the levels of different neurotransmitters and neuromodulators in the central nervous system [7,8]. Citicoline has great neuroprotective properties mediated through various mechanisms. These include the maintenance of sphingomyelin and cardiolipin levels (essential for mitochondrial electron transport in the inner mitochondrial membrane), restoration of phosphatidylcholine levels, increased activity of glutathione reductase and glutathione synthesis, reduction of lipid peroxidation, and restoration of $Na+/K+$ ATPase activity [9]. Moreover, citicoline enhances the levels of acetylcholine, dopamine, noradrenaline, and serotonin in various brain regions [9], and it stimulates dopamine release in the retina [10].

Considering these properties, citicoline has been researched as a possible promising treatment for several neurological conditions, including glaucoma, brain ischemia, and Parkinson's and Alzheimer's diseases. [3,11–13].

Nowadays, citicoline is globally available as a dietary supplement and is used as a drug in many countries. It can be given through intravenous or oral administration, with very good bioavailability. Once absorbed, is quickly metabolized to cytidine and choline and distributed throughout the body; it crosses the blood–brain barrier and reaches the central nervous system, where it is incorporated into the membrane phospholipid fraction [14]. Citicoline demonstrates minimal toxicity, making it a safe molecule with few adverse effects. The only reported side effect is digestive intolerance following oral administration [15].

The proven daily therapeutic dosage of citicoline in humans is 500–2000 mg (7–28 mg/kg) [15], and it is also currently available for topical treatment and can be administered as eye drops to enhance patient compliance and adherence [3]. Citicoline appears to be involved in mitigating RGC dysfunction and preventing their apoptosis. Citicoline showed antiapoptotic effects on damaged RGCs and enhanced axon regeneration in a mouse retinal explant [16]. Moreover, several trials have also demonstrated the therapeutic effectiveness of citicoline therapy in glaucoma patients. The citicoline treatment for 2–8 years in glaucoma patients with moderate visual defects improved retinal function and neural conduction. The continuation of the treatment significantly slowed, stabilized, or even improved glaucomatous visual dysfunction [17]. Similarly, a study by Ottobelli et al. confirmed the enduring benefit of oral citicoline supplementation, suggesting that this intervention could considerably attenuate the glaucoma progression [18]. The role of citicoline was also investigated in association to other neuroprotective products. Melecchi and colleagues reported that citicoline combined with niacin was effective in restoring RGC activity in an animal model of induced ocular hypertension. Moreover, the combination of these substances showed better efficacy over each single compound in reducing inflammatory and oxidative stress markers and preserving mitochondrial function [19]. Similarly, Mastropasqua et al. described a synergistic effect of citicoline, coenzyme Q10, and vitamin B3, which improved mitochondrial activity, reduced inflammation and oxidation, and exhibited neuroprotective properties in vitro [20].

Research on citicoline's role in glaucoma is expanding and, overall, the results consistently underscore citicoline as a safe compound with beneficial effects on visual function. However, further studies are essential to clarify the dose–response relationship and support the demonstrated clinical benefits of this interesting neuroprotective molecule.

2.2. Homotaurine

Homotaurine (also known as tramiprosate, 3-amino-1-propanesulfonic acid, or 3-APS) is a naturally sourced amino sulfonate compound identified in marine red algae, originally extracted from this source [21].

This compound is recognized for its potential to enhance the transmission of nervous impulses in the central nervous system and its neuromodulatory effects [22]. Homotaurine has the ability to interfere with various biological pathways in both in vitro and in vivo experimental models. It has been discovered to possess cytoprotective, neuroprotective, and neurotropic activities through a range of different mechanisms. It is also an analogue of GABA (4-aminobutyrate, γ-aminobutyric acid), thus exerting potent agonistic activity on GABA receptors, with a preference for GABA type A receptors. This characteristic contributes to its anti-nociceptive and analgesic activities, likely mediated by opioid and cholinergic mechanisms [23]. As a sulfur-containing amino acid, homotaurine could have a protective effect against cellular damage, especially in defense against oxidative damage to DNA caused by free radicals [24]. Additionally, it possesses the ability to prevent the formation of β-amyloid plaques, which are implicated in the apoptosis of neuronal cells and various neurodegenerative processes in the central nervous system [22]. This effect extends not only to the central nervous system but also to the ophthalmic field. The existing literature has brought attention to the potential involvement of amyloid in the induction of RGC apoptosis in experimental glaucoma models [25], suggesting that homotaurine could serve as a potentially effective treatment for glaucoma. In a recent study, it was found that the combined formulation of citicoline and homotaurine exhibits potent synergistic neuroprotective effects in cultured retinal cells, reducing the proapoptotic consequences linked to exposure to both glutamate and elevated glucose levels [26]. In another study, a randomized controlled multicentric trial demonstrated that the daily oral intake of the fixed combination of citicoline and homotaurine for 4 months led to an improvement in the function of inner retinal cells. This improvement occurred independently of intraocular pressure (IOP) reduction and positively impacted both the visual field and the perception of quality of life [27].

2.3. Coenzyme Q10

Coenzyme Q10 (CoQ10), also known as ubiquinone or ubidecarenone, is a 1,4-benzoquinone and Q represents the quinone chemical group. It is a naturally occurring hydrophobic molecule synthesized endogenously in every cell of animals and plants. Intracellular synthesis is the main source, but a small portion is introduced through the diet. The richest nutritional sources of CoQ10 are liver and other animal organs, as well as meat, fish, nuts, and some oils, while much lower levels can be found in dairy products, vegetables, fruits, and cereals [28]. CoQ10 is a ubiquitous compound essential for various functions associated with energy metabolism. It is an important cofactor of the mitochondrial electron transport chain, acting as a mobile electron and proton transporter from complex I (NADH: ubiquinone reductase) and complex II (succinate: ubiquinone reductase) to complex III (ubiquinone cytochrome c oxidase) in the inner mitochondrial membrane [29]. In addition, when CoQ10 turns from its oxidized form, ubiquinone, to the fully reduced form, ubiquinol, it acts as a potent lipid-soluble antioxidant and scavenger of free radicals. It directly eliminates free radicals or recycles and regenerates other antioxidants such as ascorbic acid (vitamin C) and tocopherol (vitamin E) [30]. In this way, it protects membrane lipids, proteins, and mitochondrial DNA from oxidative damage. Considering that dysfunctional energy metabolism and oxidative stress could be the main causes of the pathogenesis of many pathological conditions, including neurodegenerative diseases, CoQ10 has been utilized in the treatment of cardiac, neurologic, oncologic, and immunologic disorders [31,32]. The levels of CoQ10 decrease with age in the brain and various tissues in animals and humans. As a result, CoQ10 also plays an effective therapeutic role in age-related neurodegenerative disorders, such as Alzheimer's and Parkinson's disease, multiple sclerosis, epilepsy, depression, stroke, and glaucoma [32,33]. Due to its significant molecular weight and hydrophobic properties, the topical application of CoQ10 has poor intraocular penetration and limited bioavailability. Additionally, CoQ10 is a substrate of P-glycoprotein, an efflux membrane transporter expressed on RGCs and corneal epithelial cells. To avoid this, CoQ10 is often combined with vitamin E, which improves its bioavailability by inhibiting P-glycoprotein [34,35].

Evidence of mitochondrial dysfunction in neurodegenerative diseases comes from animal models, studies on patients' mitochondria, and assessments of oxidative stress markers. Therefore, the potential neuroprotective effect of CoQ10 has been demonstrated in several in vitro studies and animal models [36]. In glaucoma-related models, topical treatment with CoQ10 or its integration into the diet has demonstrated the ability to protect RGCs against oxidative stress and to promote RGC survival by inhibiting RGC apoptosis [37,38]. In a mechanical optic nerve injury rat model, topical treatment with a combination of CoQ10 and vitamin E increased the number of RGCs, inhibiting apoptosis and astrocyte and microglial cell activation [39]. Furthermore, several studies highlighted the neuroprotective effect of CoQ10 on the retina. In fact, topical treatment with CoQ10 in a rat model of transient IOP elevation reduced extracellular glutamate levels, decreased retinal damage, and avoided apoptotic cell death [40]. In a mouse model of retinal ischemia/reperfusion injury, dietary supplementation with ubiquinol (the reduced form of CoQ10) enhanced the survival of RGCs by preventing cell death mediated by apoptosis. Additionally, it inhibited microglial cell and astrocyte activation in the retina [41]. In addition, in a 12-month clinical trial, vitamin E and CoQ10 eye drops improved inner retinal function and enhanced visual cortical responses in primary open-angle glaucoma patients [42].

2.4. Epigallocatechin-3-Gallate

Epigallocatechin-3-gallate (EGCG) is a type of catechin, a polyphenolic compound highly abundant in green tea, comprising 50–70% of its catechins. Due to its prominence in tea, much of the research on green tea centers around EGCG. However, clinical use of EGCG still faces several challenges. When taken orally, it has low bioavailability, estimated to be between 0.1% and 0.3% in both rats and humans. It enters the bloodstream at a very low micromolar concentration and disappears from the plasma within several hours (<8 h) due to fast metabolism (glucuronidation, methylation, and sulfation) and microbial metabolism. For this reason, finding effective ways to deliver EGCG to specific target sites remains a complex issue [43,44]. Several studies have demonstrated that EGCG is a potent antioxidant with multifunctional properties, including anti-inflammatory [45] and vasodilator effects, which all contribute to its neuroprotective action. Animal studies have demonstrated that EGCG also possesses anti-aging properties by functioning as a scavenger for free radicals [46]. Moreover, cancer chemopreventive/chemotherapeutic effects have also been demonstrated [47].

In an interventional study involving a mouse model with optic nerve crush, systemic treatment with EGCG demonstrated protective effects on RGCs after this event, suggesting that EGCG could be a promising therapeutic agent for optic nerve diseases, including glaucoma [48].

2.5. Vitamins

Vitamins constitute a heterogeneous group of organic compounds classified as micronutrients, as they are required by the body in limited quantities, typically in the range of milligrams or micrograms. Vitamins are generally classified based on their chemical solubility properties: fat-soluble vitamins are A, D, E, and K and water-soluble vitamins include B complex vitamins and vitamin C. Vitamins play a crucial role in regulating numerous chemical reactions within our body and can act as coenzymes, biological antioxidants, cofactors in redox reactions, or hormones. The primary mechanism by which vitamins may have neuroprotective benefits is probably due to their antioxidant activity [49–52].

Several studies have explored the relationship between dietary or supplement intake of antioxidants and glaucoma risk, with controversial results.

In a cross-sectional study conducted as part of the National Health and Nutrition Examination Survey in the United States during 2005–2006, involving 2912 participants, Wang and colleagues focused on the association between glaucoma prevalence and supplement intake, as well as serum levels of vitamins A, C, and E. The study found no association between either supplementary consumption or serum levels of vitamins A and E with glaucoma prevalence. Interestingly, both low- and high-dose supplementary consumption of vitamin C were associated with decreased odds of glaucoma, while serum levels of vitamin C did not correlate with glaucoma prevalence [53]. A systematic review found that blood levels of vitamins (A, B complex, C, D, and E) did not show an association with open-angle glaucoma, but this study highlighted a positive association between the dietary intake of vitamins A and C and open-angle glaucoma [54]. Similarly, a meta-analysis did not find a significative association between serum vitamin B6, vitamin B12, and vitamin D levels and different types of glaucoma [55].

In a prospective study, which included 116,484 participants aged $\geq$ 40 years, no significant association was found between dietary intake of antioxidant vitamins (A, C, and E) and carotenoids and the risk of primary open-angle glaucoma over an average follow-up period of 9.1 years [56]. Conversely, in a cross-sectional study involving 1155 participants, increased consumption of specific fruits and vegetables containing vitamins A, B2, C, and carotenoids was linked to a reduced glaucoma risk in old women [57]. In The Rotterdam Study, a prospective study involving a cohort of 3502 participants aged 55 years and older, no significant association between the intake of most evaluated antioxidant carotenoids and vitamins (C and E) and open-angle glaucoma was found. However, compared to the group with a low consumption, those with a high intake of vitamin B1 and retinol equivalents showed approximately a twofold decreased incidence of open-angle glaucoma [58]. In a randomized controlled trial carried out on older adults, the use of oral antioxidant supplementation, which included B-group vitamins;, vitamins A, C, and E; carotenoids; and antioxidant minerals, with or without omega-3 fatty acids, over a 2-year follow-up did not prevent visual field loss or thinning of the retinal nerve fiber layer or ganglion cell complex. This suggests that such supplementation does not appear to be beneficial as an adjuvant treatment for mild to moderate primary open-angle glaucoma in the short term [59].

Considering all these findings, the role of vitamins as neuroprotective agents in glaucoma management is still controversial.

2.5.1. Vitamin B1

Vitamin B1, also known as thiamin, is an essential cofactor, indispensable for the normal growth and development of the body, playing a crucial role in various biochemical and physiological processes. Vitamin B1 is abundant in foods such as meat, whole grains, eggs, fish, legumes, and nuts [60]. Vitamin B1 deficiency rarely manifests as optic neuropathy, typically presenting as bilateral, severe involvement with associated optic disc swelling [61,62]. The Rotterdam Study suggested a protective effect of thiamine against open-angle glaucoma [58], whereas the study by Giaconi et al. did not report any association between vitamin B1 and open-angle glaucoma [63].

2.5.2. Vitamin B2

Riboflavin, also known as vitamin B2, plays a vital role in cellular processes, serving as a component of coenzymes like flavin mononucleotide and flavin adenine dinucleotide involved in electron transport. Rich sources of riboflavin include poultry, fish, eggs, dairy products, and various plant foods [64]. A study by Coleman et al. observed a decreased risk of glaucoma diagnosis in women consuming at least 2 mg/day of vitamin B2 from natural food sources [57].

2.5.3. Vitamin B3

Nicotinamide is a water-soluble amide that, together with nicotinic acid, forms the niacin and/or vitamin B3 complex. It is a precursor to nicotinamide adenine dinucleotide (NAD+), playing a crucial role in essential cellular functions. As a key component of the glycolysis pathway, nicotinamide contributes to NAD+ production for ATP generation, influencing cellular energetics and various metabolic processes [65]. NAD+ is a crucial coenzyme in hydride-transfer enzymes, essential for energy production and the synthesis of fatty acids, cholesterol, and steroids. It participates in oxidation–reduction reactions as a hydride donor (NADH and NADPH) and acceptor (NAD+ and NADP). NAD+ primarily acts in catabolic reactions, breaking down carbohydrates, fats, proteins, and alcohol for energy, while NADP is involved in anabolic reactions, contributing to the synthesis of cellular macromolecules [66].

Meat, eggs, fish, dairy, coffee, tea, and niacin-fortified cereals are particularly rich sources of nicotinamide, while it is found in lesser amounts in vegetables. Nicotinamide can also be produced from dietary tryptophan, which is an essential amino acid [67]. Nicotinamide, classified as a food additive product rather than a pharmaceutical product, exhibits good bioavailability when administered orally. It distributes effectively across all body tissues, undergoes metabolism in the liver, and is excreted through the kidneys. The recommended dietary intake of nicotinamide is approximately 15 mg/day. Adverse effects from excessive intake, even at pharmacologically high doses, are uncommon. [68]. Nicotinamide also has anti-inflammatory effects; photoprotective effects on the skin; and reduces pigmentation, wrinkles, ultra-violet induced immunosuppression, and sebum production [69]. Moreover, nicotinamide has long been linked to neuronal development, survival, and function in the central nervous system. It contributes to neuronal death as well as neuroprotection, and a number of studies point to its significance in neurological disorders and neurodegenerative illnesses [70].

The enzyme nicotinamide phosphoribosyl transferase is responsible for synthesizing nicotinamide mononucleotide from nicotinamide. Its involvement in the metabolic pathway for NAD biosynthesis suggests its importance in cells sensitive to declining NAD levels, particularly neurons [71]. Changes in NAD homeostasis have been observed with aging [72], suggesting that nicotinamide may play a crucial role in neuronal maturation and neuroprotection by influencing NAD+ levels within neurons. Furthermore, nicotinamide contributes to DNA stability and preserves membrane integrity, preventing cellular injury, phagocytosis, apoptosis, and the formation of vascular clots [73]. The multitude of intracellular systems affected by nicotinamide levels complicates the identification of precise mechanisms of action for this dietary metabolite. However, it seems that the pivotal way in which nicotinamide might act is by restoring ATP levels in neurons. Furthermore, it seems to be implicated in three key neurodegenerative conditions: Alzheimer's, Parkinson's, and Huntington's disease [74–76]. In the ophthalmic field, a nicotinamide-supplemented diet decreased mitochondrial susceptibility and greatly prevented RGCs from degenerating, according to research on mice [77,78].

In a recent study, a cohort of individuals with primary open-angle glaucoma showed a notably lower concentration of nicotinamide compared to the control group [79]. In addition, in a crossover, double-masked, randomized clinical trial involving 57 participants with glaucoma under IOP-lowering medications, oral nicotinamide supplementation resulted in an early enhancement of inner retinal function [80]. All these findings seem to suggest that nicotinamide could represent a promising molecule for neuroprotection in glaucoma.

2.5.4. Vitamin B6, Vitamin B9, and Vitamin B12

Vitamin B6 comprises a group of six water-soluble chemical compounds, and pyridoxal phosphate is the active form. B6 is a vitamin found in poultry, fish, and plant-based foods. Pyridoxal phosphate acts as a cofactor for approximately 160 reactions in the body, including gluconeogenesis and glycogenolysis to amino acid and lipids biosynthesis and metabolism [81]. Furthermore, vitamin B6 is involved in regulating homocysteine levels, an amino acid also associated with oxidative stress and apoptosis in RGCs [82].

Vitamin B9, also known as folic acid or folate, is essential for the synthesis of DNA and RNA, and plays a key role in the breakdown of homocysteine. Good sources of vitamin B9 include plants foods, such as leafy greens and legumes. Insufficient folate in adults is linked to cognitive decline and visual system complications, including nutritional amblyopia and optic disc disorders. In fact, low serum folate correlates with nutritional optic neuropathy, leading to gradual visual loss and symptoms like central scotoma and altered color perception [62,83].

Vitamin B12, or cobalamin, is obtained only through the intake of animal-sourced foods, such as eggs, fish, and meat. Vitamin B12 is essential in the metabolism of carbohydrates, lipids, and proteins, DNA synthesis, hematopoiesis, and the maintenance of the integrity of the peripheral and central nervous systems. The primary cause of vitamin B12 deficiency is prolonged dietary deprivation without adequate supplementation [84]. Vitamin B12 deficiency can lead to pernicious anemia, high homocysteine levels, and damage to the nervous system. Optic neuropathy may occur before hematologic abnormalities and be the first sign of a cobalamin deficit. [62]. A study involving patients with open-angle glaucoma exhibited significantly lower serum levels of vitamin B12 compared to controls [85]. On the other hand, other studies did not report significant differences in plasma levels of vitamin B6 or serum levels of vitamins B9 and B12 between open-angle glaucoma patients and controls [86,87]. However, lower levels of vitamin B9 and B12 are significantly linked to higher homocysteine levels, which has been associated with oxidative stress and apoptosis in RGCs. In fact, increased levels of homocysteine have been reported in the aqueous humor and plasma of patients with primary open-angle glaucoma. In addition, reduced levels of vitamin B6, B9, and B12 were also linked to increased homocysteine levels in individuals with pseudoexfoliation glaucoma [88].

2.5.5. Vitamin C

Vitamin C, or ascorbic acid, is a potent antioxidant exerting beneficial effects on redox oxidative pathways, inflammaging, endothelial integrity, and lipoprotein metabolism. Vitamin C is synthesized from glucose in the liver of many mammalian species; however, humans have evolutionarily lost this synthetic ability, making it necessary to obtain vitamin C through the diet [89], and fruits and vegetables are the main sources of vitamin C. Concerning its neuroprotective properties, the studies investigating the association between blood levels of vitamin C and glaucoma showed conflicting results. In patients with normal tension glaucoma, lower serum levels of vitamin C were reported compared to controls [90], but in patients with open-angle glaucoma no significant differences were observed [91]. Conversely, a cross-sectional study involving 2912 participants aged > 40 highlighted weak evidence that supplemental vitamin C intake might possibly be associated with a decreased risk of glaucoma [53].

2.5.6. Vitamin A

Vitamin A (retinol) acts as a significant dietary antioxidant and is abundant in various sources, including dairy products, fish, meat, and plants. The biological activity of vitamin A is also exhibited by carotenoids, which act as provitamin A. Among these, β-carotene is the most active. β-carotene is a potent antioxidant, reducing the accumulation of reactive oxygen species, including hydrogen peroxide and lipid peroxide radicals [92]. Because β-carotene may reduce oxidative stress and counteract lipid peroxidation, it plays a major role in brain-related disorders [93]. Particularly, in brain diseases linked to reactive oxygen species, therapy with β-carotene may decrease neuronal loss since oxidative stress strongly contributes to neuronal death during neurotoxicity [94].

Five studies have examined the relationship between blood vitamin A levels and glaucoma, all showing conflicting results. In fact, one study reported higher vitamin A levels in patients with primary open-angle glaucoma compared to those with normal tension glaucoma [86], while another study similarly found higher levels compared to controls [95]. Conversely, three other studies did not identify significant differences in vitamin A concentration between individuals with glaucoma and healthy subjects [53,90,96].

Despite these conflicting results, The Rotterdam Study meta-analysis has found that individuals with a high intake of retinol equivalents have approximately half the risk of developing open-angle glaucoma compared to those with a low intake of these nutrients [58], suggesting a potential favorable association of dietary retinol intake in patients with open-angle glaucoma.

2.5.7. Vitamin E

Vitamin E is a fat-soluble vitamin with eight identified isoforms that include four tocopherols and four tocotrienols designated as α-, β-, γ-, and δ-. The most studied isoform is α-tocopherol (αT). It is a potent antioxidant agent against oxidative stress damage caused by free radicals, preventing the oxidation of polyunsaturated fatty acids in cell membranes by donating hydrogen from the phenolic group on the chromanol ring. All forms of vitamin E have robust antioxidant activities, thanks to their similar phenolic moieties [97]. Vitamin E in its natural state is produced by plants, with αT being primarily concentrated in certain seeds. Notably, αT is abundantly found in peanuts, almonds, and sunflower seeds. Consequently, this form of vitamin E is prevalent in various food oils such as corn, soybean, and peanut oil [98]. Vitamin E is an essential micronutrient and in the intestinal tract, dietary tocopherols and tocotrienols are absorbed with dietary fats. In the liver, the αT isoform has a greater affinity for the αT transfer protein, which facilitates the incorporation of αT into lipoproteins. This process promotes the transportation of vitamin E to various tissues through circulation [99]. The current recommended daily intake of vitamin E for adults is set at 15 mg, for both males and females. Vitamin E plays a crucial role as an antioxidant in various tissues, including the eye. In fact, in rat models with increased IOP, those with a vitamin-E-deficient diet had significantly higher RGC death due to increased lipid peroxidation compared to rats following a diet containing vitamin E [100]. In humans, the reduction of glaucoma progression was observed with daily vitamin E integration [101], in addition to a neuroprotective effect of αT oral supplement against glaucomatous damage [102].

2.6. Forskolin

Forskolin is a diterpene abundant in the leaves, roots, and tubers of Coleus forskohlii, a medicinal plant native to India and Southeast Asia. It is a natural active compound that acts as a second messenger, stimulating cyclic adenosine monophosphate (cAMP) through direct activation of adenylate cyclase. In cells treated with forskolin, the intracellular concentration of the second messenger cAMP increases rapidly [103]. Several in vitro and in vivo studies highlight forskolin as a neuroprotective agent, considering its efficacy in lowering IOP in animals and humans [104,105] as well as its protective effect on RGCs against insults associated with glaucoma [106]. Therefore, forskolin may exert beneficial indirect neuroprotective effects on RGCs by reducing the IOP. In a double-blind, randomized, controlled trial, patients with primary open-angle glaucoma who were treated with forskolin 1% eye drops (two drops three times a day) for 4 weeks exhibited a notable reduction in IOP [107]. This could be explained by the hypotensive effect of forskolin, which leads to decreased aqueous humor accumulation [52]. In another clinical study, a dietary supplement containing forskolin given to patients with primary open-angle glaucoma was able to reduce IOP and enhance their pattern electroretinogram amplitude. This could suggest a positive impact on the survival and/or function of RGCs [108].

It seems that some of neuroprotective effects of forskolin are mediated by the activation and enhancement of neurotrophins' activity. Meyer-Franke et al. showed that forskolin added to a culture medium containing brain-derived neurotrophic factor (BDNF), ciliary-derived neurotrophic factor (CTNF), and insulin-like growth factor-1 (IGF-1) increased the RGC lifespan [106]. Similarly, when included in a combined treatment with BDNF and CTNF, forskolin significantly enhanced the survival of axotomized RGCs in the cat retina [109].

In animal studies, a dietary supplementation of forskolin, homotaurine, spearmint, and vitamins B showed protect effects against RGC loss in rodent models of optic nerve injury [110] and glaucoma [111]. The forskolin supplement mixture was able to reduce inflammatory cytokines, leading to decreased apoptotic markers, sparing RGCs and preserving visual function, without impacting IOP in glaucomatous rodents [111].

2.7. Ribes Nigrum

Ribes nigrum, commonly known as blackcurrant, is a plant belonging to the Grossulariaceae family that contains 160 species, native to Europe and Asian Russia. Some species of Ribes have been employed in traditional and local medicine for the treatment of glaucoma, cardiovascular disease, hepatitis, hyperlipidemia, hypertension, and other health issues [112]. Blackcurrant is a good source of polyphenols, containing four different types of anthocyanins, which are the subject of research in studies on glaucoma progression. In a randomized, placebo-controlled study, Ohguro and colleagues investigated the influence of the blackcurrant anthocyanins (BCACs) on the disease progression of open-angle glaucoma in 38 patients treated using antiglaucoma drops. For a period of 24 months, participants were administered BCACs (50 mg/day, n = 19) or placebos (n = 19) orally once a day. The trial results showed that the BCAC-treated group exhibited a significant improvement in ocular blood flow and in the visual field, whereas no significant changes were observed in systemic and ocular conditions, including IOP [113]. In another study by Ohguro et al., the effects of oral administration of BCACs on IOP were investigated in both healthy subjects and patients with glaucoma. A double-blind, placebo-controlled crossover study was conducted with 12 healthy subjects treated once daily with oral BCACs (50 mg) and 21 primary open-angle glaucoma patients (BCACs, n = 12; placebo, n = 9) treated with a single antiglaucomatous drug. They observed a significative decrease in mean IOP values (at 4 weeks, $p = 0.039$), not only in healthy participants but also in glaucoma patients using BCACs ($p = 0.027$) over 2 years [114]. The results of these studies seem to suggest that the administration of BCACs may be a safe and promising supplement for healthy subjects and glaucomatous patients already treated with antiglaucomatous drugs.

2.8. Berberine

Berberine is a quaternary ammonium salt classified within the benzylisoquinoline alkaloids. It occurs natural in some plants of the *Berberis* genus, typically in the roots, rhizomes, stems, and bark. Berberine is widely utilized in various traditional medical systems, including Ayurvedic, Chinese, and Iranian medicine [115]. Berberine, exhibiting a variety of pharmacological activities, shows anti-heart failure, antioxidant, antimicrobial, anti-inflammatory, hypocholesterolemic, antitumor, and immunomodulatory properties [116–119]. Although its clinical uses are limited due to its poor solubility and bioavailability (less than 1%) [120], ongoing preclinical studies are driving exploration towards new potential applications. In recent years, many studies have investigated the role of berberine in central nervous system diseases. These investigations have revealed that berberine can effectively cross the blood–brain barrier, exerting positive effects on brain functions [121–123]. Berberine has demonstrated significant neuroprotective properties in studies carried out in vitro and on animal models against drug- and toxin-induced neurotoxicity, ischemia-reperfusion damage, and chronic neurodegenerative conditions such as Alzheimer's and Parkinson's diseases, depression, schizophrenia, epilepsy, and anxiety [122,124–126]. The neuroprotective effects of berberine are mediated by intricate molecular mechanisms that involve several biological functions, including antioxidant, anti-inflammatory, and antiapoptotic actions [127]. Currently, human studies reporting the pharmacological effects of berberine on neurodegenerative diseases are limited. Moreover, most studies on the use of berberine in treating neurodegenerative diseases have focused on Alzheimer's and Parkinson's diseases [128], with only a few involving other conditions. Therefore, its mechanism of action has been explored in vitro and in animal models, but much remains to be clarified in humans. Berberine could be a valuable potential therapeutic target for various neurodegenerative diseases, including glaucoma, but further research is still needed to fully understand the bioavailability, efficacy, and dosage of berberine in clinical studies.

2.9. Ginkgo Biloba

Ginkgo Biloba is a tree native to East Asia and belongs to the *Gymnosperm* species. It is a very ancient tree, first appearing approximately 250 million years ago, considered a "living fossil". These trees have been used in traditional Chinese and Japanese medicine for centuries, with ginkgo seeds recognized for their therapeutic properties, while the leaves were commonly used in teas for medicinal purposes [129].

The plant's composition includes bioactive compounds like flavonoids (e.g., quercetin and kaempferol), bioflavonoids, organic acids (e.g., ginkgolic acid), and terpene lactones (e.g., ginkgolides A, B, and C), expanding its utility across several biological systems. Most randomized, controlled trials utilize the standardized extract of Ginkgo biloba (GBE) leaves, EGb761. This extract, containing flavonoids (24%), terpene lactones (6%), and a low concentration of ginkgolic acids (0.0005%), has been shown to support age-related conditions including neurodegenerative disorders, cognitive decline, and glaucoma [130]. Its potential use is justified by its demonstrated neuroprotective and antioxidant properties, along with its ability to increase blood flow through vasodilation and reduce blood viscosity [131]. For glaucoma management, the effects of GBE on RGCs have been predominantly studied in animal models. Two studies have demonstrated that administering GBE daily for 4 weeks after an optic nerve crush injury led to increased survival rates of RGCs [132,133]. In another study conducted in vivo, the impact of GBE on increased IOP and RGC density was also evaluated, showing that both pretreatment and early posttreatment with EGb761 effectively exhibited neuroprotective effects in a rat model of chronic glaucoma [134]. Clinical studies involving GBE focused on two distinct outcomes: enhancement of blood flow or improvement in the visual field. In studies focusing on blood flow improvements, Park et al. found increased peripapillary blood flow in normal tension glaucoma patients after 4 weeks of GBE (80 mg twice daily) oral administration [135]. Similarly, the effects of GBE on ocular blood flow were affirmed in open angle glaucoma patients treated for 4 weeks with an antioxidant dietary supplement containing 120 mg/day of GBE [136]. On the other hand, there are conflicting results in studies regarding the effect of GBE on visual field outcomes [130]. Quaranta et al. carried out a study in Italy involving 27 patients with normal tension glaucoma, assessing visual field outcomes following GBE supplementation. Significant improvements were observed in visual field indices with 40 mg GBE three times/daily for 4 weeks compared to a placebo, suggesting potential benefits on retinal sensitivity and cognitive function. However, these effects were only temporary and did not persist after the washout period [137]. Another study also investigated GBE effects on visual field and contrast sensitivity in 28 Chinese patients with normal tension glaucoma but found no significant differences compared to a placebo [138]. Given the inconsistent findings in the existing literature, further research is warranted to determine the efficacy of GBE in glaucoma treatment and management. Additionally, it is also important to note that none of the current studies on GBE address the treatment and management of primary open-angle glaucoma, which is the most common clinical form.

3. Discussion

This review evaluated the neuroprotective properties of several nutrients in contemporary ophthalmology and medicine, as summarized in Tables 1 and 2. Most of the molecules analyzed in this review carry out their neuroprotective action through a predominantly antioxidant action, protecting RGCs from oxidative stress, thus reducing their apoptosis and improving their visual function. The increasing prevalence of these dietary supplements in the published scientific literature heralds a new era in the treatment of many medical conditions, such as glaucoma, neurodegenerative diseases, and other ocular disorders. Nutrient-rich substances are an appealing inclusive choice in medical therapy because of their low cost, simple absorption, and lack of major negative effects when taken as prescribed. These supplements undoubtedly cannot take the place of conventional medical and surgical care, but they can have a synergistic beneficial impact that increases the effectiveness of gold-standard therapies and helps stabilize the patient's overall health.

Furthermore, it is interesting to note how some of the molecules discussed in this review, in addition to their properties already analyzed, could have a further neuroprotective effect by stimulating the metabolic pathway of vascular endothelial growth factor (VEGF). In fact, it has been demonstrated in vitro and in animal models that coenzyme Q10, forskolin, and berberine can promote angiogenesis in cerebral ischemic areas [139–141]. However, to date, no in vivo clinical studies have yet been carried out on human models and, in particular, for glaucoma.

Another interesting aspect to consider about these molecules, in addition to the aforesaid therapeutic and neuroprotective effects, is their safe profile, which could make them easily and further usable in clinical practice. In fact, to date, only citicoline, homotaurine, coenzyme Q10, and Gingko biloba have been shown to have minimal side effects, mainly linked to digestive intolerance and at high doses. Furthermore, some of the discussed compounds, such as coenzyme Q10, forskolin, and Gingko biloba, can interfere with the action of some drugs, such as antihypertensive, antiplatelet, and anticoagulant drugs [142,143].

In addition, given the demonstrated effect of forskolin and Ribes nigrum on IOP reduction, it could be challenging to carry out clinical studies to demonstrate the effect of these two molecules or other ones in managing the IOP increase following intravitreal injections [144–146], since, to date, there are no data published in the scientific literature.

In Table 3, we summarized other minor naturally-derived molecules with potential neuroprotective properties, but future studies are needed to better understand their potential role and use in clinical practice.

This narrative review has some limitations including its narrative and non-systematic nature and having used a single scientific database (PubMed) for its drafting. Furthermore, in this review, only some of the main naturally derived molecules currently utilized in clinical practice for neuroprotection in case of glaucoma have been covered.

Table 1. Summary of the main effects of the discussed neuroprotective molecules.

Active Compounds	Daily Therapeutic Dosage	Prescription Duration	Neuroprotective Effects	Administration	Bioavailability	Adverse Effect and Contraindications
Citicoline	500–2000 mg	2 weeks–4 months	Possible mitigation of RGC dysfunction and prevention of their apoptosis Improved retinal function and neural conduction Improved glaucomatous visual dysfunction	Oral Eye drops	High	Minimal toxicity, predominantly digestive intolerance
Homotaurine	50–100 g	2 weeks–4 months	Possible mitigation of RGC dysfunction and prevention of their apoptosis Improved retinal function	Oral	Moderate	Minimal toxicity, predominantly digestive intolerance
Coenzyme Q10	90–200 mg	Weeks–months	Protect RGCs against oxidative stress Promote RGC survival by inhibiting RGC apoptosis Enhance visual cortical responses in OAG	Oral Eye drops	Moderate/high, depending on the formulation	Minimal toxicity, predominantly digestive intolerance May increase the metabolism of warfarin May cause an excessive decrease in blood pressure when taken together with antihypertensive drugs May reduce the effectiveness of some pro-oxidant chemotherapy treatments
Forskolin	20–50 mg	Weeks–months	Decrease IOP Protective effect on RGCs	Oral Eye drops	Not available	Limited data May interact with antihypertensive drugs
Epigallocatechin-3-gallate	300 mg	Weeks–months	Antioxidant activity Protective effects on RGCs after optic nerve crush	Oral	Very Low	Limited data
Ribes nigrum	50 mg	Weeks–months	Improvement in ocular blood flow and in the visual field Decrease in mean IOP values	Oral	Not available	Limited data
Berberine	500–1500 mg	Weeks–months	Not fully demonstrated	Oral	Very low	Limited data
Ginkgo Biloba	80–600 mg	Weeks–months	Antioxidant activity Anti-inflammatory effects Increase ocular blood flow	Oral	Moderate/High	Minimal toxicity, predominantly digestive intolerance May cause bleeding with concomitant use of antiplatelet or anticoagulant drugs

RGCs: retinal ganglion cells; IOP: intraocular pressure; OAG: open angle glaucoma.

Table 2. Summary of the main neuroprotective effects of vitamins.

Vitamin	Vitamer Chemical Name	Recommended Daily Intake for Adults *	Sources	Neuroprotective Effects
B1	Thiamin	1.2 mg for man 1.1 mg for women	Cereal grain, meat, egg, fish, legume, nut	Possible protective effect against open-angle glaucoma
B2	Riboflavin	1.3 mg for man 1.1 mg for women	Poultry, fish, egg, dairy products, plant foods	Associated with lower risk of glaucoma diagnosis
B3	Niacin	16 mg for man 14 mg for women	Meat, egg, fish, dairy, coffee, tea	Protect retinal ganglion cells from degeneration Enhance inner retinal function
B6 B9 B12	Pyridoxin Folate Cobalamine	1–1.7 mg 400 mcg 2.4 mcg	Poultry, fish, plant-based foods Dark green leafy vegetables, nut, avocado Meat, fish, eggs	Regulators of homocysteine levels
C	Ascorbic acid	90 mg for men 75 mg for women	Fruits and vegetables	Antioxidant activity associated with lower risk of glaucoma diagnosis
A	Retinol	900 mcg 700 mcg	Carrot, tomato, butter, cream cheese, egg, fish	Antioxidant activity Associated with lower risk of open-angle glaucoma diagnosis
E	Tocopherol	15 mg	Peanuts, almonds, sunflower seeds	Antioxidant activity Associated with lower progression of glaucoma

* Institute of Medicine (US) Standing Committee on the Scientific Evaluation of Dietary Reference Intakes and its Panel on Folate, Other B Vitamins, and Choline. *Dietary Reference Intakes for Thiamin, Riboflavin, Niacin, Vitamin B6, Folate, Vitamin B12, Pantothenic Acid, Biotin, and Choline.* Washington, DC: National Academies Press (US); 1998.

Table 3. Summary of minor plant-derived neuroprotective compounds.

Active Compounds	Daily Therapeutic Dosage	Neuroprotective Effects	Administration	Bioavailability	Adverse Effect and Contraindications
Crocetin [147]	In rats, 50–100 mg/kg	Antioxidant activity ROS scavenger	Oral	Low	No adverse effects demonstrated No adverse effects are available in long-term administration
Hesperidin [148,149]	50 mg	Antioxidant activity Possible protection of RGCs against oxidative stress Possible prevention of RGCs' death	Oral Intravitreal	Low	Low toxicity at a wide range of doses
Lycium barbarum [150]	In rats, 1 mg/kg	In animal model Antioxidant activity Anti-inflammatory effects Possible prevention of RGCs' loss Preservation of retinal structure and function	Oral	Not available	No adverse effects demonstrated Possible interaction with warfarin
Tamarindus Indica [151,152]	In rats, 100–5000 mg/kg	Antioxidant activity	Oral	Not available	No toxic reported Potentially increases the bioavailability of aspirin
Resveratrol [153,154]	In rats, 20–250 mg/kg	Potential prevention retinal damage and RGC apoptosis Antioxidant activity Anti-inflammatory effects	Oral Intragastric Intraperitoneal	Low	No adverse effects demonstrated Alteration or inhibition of CYP3A4 enzyme activity May interact with blood thinners like warfarin, increasing the risk of bleeding
Scutellaria baicalensis Georgi [155]		Only in animal models in vitro Blood pressure level reduction Antioxidative effects Anti-inflammatory effects	Intraperitoneal	Not available	Limited data
Vaccinium myrtillus [156]	In rats 100–500 mg/kg	Blood pressure level reduction Strong antioxidative effects Anti-inflammatory effects	Oral	Not available	Rare allergic reaction

4. Conclusions

In conclusion, the treatment of neurodegenerative diseases, including glaucoma, may benefit from the integrative use of antioxidants, vitamins, organic compounds, and micronutrients as IOP-independent techniques [156]. Nonetheless, to fully use the neuroprotective qualities of these supplements as adjuvant therapeutic alternatives in treatment regimens, further research and even large-scale multicenter clinical studies are consistently needed to confirm their efficacy. Lastly, it is critical to remember that therapeutic medications in the form of eye drops, such as prostaglandin analogs and beta blockers, remain the first-choice therapeutic for glaucoma [157].

Author Contributions: A.D., L.V., F.L., G.A., A.C. and V.G. analyzed the literature and wrote the original draft. A.P. and G.G. conceived the article and reviewed the manuscript. All authors have read and agreed to the published version of the manuscript.

Funding: This research received no external funding.

Institutional Review Board Statement: Not applicable.

Informed Consent Statement: Not applicable.

Data Availability Statement: The data can be shared upon request.

Conflicts of Interest: The authors declare no conflicts of interest.

References

1. Boccaccini, A.; Cavaterra, D.; Carnevale, C.; Tanga, L.; Marini, S.; Bocedi, A.; Lacal, P.M.; Manni, G.; Graziani, G.; Sbardella, D.; et al. Novel frontiers in neuroprotective therapies in glaucoma: Molecular and clinical aspects. *Mol. Asp. Med.* **2023**, *94*, 101225. [CrossRef]
2. Tham, Y.-C.; Li, X.; Wong, T.Y.; Quigley, H.A.; Aung, T.; Cheng, C.-Y. Global prevalence of glaucoma and projections of glaucoma burden through 2040: A systematic review and meta-analysis. *Ophthalmology* **2014**, *121*, 2081–2090. [CrossRef] [PubMed]
3. Chitu, I.; Tudosescu, R.; Leasu-Branet, C.; Voinea, L.-M. Citicoline—A neuroprotector with proven effects on glaucomatous disease. *Romanian J. Ophthalmol.* **2017**, *61*, 152–158. [CrossRef] [PubMed]
4. Parisi, V.; Centofanti, M.; Ziccardi, L.; Tanga, L.; Michelessi, M.; Roberti, G.; Manni, G. Treatment with citicoline eye drops enhances retinal function and neural conduction along the visual pathways in open angle glaucoma. *Graefe's Arch. Clin. Exp. Ophthalmol.* **2015**, *253*, 1327–1340. [CrossRef]
5. Villoslada, P.; Steinman, L. New targets and therapeutics for neuroprotection, remyelination and repair in multiple sclerosis. *Expert Opin. Investig. Drugs* **2020**, *29*, 443–459. [CrossRef] [PubMed]
6. Levin, L.A.; Patrick, C.; Choudry, N.B.; Sharif, N.A.; Goldberg, J.L. Neuroprotection in neurodegenerations of the brain and eye: Lessons from the past and directions for the future. *Front. Neurol.* **2022**, *13*, 964197. [CrossRef]
7. Secades, J.J.; Frontera, G. CDP-choline: Pharmacological and clinical review. *Methods Find. Exp. Clin. Pharmacol.* **1995**, *17* (Suppl. B), 1–54. [PubMed]
8. Weiss, G.B. Metabolism and actions of CDP-choline as an endogenous compound and administered exogenously as citicoline. *Life Sci.* **1995**, *56*, 637–660. [CrossRef]
9. Adibhatla, R.M.; Hatcher, J.F.; Dempsey, R.J. Citicoline: Neuroprotective mechanisms in cerebral ischemia. *J. Neurochem.* **2002**, *80*, 12–23. [CrossRef] [PubMed]
10. Rejdak, R.; Toczołowski, J.; Solski, J.; Duma, D.; Grieb, P. Citicoline treatment increases retinal dopamine content in rabbits. *Ophthalmic Res.* **2002**, *34*, 146–149. [CrossRef] [PubMed]
11. Fioravanti, M.; Yanagi, M. Cytidinediphosphocholine (CDP choline) for cognitive and behavioural disturbances associated with chronic cerebral disorders in the elderly. *Cochrane Database Syst. Rev.* **2000**, *2*, CD000269. [CrossRef]
12. Eberhardt, R.; Birbamer, G.; Gerstenbrand, F.; Rainer, E.; Traegner, H. Citicoline in the treatment of Parkinson's disease. *Clin Ther.* **1990**, *12*, 489–495. [PubMed]
13. Gandolfi, S.; Marchini, G.; Caporossi, A.; Scuderi, G.; Tomasso, L.; Brunoro, A. Cytidine 5′-Diphosphocholine (Citicoline): Evidence for a Neuroprotective Role in Glaucoma. *Nutrients* **2020**, *12*, 793. [CrossRef] [PubMed]
14. Secades, J.J.; Lorenzo, J.L. Citicoline: Pharmacological and clinical review, 2006 update. *Methods Find. Exp. Clin. Pharmacol.* **2006**, *28* (Suppl. B), 1–56. [PubMed]
15. Grieb, P. Neuroprotective Properties of Citicoline: Facts, Doubts and Unresolved Issues. *CNS Drugs* **2014**, *28*, 185–193. [CrossRef]
16. Oshitari, T.; Fujimoto, N.; Adachi-Usami, E. Citicoline has a protective effect on damaged retinal ganglion cells in mouse culture retina. *Neuroreport* **2002**, *13*, 2109–2111. [CrossRef] [PubMed]
17. Parisi, V.; Coppola, G.; Centofanti, M.; Oddone, F.; Angrisani, A.M.; Ziccardi, L.; Ricci, B.; Quaranta, L.; Manni, G. Evidence of the neuroprotective role of citicoline in glaucoma patients. *Prog. Brain Res.* **2008**, *173*, 541–554. [CrossRef]

18. Ottobelli, L.; Manni, G.; Centofanti, M.; Iester, M.; Allevena, F.; Rossetti, L. Citicoline oral solution in glaucoma: Is there a role in slowing disease progression? *Ophthalmologica* **2013**, *229*, 219–226. [CrossRef]
19. Melecchi, A.; Amato, R.; Monte, M.D.; Rusciano, D.; Bagnoli, P.; Cammalleri, M. Restored retinal physiology after administration of niacin with citicoline in a mouse model of hypertensive glaucoma. *Front. Med.* **2023**, *10*, 1230941. [CrossRef]
20. Mastropasqua, L.; Agnifili, L.; Ferrante, C.; Sacchi, M.; Figus, M.; Rossi, G.C.M.; Brescia, L.; Aloia, R.; Orlando, G. Citicoline/Coenzyme Q10/Vitamin B3 Fixed Combination Exerts Synergistic Protective Effects on Neuronal Cells Exposed to Oxidative Stress. *Nutrients* **2022**, *14*, 2963. [CrossRef]
21. Wright, T. Tramiprosate. *Drugs Today* **2006**, *42*, 291–298. [CrossRef]
22. Caltagirone, C.; Ferrannini, L.; Marchionni, N.; Nappi, G.; Scapagnini, G.; Trabucchi, M. The potential protective effect of tramiprosate (homotaurine) against Alzheimer's disease: A review. *Aging Clin. Exp. Res.* **2012**, *24*, 580–587. [CrossRef]
23. De Valderas, R.M.; Serrano, M.I.; Serrano, J.S.; Fernandez, A. Effect of homotaurine in experimental analgesia tests. *Gen. Pharmacol. Vasc. Syst.* **1991**, *22*, 717–721. [CrossRef] [PubMed]
24. Messina, S.A.; Dawson, R.J. Attenuation of oxidative damage to DNA by taurine and taurine analogs. *Adv. Exp. Med. Biol.* **2000**, *483*, 355–367. [CrossRef] [PubMed]
25. Parisi, V.; Oddone, F.; Ziccardi, L.; Roberti, G.; Coppola, G.; Manni, G. Citicoline and Retinal Ganglion Cells: Effects on Morphology and Function. *Curr. Neuropharmacol.* **2018**, *16*, 919–932. [CrossRef]
26. Davinelli, S.; Chiosi, F.; Di Marco, R.; Costagliola, C.; Scapagnini, G. Cytoprotective Effects of Citicoline and Homotaurine against Glutamate and High Glucose Neurotoxicity in Primary Cultured Retinal Cells. *Oxidative Med. Cell. Longev.* **2017**, *2017*, 2825703. [CrossRef]
27. Rossi, G.C.M.; Rolle, T.; De Silvestri, A.; Sisto, D.; Mavilio, A.; Mirabile, A.V.; Paviglianiti, A.; Strano, B.; Picasso, E.; Pasinetti, G.M.; et al. Multicenter, Prospective, Randomized, Single Blind, Cross-Over Study on the Effect of a Fixed Combination of Citicoline 500 mg Plus Homotaurine 50 mg on Pattern Electroretinogram (PERG) in Patients with Open Angle Glaucoma on Well Controlled Intraocular Pressure. *Front. Med.* **2022**, *9*, 882335. [CrossRef]
28. Kamei, M.; Fujita, T.; Kanbe, T.; Sasaki, K.; Oshiba, K.; Otani, S.; Matsui-Yuasa, I.; Morisawa, S. The distribution and content of ubiquinone in foods. *Int. J. Vitam. Nutr. Res.* **1986**, *56*, 57–63.
29. Trumpower, B.L. New concepts on the role of ubiquinone in the mitochondrial respiratory chain. *J. Bioenerg. Biomembr.* **1981**, *13*, 1–24. [CrossRef] [PubMed]
30. Crane, F.L. Biochemical Functions of Coenzyme Q_{10}. *J. Am. Coll. Nutr.* **2001**, *20*, 591–598. [CrossRef]
31. Greenberg, S.; Frishman, W.H. Co-Enzyme Q_{10}: A New Drug for Cardiovascular Disease. *J. Clin. Pharmacol.* **1990**, *30*, 596–608. [CrossRef] [PubMed]
32. Bagheri, S.; Haddadi, R.; Saki, S.; Kourosh-Arami, M.; Rashno, M.; Mojaver, A.; Komaki, A. Neuroprotective effects of coenzyme Q10 on neurological diseases: A review article. *Front. Neurosci.* **2023**, *17*, 1188839. [CrossRef]
33. Henchcliffe, C.; Spindler, M.; Beal, M.F. Coenzyme Q10 effects in neurodegenerative disease. *Neuropsychiatr. Dis. Treat.* **2009**, *5*, 597–610. [CrossRef] [PubMed]
34. Itagaki, S.; Ochiai, A.; Kobayashi, M.; Sugawara, M.; Hirano, T.; Iseki, K. Interaction of Coenzyme Q10 with the Intestinal Drug Transporter P-Glycoprotein. *J. Agric. Food Chem.* **2008**, *56*, 6923–6927. [CrossRef]
35. Adornetto, A.; Rombolà, L.; Morrone, L.A.; Nucci, C.; Corasaniti, M.T.; Bagetta, G.; Russo, R. Natural Products: Evidence for Neuroprotection to Be Exploited in Glaucoma. *Nutrients* **2020**, *12*, 3158. [CrossRef] [PubMed]
36. Beal, M.F. Coenzyme Q_{10} administration and its potential for treatment of neurodegenerative diseases. *BioFactors* **1999**, *9*, 261–266. [CrossRef] [PubMed]
37. Lee, D.; Kim, K.-Y.; Shim, M.S.; Kim, S.Y.; Ellisman, M.H.; Weinreb, R.N.; Ju, W.-K. Coenzyme Q10 ameliorates oxidative stress and prevents mitochondrial alteration in ischemic retinal injury. *Apoptosis* **2014**, *19*, 603–614. [CrossRef] [PubMed]
38. Lee, D.; Shim, M.S.; Kim, K.-Y.; Noh, Y.H.; Kim, H.; Kim, S.Y.; Weinreb, R.N.; Ju, W.-K. Coenzyme Q10 Inhibits Glutamate Excitotoxicity and Oxidative Stress–Mediated Mitochondrial Alteration in a Mouse Model of Glaucoma. *Investig. Ophthalmol. Vis. Sci.* **2014**, *55*, 993–1005. [CrossRef]
39. Acar, S.E.; Sarıcaoğlu, M.S.; Çolak, A.; Aktaş, Z.; Dinçel, A.S. Neuroprotective effects of topical coenzyme Q10 + vitamin E in mechanic optic nerve injury model. *Eur. J. Ophthalmol.* **2020**, *30*, 714–722. [CrossRef]
40. Russo, R.; Cavaliere, F.; Rombola, L.; Gliozzi, M.; Cerulli, A.; Nucci, C.; Fazzi, E.; Bagetta, G.; Corasaniti, M.T.; Morrone, L.A. Rational basis for the development of coenzyme Q10 as a neurotherapeutic agent for retinal protection. *Prog. Brain Res.* **2008**, *173*, 575–582. [CrossRef] [PubMed]
41. Ju, W.-K.; Shim, M.S.; Kim, K.-Y.; Bu, J.H.; Park, T.L.; Ahn, S.; Weinreb, R.N. Ubiquinol promotes retinal ganglion cell survival and blocks the apoptotic pathway in ischemic retinal degeneration. *Biochem. Biophys. Res. Commun.* **2018**, *503*, 2639–2645. [CrossRef] [PubMed]
42. Parisi, V.; Centofanti, M.; Gandolfi, S.; Marangoni, D.; Rossetti, L.; Tanga, L.; Tardini, M.; Traina, S.; Ungaro, N.; Vetrugno, M.; et al. Effects of Coenzyme Q10 in Conjunction with Vitamin E on Retinal-Evoked and Cortical-Evoked Responses in Patients with Open-Angle Glaucoma. *Eur. J. Gastroenterol. Hepatol.* **2014**, *23*, 391–404. [CrossRef] [PubMed]
43. Khan, N.; Mukhtar, H. Tea Polyphenols in Promotion of Human Health. *Nutrients* **2018**, *11*, 39. [CrossRef]
44. Pervin, M.; Unno, K.; Takagaki, A.; Isemura, M.; Nakamura, Y. Function of Green Tea Catechins in the Brain: Epigallocatechin Gallate and Its Metabolites. *Int. J. Mol. Sci.* **2019**, *20*, 3630. [CrossRef] [PubMed]

45. Tedeschi, E.; Suzuki, H.; Menegazzi, M. Antiinflammatory Action of EGCG, the Main Component of Green Tea, through STAT-1 Inhibition. *Ann. N. Y. Acad. Sci.* **2002**, *973*, 435–437. [CrossRef]
46. Namita, P.; Mukesh, R.; Vijay, K. Camellia Sinensis (Green Tea): A Review. 2012. Available online: https://api.semanticscholar.org/CorpusID:43669711 (accessed on 01 August 2012).
47. Khan, N.; Mukhtar, H. Multitargeted therapy of cancer by green tea polyphenols. *Cancer Lett.* **2008**, *269*, 269–280. [CrossRef] [PubMed]
48. Xie, J.; Jiang, L.; Zhang, T.; Jin, Y.; Yang, D.; Chen, F. Neuroprotective effects of Epigallocatechin-3-gallate (EGCG) in optic nerve crush model in rats. *Neurosci. Lett.* **2010**, *479*, 26–30. [CrossRef] [PubMed]
49. Lee, K.H.; Cha, M.; Lee, B.H. Neuroprotective Effect of Antioxidants in the Brain. *Int. J. Mol. Sci.* **2020**, *21*, 7152. [CrossRef] [PubMed]
50. Lawler, T.; Liu, Y.; Christensen, K.; Vajaranant, T.S.; Mares, J. Dietary Antioxidants, Macular Pigment, and Glaucomatous Neurodegeneration: A Review of the Evidence. *Nutrients* **2019**, *11*, 1002. [CrossRef]
51. Sandeep; Sahu, M.R.; Rani, L.; Kharat, A.S.; Mondal, A.C. Could Vitamins Have a Positive Impact on the Treatment of Parkinson's Disease? *Brain Sci.* **2023**, *13*, 272. [CrossRef]
52. Rusciano, D.; Pezzino, S.; Mutolo, M.G.; Giannotti, R.; Librando, A.; Pescosolido, N. Neuroprotection in Glaucoma: Old and New Promising Treatments. *Adv. Pharmacol. Sci.* **2017**, *2017*, 4320408. [CrossRef]
53. Wang, S.Y.; Singh, K.; Lin, S.C. Glaucoma and vitamins A, C, and E supplement intake and serum levels in a population-based sample of the United States. *Eye* **2013**, *27*, 487–494. [CrossRef] [PubMed]
54. Ramdas, W.D.; Schouten, J.; Webers, C.A.B. The Effect of Vitamins on Glaucoma: A Systematic Review and Meta-Analysis. *Nutrients* **2018**, *10*, 359. [CrossRef] [PubMed]
55. Li, S.; Li, D.; Shao, M.; Cao, W.; Sun, X. Lack of Association between Serum Vitamin B_6, Vitamin B_{12}, and Vitamin D Levels with Different Types of Glaucoma: A Systematic Review and Meta-Analysis. *Nutrients* **2017**, *9*, 636. [CrossRef]
56. Kang, J.H.; Pasquale, L.R.; Willett, W.; Rosner, B.; Egan, K.M.; Faberowski, N.; Hankinson, S.E. Antioxidant Intake and Primary Open-Angle Glaucoma: A Prospective Study. *Am. J. Epidemiology* **2003**, *158*, 337–346. [CrossRef] [PubMed]
57. Coleman, A.L.; Stone, K.L.; Kodjebacheva, G.; Yu, F.; Pedula, K.L.; Ensrud, K.E.; Cauley, J.A.; Hochberg, M.C.; Topouzis, F.; Badala, F.; et al. Glaucoma Risk and the Consumption of Fruits and Vegetables Among Older Women in the Study of Osteoporotic Fractures. *Am. J. Ophthalmol.* **2008**, *145*, 1081–1089. [CrossRef] [PubMed]
58. Ramdas, W.D.; Wolfs, R.C.; Kiefte-de Jong, J.C.; Hofman, A.; de Jong, P.T.; Vingerling, J.R.; Jansonius, N.M. Nutrient intake and risk of open-angle glaucoma: The Rotterdam Study. *Eur. J. Epidemiol.* **2012**, *27*, 385–393. [CrossRef] [PubMed]
59. Garcia-Medina, J.J.; Garcia-Medina, M.; Garrido-Fernandez, P.; Galvan-Espinosa, J.; Garcia-Maturana, C.; Zanon-Moreno, V.; Pinazo-Duran, M.D. A two-year follow-up of oral antioxidant supplementation in primary open-angle glaucoma: An open-label, randomized, controlled trial. *Acta Ophthalmol.* **2015**, *93*, 546–554. [CrossRef]
60. Liu, D.; Ke, Z.; Luo, J. Thiamine Deficiency and Neurodegeneration: The Interplay Among Oxidative Stress, Endoplasmic Reticulum Stress, and Autophagy. *Mol. Neurobiol.* **2017**, *54*, 5440–5448. [CrossRef]
61. Gratton, S.; Lam, B. Visual loss and optic nerve head swelling in thiamine deficiency without prolonged dietary deficiency. *Clin. Ophthalmol.* **2014**, *8*, 1021–1024. [CrossRef] [PubMed]
62. Roda, M.; di Geronimo, N.; Pellegrini, M.; Schiavi, C. Nutritional Optic Neuropathies: State of the Art and Emerging Evidences. *Nutrients* **2020**, *12*, 2653. [CrossRef] [PubMed]
63. Giaconi, J.A.; Yu, F.; Stone, K.L.; Pedula, K.L.; Ensrud, K.E.; Cauley, J.A.; Hochberg, M.C.; Coleman, A.L. The Association of Consumption of Fruits/Vegetables with Decreased Risk of Glaucoma Among Older African-American Women in the Study of Osteoporotic Fractures. *Arch. Ophthalmol.* **2012**, *154*, 635–644. [CrossRef]
64. Pinto, J.T.; Zempleni, J. Riboflavin. *Adv. Nutr. Int. Rev. J.* **2016**, *7*, 973–975. [CrossRef] [PubMed]
65. Rennie, G.; Chen, A.C.; Dhillon, H.; Vardy, J.; Damian, D.L. Nicotinamide and neurocognitive function. *Nutr. Neurosci.* **2015**, *18*, 193–200. [CrossRef] [PubMed]
66. Belenky, P.; Bogan, K.L.; Brenner, C. NAD+ metabolism in health and disease. *Trends Biochem. Sci.* **2007**, *32*, 12–19. [CrossRef] [PubMed]
67. Bogan, K.L.; Brenner, C. Nicotinic Acid, Nicotinamide, and Nicotinamide Riboside: A Molecular Evaluation of NAD^+ Precursor Vitamins in Human Nutrition. *Annu. Rev. Nutr.* **2008**, *28*, 115–130. [CrossRef] [PubMed]
68. Knip, M.; Douek, I.F.; Moore, W.P.T.; Gillmor, H.A.; McLean, A.E.M.; Bingley, P.J.; Gale, E.A.M.; for the ENDIT Group. Safety of high-dose nicotinamide: A review. *Diabetologia* **2000**, *43*, 1337–1345. [CrossRef]
69. Rolfe, H.M. A review of nicotinamide: Treatment of skin diseases and potential side effects. *J. Cosmet. Dermatol.* **2014**, *13*, 324–328. [CrossRef] [PubMed]
70. Gasperi, V.; Sibilano, M.; Savini, I.; Catani, M.V. Niacin in the Central Nervous System: An Update of Biological Aspects and Clinical Applications. *Int. J. Mol. Sci.* **2019**, *20*, 974. [CrossRef]
71. Fricker, R.A.; Green, E.L.; Jenkins, S.I.; Griffin, S.M. The Influence of Nicotinamide on Health and Disease in the Central Nervous System. *Int. J. Tryptophan Res.* **2018**, *11*, 1178646918776658. [CrossRef]
72. Gomes, A.P.; Price, N.L.; Ling, A.J.Y.; Moslehi, J.J.; Montgomery, M.K.; Rajman, L.; White, J.P.; Teodoro, J.S.; Wrann, C.D.; Hubbard, B.P.; et al. Declining NAD+ Induces a Pseudohypoxic State Disrupting Nuclear-Mitochondrial Communication during Aging. *Cell* **2013**, *155*, 1624–1638. [CrossRef] [PubMed]

73. Maiese, K.; Chong, Z.Z. Nicotinamide: Necessary nutrient emerges as a novel cytoprotectant for the brain. *Trends Pharmacol. Sci.* **2003**, *24*, 228–232. [CrossRef] [PubMed]
74. Chen, J.; Chopp, M. Niacin, an old drug, has new effects on central nervous system disease. *Open Drug Discov. J.* **2010**, *2*, 181–186.
75. Williams, A.; Ramsden, D. Nicotinamide: A double edged sword. *Park. Relat. Disord.* **2005**, *11*, 413–420. [CrossRef] [PubMed]
76. Beal, M.F.; Henshaw, D.R.; Jenkins, B.G.; Rosen, B.R.; Schulz, J.B. Coenzyme Q_{10} and nicotinamide block striatal lesions produced by the mitochondrial toxin malonate. *Ann. Neurol.* **1994**, *36*, 882–888. [CrossRef] [PubMed]
77. Williams, P.A.; Harder, J.M.; Foxworth, N.E.; Cochran, K.E.; Philip, V.M.; Porciatti, V.; Smithies, O.; John, S.W.M. Vitamin B_3 modulates mitochondrial vulnerability and prevents glaucoma in aged mice. *Science* **2017**, *355*, 756–760. [CrossRef]
78. Williams, P.A.; Harder, J.M.; Cardozo, B.H.; Foxworth, N.E.; John, S.W.M. Nicotinamide treatment robustly protects from inherited mouse glaucoma. *Commun. Integr. Biol.* **2018**, *11*, e1356956. [CrossRef]
79. Nzoughet, J.K.; de la Barca, J.M.C.; Guehlouz, K.; Leruez, S.; Coulbault, L.; Allouche, S.; Bocca, C.; Muller, J.; Amati-Bonneau, P.; Gohier, P.; et al. Nicotinamide Deficiency in Primary Open-Angle Glaucoma. *Investig. Ophthalmol. Vis. Sci.* **2019**, *60*, 2509–2514. [CrossRef]
80. Hui, F.; Tang, J.; Williams, P.A.; McGuinness, M.B.; Hadoux, X.; Casson, R.J.; Coote, M.; Trounce, I.A.; Martin, K.R.; van Wijngaarden, P.; et al. Improvement in inner retinal function in glaucoma with nicotinamide (vitamin B3) supplementation: A crossover randomized clinical trial. *Clin. Exp. Ophthalmol.* **2020**, *48*, 903–914. [CrossRef] [PubMed]
81. Stach, K.; Stach, W.; Augoff, K. Vitamin B6 in Health and Disease. *Nutrients* **2021**, *13*, 3229. [CrossRef]
82. Ho, P.; Ho, P.I.; Ashline, D.; Dhitavat, S.; Ortiz, D.; Collins, S.C.; Shea, T.B.; Rogers, E. Folate deprivation induces neurodegeneration: Roles of oxidative stress and increased homocysteine. *Neurobiol. Dis.* **2003**, *14*, 32–42. [CrossRef] [PubMed]
83. De Silva, P.; Jayamanne, G.; Bolton, R. Folic acid deficiency optic neuropathy: A case report. *J. Med. Case Rep.* **2008**, *2*, 299. [CrossRef]
84. Langan, R.C.; Goodbred, A.J. Vitamin B12 Deficiency: Recognition and Management. *Am. Fam. Physician* **2017**, *96*, 384–389. [PubMed]
85. Coban, D.T.; Ariturk, N.; Elmacioglu, F.; Ulus, C.A. The relationship between glaucoma and serum vitamin B12, folic acid levels and nutrition. *Acta Medica Mediterr.* **2015**, *31*, 281–286.
86. Belmonte, A.; Tormo, C.; Lopez, N.; Villalba, C.; Fernandez, C.; Hernandez, F.B. Vitamins A, E, B12 and folate levels in different types of glaucoma. *Clin. Chem. Lab. Med.* **2011**, *49*, 816.
87. Cumurcu, T.; Sahin, S.; Aydin, E. Serum homocysteine, vitamin B 12 and folic acid levels in different types of glaucoma. *BMC Ophthalmol.* **2006**, *6*, 6. [CrossRef] [PubMed]
88. Roedl, J.B.; Bleich, S.; Reulbach, U.; Rejdak, R.; Naumann, G.O.H.; Kruse, F.E.; Schlötzer-Schrehardt, U.; Kornhuber, J.; Jünemann, A.G.M. Vitamin deficiency and hyperhomocysteinemia in pseudoexfoliation glaucoma. *J. Neural Transm.* **2007**, *114*, 571–575. [CrossRef]
89. Monacelli, F.; Acquarone, F.M.E.; Giannotti, C.; Borghi, R.; Nencioni, A. Vitamin C, Aging and Alzheimer's Disease. *Nutrients* **2017**, *9*, 670. [CrossRef]
90. Yuki, K.; Murat, D.; Kimura, I.; Ohtake, Y.; Tsubota, K. Reduced-serum vitamin C and increased uric acid levels in normal-tension glaucoma. *Graefe's Arch. Clin. Exp. Ophthalmol.* **2010**, *248*, 243–248. [CrossRef] [PubMed]
91. Asregadoo, E.R. Blood levels of thiamine and ascorbic acid in chronic open-angle glaucoma. *Ann. Ophthalmol.* **1979**, *11*, 1095–1100. [PubMed]
92. Park, H.-A.; Hayden, M.M.; Bannerman, S.; Jansen, J.; Crowe-White, K.M. Anti-Apoptotic Effects of Carotenoids in Neurodegeneration. *Molecules* **2020**, *25*, 3453. [CrossRef] [PubMed]
93. Hira, S.; Saleem, U.; Anwar, F.; Sohail, M.F.; Raza, Z.; Ahmad, B. β-Carotene: A Natural Compound Improves Cognitive Impairment and Oxidative Stress in a Mouse Model of Streptozotocin-Induced Alzheimer's Disease. *Biomolecules* **2019**, *9*, 441. [CrossRef] [PubMed]
94. Chen, P.; Li, L.; Gao, Y.; Xie, Z.; Zhang, Y.; Pan, Z.; Tu, Y.; Wang, H.; Han, Q.; Hu, X.; et al. β-carotene provides neuro protection after experimental traumatic brain injury via the Nrf2–ARE pathway. *J. Integr. Neurosci.* **2019**, *18*, 153–161. [CrossRef] [PubMed]
95. Engin, K.N.; Yemişci, B.; Yiğit, U.; Ağaçhan, A.; Coşkun, C. Variability of serum oxidative stress biomarkers relative to biochemical data and clinical parameters of glaucoma patients. *Mol. Vis.* **2010**, *16*, 1260–1271. [PubMed]
96. López-Riquelme, N.; Villalba, C.; Tormo, C.; Belmonte, A.; Fernandez, C.; Torralba, G.; Hernández, F. Endothelin-1 levels and biomarkers of oxidative stress in glaucoma patients. *Int. Ophthalmol.* **2015**, *35*, 527–532. [CrossRef]
97. Mustacich, D.J.; Bruno, R.S.; Traber, M.G. Vitamin E. *Vitam. Horm.* **2007**, *76*, 1–21. [CrossRef] [PubMed]
98. McLaughlin, P.J.; Weihrauch, J.L. Vitamin E content of foods. *J. Am. Diet. Assoc.* **1979**, *75*, 647–665. [CrossRef] [PubMed]
99. Traber, M.G. Vitamin E Regulatory Mechanisms. *Annu. Rev. Nutr.* **2007**, *27*, 347–362. [CrossRef]
100. Ko, M.-L.; Peng, P.-H.; Hsu, S.-Y.; Chen, C.-F. Dietary Deficiency of Vitamin E Aggravates Retinal Ganglion Cell Death in Experimental Glaucoma of Rats. *Curr. Eye Res.* **2010**, *35*, 842–849. [CrossRef]
101. Cellini, M.; Caramazza, N.; Mangiafico, P.; Possati, G.L.; Caramazza, R. Fatty acid use in glaucomatous optic neuropathy treatment. *Acta Ophthalmol. Scand.* **1998**, *76*, 41–42. [CrossRef]
102. Engin, K.; Engin, G.; Kucuksahin, H.; Oncu, M.; Guvener, B. Clinical Evaluation of the Neuroprotective Effect of α-Tocopherol against Glaucomatous Damage. *Eur. J. Ophthalmol.* **2007**, *17*, 528–533. [CrossRef] [PubMed]
103. Seamon, K.B.; Daly, J.W. Forskolin: A unique diterpene activator of cyclic AMP-generating systems. *J. Cycl. Nucleotide* **1981**, *7*, 201–224.

104. Caprioli, J.; Sears, M. Forskolin lowers intraocular pressure in rabbits, monkeys, and man. *Lancet* **1983**, *321*, 958–960. [CrossRef] [PubMed]
105. Caprioli, J.; Sears, M.; Bausher, L.; Gregory, D.; Mead, A. Forskolin lowers intraocular pressure by reducing aqueous in-flow. *Investig. Ophthalmol. Vis. Sci.* **1984**, *25*, 268–277.
106. Meyer-Franke, A.; Kaplan, M.R.; Pfieger, F.W.; Barres, B.A. Characterization of the signaling interactions that promote the survival and growth of developing retinal ganglion cells in culture. *Neuron* **1995**, *15*, 805–819. [CrossRef]
107. Majeed, M.; Nagabhushanam, K.; Natarajan, S.; Vaidyanathan, P.; Karri, S.K. A Double-blind, Randomized Clinical Trial to Evaluate the Efficacy and Safety of Forskolin Eye Drops 1% in the Treatment of Open Angle Glaucoma ? A Comparative Study. *J. Clin. Trials* **2014**, *4*, 1000184. [CrossRef]
108. Sisto, D.; Lavermicocca, N.; Errico, D.; Rusciano, D. Oral administration of forskolin and rutin contributes to reduce in-traocular pressure and improve PERG (Pattern Electroretinogram) amplitude in glaucomatous patients. *JSM Biotechnol. Bioeng.* **2014**, *2*, 1036.
109. Watanabe, M.; Tokita, Y.; Kato, M.; Fukuda, Y. Intravitreal injections of neurotrophic factors and forskolin enhance survival and axonal regeneration of axotomized beta ganglion cells in cat retina. *Neuroscience* **2003**, *116*, 733–742. [CrossRef]
110. Locri, F.; Cammalleri, M.; Monte, M.D.; Rusciano, D.; Bagnoli, P. Protective Efficacy of a Dietary Supplement Based on Forskolin, Homotaurine, Spearmint Extract, and Group B Vitamins in a Mouse Model of Optic Nerve Injury. *Nutrients* **2019**, *11*, 2931. [CrossRef]
111. Cammalleri, M.; Monte, M.D.; Amato, R.; Bagnoli, P.; Rusciano, D. A Dietary Combination of Forskolin with Homotaurine, Spearmint and B Vitamins Protects Injured Retinal Ganglion Cells in a Rodent Model of Hypertensive Glaucoma. *Nutrients* **2020**, *12*, 1189. [CrossRef]
112. Sun, Q.; Wang, N.; Xu, W.; Zhou, H. Genus Ribes Linn. (Grossulariaceae): A comprehensive review of traditional uses, phytochemistry, pharmacology and clinical applications. *J. Ethnopharmacol.* **2021**, *276*, 114166. [CrossRef] [PubMed]
113. Ohguro, H.; Ohguro, I.; Katai, M.; Tanaka, S. Two-Year Randomized, Placebo-Controlled Study of Black Currant Anthocyanins on Visual Field in Glaucoma. *Ophthalmologica* **2012**, *228*, 26–35. [CrossRef]
114. Ohguro, H.; Ohguro, I.; Yagi, S. Effects of Black Currant Anthocyanins on Intraocular Pressure in Healthy Volunteers and Patients with Glaucoma. *J. Ocul. Pharmacol. Ther.* **2013**, *29*, 61–67. [CrossRef]
115. Cheng, Z.; Kang, C.; Che, S.; Su, J.; Sun, Q.; Ge, T.; Guo, Y.; Lv, J.; Sun, Z.; Yang, W.; et al. Berberine: A Promising Treatment for Neurodegenerative Diseases. *Front. Pharmacol.* **2022**, *13*, 845591. [CrossRef] [PubMed]
116. Li, Z.; Geng, Y.-N.; Jiang, J.-D.; Kong, W.-J. Antioxidant and Anti-Inflammatory Activities of Berberine in the Treatment of Diabetes Mellitus. *Evid. Based Complement. Altern. Med.* **2014**, *2014*, 289264. [CrossRef]
117. Song, D.; Hao, J.; Fan, D. Biological properties and clinical applications of berberine. *Front. Med.* **2020**, *14*, 564–582. [CrossRef] [PubMed]
118. Tian, E.; Sharma, G.; Dai, C. Neuroprotective Properties of Berberine: Molecular Mechanisms and Clinical Implications. *Antioxidants* **2023**, *12*, 1883. [CrossRef] [PubMed]
119. Imenshahidi, M.; Hosseinzadeh, H. Berberine and barberry (*Berberis vulgaris*): A clinical review. *Phytotherapy Res.* **2019**, *33*, 504–523. [CrossRef] [PubMed]
120. Khoshandam, A.; Imenshahidi, M.; Hosseinzadeh, H. Pharmacokinetic of berberine, the main constituent of *Berberis vulgaris* L.: A comprehensive review. *Phytotherapy Res.* **2022**, *36*, 4063–4079. [CrossRef] [PubMed]
121. Ahmed, T.; Gilani, A.-U.; Abdollahi, M.; Daglia, M.; Nabavi, S.M. Berberine and neurodegeneration: A review of literature. *Pharmacol. Rep.* **2015**, *67*, 970–979. [CrossRef]
122. Pires, E.N.S.; Frozza, R.L.; Hoppe, J.B.; Menezes, B.d.M.; Salbego, C.G. Berberine was neuroprotective against an in vitro model of brain ischemia: Survival and apoptosis pathways involved. *Brain Res.* **2014**, *1557*, 26–33. [CrossRef]
123. Fan, J.; Zhang, K.; Jin, Y.; Li, B.; Gao, S.; Zhu, J.; Cui, R. Pharmacological effects of berberine on mood disorders. *J. Cell. Mol. Med.* **2019**, *23*, 21–28. [CrossRef]
124. Kulkarni, S.K.; Dhir, A. Berberine: A plant alkaloid with therapeutic potential for central nervous system disorders. *Phytother. Res.* **2010**, *24*, 317–324. [CrossRef] [PubMed]
125. Fan, J.; Li, B.; Ge, T.; Zhang, Z.; Lv, J.; Zhao, J.; Wang, P.; Liu, W.; Wang, X.; Mlyniec, K.; et al. Berberine produces antidepressant-like effects in ovariectomized mice. *Sci. Rep.* **2017**, *7*, 1310. [CrossRef] [PubMed]
126. Yuan, N.-N.; Cai, C.-Z.; Wu, M.-Y.; Su, H.-X.; Li, M.; Lu, J.-H. Neuroprotective effects of berberine in animal models of Alzheimer's disease: A systematic review of pre-clinical studies. *BMC Complement. Altern. Med.* **2019**, *19*, 109. [CrossRef]
127. Lin, X.; Zhang, N. Berberine: Pathways to protect neurons. *Phytother. Res.* **2018**, *32*, 1501–1510. [CrossRef]
128. Wang, Y.; Tong, Q.; Ma, S.-R.; Zhao, Z.-X.; Pan, L.-B.; Cong, L.; Han, P.; Peng, R.; Yu, H.; Lin, Y.; et al. Oral berberine improves brain dopa/dopamine levels to ameliorate Parkinson's disease by regulating gut microbiota. *Signal Transduct. Target. Ther.* **2021**, *6*, 77. [CrossRef] [PubMed]
129. Diamond, B.J.; Bailey, M.R. Ginkgo biloba: Indications, mechanisms, and safety. *Psychiatr. Clin. N. Am.* **2013**, *36*, 73–83. [CrossRef] [PubMed]
130. Kang, J.M.; Lin, S. Ginkgo biloba and its potential role in glaucoma. *Curr. Opin. Ophthalmol.* **2018**, *29*, 116–120. [CrossRef]
131. Thiagarajan, G.; Chandani, S.; Harinarayana Rao, S.; Samuni, A.M.; Chandrasekaran, K.; Balasubramanian, D. Molecular and cellular assessment of ginkgo biloba extract as a possible ophthalmic drug. *Exp. Eye Res.* **2002**, *75*, 421–430. [CrossRef]

132. Ma, K.; Xu, L.; Zhang, H.; Zhang, S.; Pu, M.; Jonas, J.B. The effect of ginkgo biloba on the rat retinal ganglion cell survival in the optic nerve crush model. *Acta Ophthalmol.* **2010**, *88*, 553–557. [CrossRef]
133. Ma, K.; Xu, L.; Zhan, H.; Zhang, S.; Pu, M.; Jonas, J.B. Dosage dependence of the effect of Ginkgo biloba on the rat retinal ganglion cell survival after optic nerve crush. *Eye* **2009**, *23*, 1598–1604. [CrossRef]
134. Hirooka, K.; Tokuda, M.; Miyamoto, O.; Itano, T.; Baba, T.; Shiraga, F. The Ginkgo biloba extract (EGb 761) provides a neuroprotective effect on retinal ganglion cells in a rat model of chronic glaucoma. *Curr. Eye Res.* **2004**, *28*, 153–157. [CrossRef] [PubMed]
135. Park, J.W.; Kwon, H.J.; Chung, W.S.; Kim, C.Y.; Seong, G.J. Short-Term Effects of *Ginkgo biloba* Extract on Peripapillary Retinal Blood Flow in Normal Tension Glaucoma. *Korean J. Ophthalmol.* **2011**, *25*, 323–328. [CrossRef]
136. Harris, A.; Gross, J.; Moore, N.; Do, T.; Huang, A.; Gama, W.; Siesky, B. The effects of antioxidants on ocular blood flow in patients with glaucoma. *Acta Ophthalmol.* **2018**, *96*, e237–e241. [CrossRef]
137. Quaranta, L.; Bettelli, S.; Uva, M.G.; Semeraro, F.; Turano, R.; Gandolfo, E. Effect of Ginkgo biloba extract on preexisting visual field damage in normal tension glaucoma. *Ophthalmology* **2003**, *110*, 359–362, discussion 362–364. [CrossRef] [PubMed]
138. Guo, X.; Kong, X.; Huang, R.; Jin, L.; Ding, X.; He, M.; Liu, X.; Patel, M.C.; Congdon, N.G. Effect of Ginkgo Biloba on Visual Field and Contrast Sensitivity in Chinese Patients with Normal Tension Glaucoma: A Randomized, Crossover Clinical Trial. *Investig. Ophthalmol. Vis. Sci.* **2014**, *55*, 110–116. [CrossRef] [PubMed]
139. Upreti, S.; Nag, T.C.; Ghosh, M.P. Trolox aids coenzyme Q10 in neuroprotection against NMDA induced damage via upregulation of VEGF in rat model of glutamate excitotoxicity. *Exp. Eye Res.* **2024**, *238*, 109740. [CrossRef] [PubMed]
140. Namkoong, S.; Kim, C.-K.; Cho, Y.-L.; Kim, J.-H.; Lee, H.; Ha, K.-S.; Choe, J.; Kim, P.-H.; Won, M.-H.; Kwon, Y.-G.; et al. Forskolin increases angiogenesis through the coordinated cross-talk of PKA-dependent VEGF expression and Epac-mediated PI3K/Akt/eNOS signaling. *Cell Signal.* **2009**, *21*, 906–915. [CrossRef] [PubMed]
141. Liu, H.; Ren, X.; Ma, C. Effect of Berberine on Angiogenesis and HIF-1α/VEGF Signal Transduction Pathway in Rats with Cerebral Ischemia—Reperfusion Injury. *J. Coll. Physicians Surg. Pak.* **2018**, *28*, 753–757. [PubMed]
142. Chua, Y.; Ang, X.; Zhong, X.; Khoo, K. Interaction between warfarin and Chinese herbal medicines. *Singap. Med. J.* **2015**, *56*, 11–18. [CrossRef] [PubMed]
143. Zhuang, W.; Liu, S.; Zhao, X.; Sun, N.; He, T.; Wang, Y.; Jia, B.; Lin, X.; Chu, Y.; Xi, S. Interaction Between Chinese Medicine and Warfarin: Clinical and Research Update. *Front. Pharmacol.* **2021**, *12*, 751107. [CrossRef] [PubMed]
144. Spini, A.; Giometto, S.; Donnini, S.; Posarelli, M.; Dotta, F.; Ziche, M.; Tosi, G.M.; Girardi, A.; Lucenteforte, E.; Gini, R.; et al. Risk of Intraocular Pressure Increase with Intravitreal Injections of Vascular Endothelial Growth Factor Inhibitors: A Cohort Study. *Arch. Ophthalmol.* **2023**, *248*, 45–50. [CrossRef] [PubMed]
145. Daka, Q.; Špegel, N.; Velkovska, M.A.; Steblovnik, T.; Kolko, M.; Neziri, B.; Cvenkel, B. Exploring the Relationship between Anti-VEGF Therapy and Glaucoma: Implications for Management Strategies. *J. Clin. Med.* **2023**, *12*, 4674. [CrossRef] [PubMed]
146. Bressler, S.B.; Almukhtar, T.; Bhorade, A.; Bressler, N.M.; Glassman, A.R.; Huang, S.S.; Jampol, L.M.; Kim, J.E.; Melia, M. For the Diabetic Retinopathy Clinical Research Network Investigators Repeated Intravitreous Ranibizumab Injections for Diabetic Macular Edema and the Risk of Sustained Elevation of Intraocular Pressure or the Need for Ocular Hypotensive Treatment. *JAMA Ophthalmol.* **2015**, *133*, 589–597. [CrossRef]
147. Guo, Z.-L.; Li, M.-X.; Li, X.-L.; Wang, P.; Wang, W.-G.; Du, W.-Z.; Yang, Z.-Q.; Chen, S.-F.; Wu, D.; Tian, X.-Y. Crocetin: A Systematic Review. *Front. Pharmacol.* **2022**, *12*, 745683. [CrossRef] [PubMed]
148. Himori, N.; Yanagimachi, M.I.; Omodaka, K.; Shiga, Y.; Tsuda, S.; Kunikata, H.; Nakazawa, T. The Effect of Dietary Antioxidant Supplementation in Patients with Glaucoma. *Clin. Ophthalmol.* **2021**, *15*, 2293–2300. [CrossRef] [PubMed]
149. Maekawa, S.; Sato, K.; Fujita, K.; Daigaku, R.; Tawarayama, H.; Murayama, N.; Moritoh, S.; Yabana, T.; Shiga, Y.; Omodaka, K.; et al. The neuroprotective effect of hesperidin in NMDA-induced retinal injury acts by suppressing oxidative stress and excessive calpain activation. *Sci. Rep.* **2017**, *7*, 6885. [CrossRef]
150. Lakshmanan, Y.; Wong, F.S.Y.; Zuo, B.; So, K.-F.; Bui, B.V.; Chan, H.H.-L. Posttreatment Intervention with *Lycium Barbarum* Polysaccharides is Neuroprotective in a Rat Model of Chronic Ocular Hypertension. *Investig. Ophthalmol. Vis. Sci.* **2019**, *60*, 4606–4618. [CrossRef] [PubMed]
151. Sookying, S.; Duangjai, A.; Saokaew, S.; Phisalprapa, P. Botanical aspects, phytochemicals, and toxicity of Tamarindus indica leaf and a systematic review of antioxidant capacities of T. indica leaf extracts. *Front. Nutr.* **2022**, *9*, 977015. [CrossRef]
152. Mustapha, A.; Yakasai, I.A.; Aguye, I.A. Effect of Tamarindus indica L. on the bioavailability of aspirin in healthy human vol-unteers. *Eur. J. Drug Metab. Pharmacokinet.* **1996**, *21*, 223–226. [CrossRef]
153. Luo, H.; Zhuang, J.; Hu, P.; Ye, W.; Chen, S.; Pang, Y.; Li, N.; Deng, C.; Zhang, X. Resveratrol Delays Retinal Ganglion Cell Loss and Attenuates Gliosis-Related Inflammation From Ischemia-Reperfusion Injury. *Investig. Opthalmol. Vis. Sci.* **2018**, *59*, 3879–3888. [CrossRef]
154. Shaito, A.; Posadino, A.M.; Younes, N.; Hasan, H.; Halabi, S.; Alhababi, D.; Al-Mohannadi, A.; Abdel-Rahman, W.M.; Eid, A.H.; Nasrallah, G.K.; et al. Potential Adverse Effects of Resveratrol: A Literature Review. *Int. J. Mol. Sci.* **2020**, *21*, 2084. [CrossRef] [PubMed]
155. Jung, S.; Kang, K.; Ji, D.; Fawcett, R.; Safa, R.; Kamalden, T.; Osborne, N. The flavonoid baicalin counteracts ischemic and oxidative insults to retinal cells and lipid peroxidation to brain membranes. *Neurochem. Int.* **2008**, *53*, 325–337. [CrossRef] [PubMed]

156. Vitiello, L.; Capasso, L.; Cembalo, G.; De Pascale, I.; Imparato, R.; De Bernardo, M. Herbal and Natural Treatments for the Management of the Glaucoma: An Update. *BioMed. Res. Int.* **2023**, *2023*, 3105251. [CrossRef]
157. Gazzard, G.; Konstantakopoulou, E.; Garway-Heath, D.; Adeleke, M.; Vickerstaff, V.; Ambler, G.; Hunter, R.; Bunce, C.; Nathwani, N.; Barton, K.; et al. Laser in Glaucoma and Ocular Hypertension (LiGHT) Trial: Six-Year Results of Primary Selective Laser Trabeculoplasty versus Eye Drops for the Treatment of Glaucoma and Ocular Hypertension. *Ophthalmology* **2023**, *130*, 139–151. [CrossRef] [PubMed]

Journal of
Clinical Medicine

MDPI

Article

No Changes in Keratometry Readings and Anterior Chamber Depth after XEN Gel Implantation in Patients with Glaucoma

Filippo Tatti, Claudia Tronci, Filippo Lixi, Giuseppe Demarinis, Sviatlana Kuzmich, Enrico Peiretti, Maurizio Fossarello and Giuseppe Giannaccare *

Department of Surgical Sciences, Eye Clinic, University of Cagliari, 09124 Cagliari, Italy; filippo.tatti@unica.it (F.T.); c.tronci5@studenti.unica.it (C.T.); f.lixi1@studenti.unica.it (F.L.); demarinis91@gmail.com (G.D.); s.kuzmich@studenti.unica.it (S.K.); enripei@hotmail.com (E.P.); maurizio.fossarello@gmail.com (M.F.)

* Correspondence: giuseppe.giannaccare@unica.it

Abstract: Background: This study aimed to compare keratometry and anterior chamber depth (ACD) changes after XEN implantation in primary open-angle glaucoma (POAG) cases over a 3-month follow-up period. **Methods:** Twenty patients with POAG who underwent XEN63 implantation, either standalone or combined with cataract surgery, were included. Preoperative data, including best-corrected visual acuity (BCVA), refraction, gonioscopy, ophthalmoscopy, intraocular pressure (IOP) evaluation, and axial length, were collected. Corneal topography and ACD measurements were assessed preoperatively and at postoperative days 1, 7, 15, 30, 60, and 90. Each patient's eye that underwent XEN surgery was included in the study group, with the fellow eye serving as a control. **Results:** In the study group, there was a significant decrease in IOP after XEN stent implantation at all investigated time intervals ($p < 0.05$). However, changes in mean ACD did not show statistically significant differences at any follow-up examination in both the study and control groups. Additionally, keratometry readings revealed no significant changes in total astigmatism or steep keratometry values in either group. **Conclusions:** XEN implantation in POAG cases resulted in a significant decrease in IOP over the 3-month follow-up period. However, there were no significant changes observed in mean ACD or keratometry readings, indicating stability in these parameters post-XEN implantation. These findings suggest that XEN implantation may be an effective option for IOP reduction without affecting corneal curvature or ACD in POAG patients.

Keywords: XEN; glaucoma surgery; astigmatism; keratometry; anterior chamber depth

1. Introduction

Glaucoma is a diverse collection of chronic, progressive optic neuropathies. The estimated prevalence of this condition is 2.9% in Europe and 3.5% worldwide among those aged 40 years and older [1]. Currently, the evidence-based and widely accepted therapeutic approach for glaucoma patients is a decrease in intraocular pressure (IOP) [2].

If the medical treatment fails to halt the progression of glaucomatous damage or adversely impacts quality of life, an assessment of alternative approaches, such as selective laser trabeculoplasty (SLT) or surgical intervention, becomes imperative [2]. Numerous factors must be taken into account when determining the most effective management. These include compliance, the stage of glaucoma, and the likelihood of success with medical or laser treatment [2].

Despite being the gold standard surgical operation, trabeculectomy (TE) is characterized by an invasive nature, comparatively high-risk profile, and the potential for complications. Among them, the encapsulation of the filtering bleb is the most prevalent, occurring in 4% to 30% of cases; it causes an altered outflow and a gradual increase in IOP [3,4]. Additional common and worrisome complications include hypotonia and flat anterior chamber (FAC) [5]. Edmunds et al. determined that the incidence of hypotony and FAC was 23.9%

and 24.3%, respectively [6]. If not appropriately managed, the aforementioned conditions may give rise to further complications, such as cataract development, synechiae, persistent choroidal detachment or hypotony maculopathy, and ultimately, prolonged or permanent visual impairment [7]. Furthermore, a partial, temporary reduction in visual acuity is often observed subsequent to trabeculectomy surgery, although the precise underlying factors contributing to this reduction have not been completely clarified. It is not only attributed to changes in blood pressure, FAC, hypotony, choroidal detachment, wipe-out syndrome, and complications related to local anaesthesia [8].

Some studies have suggested a possible correlation between changes in visual acuity following TE and refractive changes [9]. A significant incidence of astigmatism following TE surgery has been observed, exhibiting a mid-to-long persistence (10–12 months) [10,11]. A persistence of astigmatism was noted by some authors among patients who received subconjunctival MMC to reduce complications related to fibrosis [12].

Nevertheless, refractive changes could also be correlated with anterior chamber depth (ACD) modifications [13]. Indeed, during the early post-trabeculectomy period, variations in ACD may occur, and these changes could be related to fluctuations in IOP and modifications of bleb functionality [14].

The impact of minimally invasive glaucoma surgeries (MIGS) on refractive changes and ACD variations still represents an open issue that deserves further exploration. Various techniques are categorized under the acronym MIGS according to the space in which the aqueous humour is drained [15,16]. There is increasing clinical interest in the field of MIGS, specifically in newer approaches named 'minimally invasive bleb surgery' (MIBS). The latter combines the filtering properties of traditional glaucoma surgery with those of MIGS. Among these, the XEN Gel Implant (AbbVie Company, Irvine, CA, USA) is a porcine gelatine 6 mm-long tube designed to create a channel from the anterior chamber to the subconjunctival space. The stent comes preloaded in an injector and is usually inserted in the iridocorneal angle via an ab interno technique with a small corneal incision, following a subconjunctival injection of 0.1 mL mitomycin C (MMC) 0.02% [17,18].

Currently, the literature lacks sufficient information regarding the refractive effects of the XEN Gel Implant [8]. The purpose of this study is to investigate keratometry and ACD changes following XEN Gel implantation in a group of patients with glaucoma. Additionally, it seeks to establish a correlation between the ACD variations and the IOP value.

2. Materials and Methods

This study included 40 eyes of 20 glaucoma patients. For each patient, one eye underwent XEN63 implantation and the fellow eye acted as a control. The subjects were recruited from a prospective cohort conducted at a single centre (University Hospital of Cagliari, Cagliari, Italy). The patients underwent surgery between October 2022 and July 2023. The study received approval by the Institutional Review Board (IRB) of the University of Cagliari (PG/2022/341; 26 January 2022). All subjects provided written informed consent and the study was performed in accordance with the Declaration of Helsinki.

Preoperative data were collected for each patient, including best-corrected visual acuity (BCVA), refraction, examination of the anterior segment with a slit lamp, gonioscopy, ophthalmoscopy, IOP evaluation, and axial length. In addition, corneal topography and anterior chamber depth measurements were assessed using the Pentacam Comprehensive Eye Scanner (Oculus Optikgeraete GmbH, Wetzlar, Germany) and the OA-Optical Biometer TOMEY GmbH. These examinations were repeated at 1, 7, 15, 30, 60, and 90 days postoperatively. Additionally, both intraoperative and postoperative complications were gathered, as well. Numerical hypotony was regarded when the IOP was less than 6 mmHg. On the other hand, persistent hypotony was defined as an IOP less than 6 mmHg that was present at two consecutive postoperative visits that were more than 15 days apart.

2.1. Surgical Procedures

In all cases, XEN Gel implantation was performed under topical anesthesia by the same surgeon (F.T.). The operating field was prepared with adequate skin disinfection and sterile field dressing. In brief, an ab interno gel stent implantation (XEN63) was performed in the upper nasal quadrant following a subconjunctival injection of mitomycin C (0.1 mL, 0.02%). The AC was filled with a cohesive viscoelastic gel, the injector needle was inserted through a 1.8 mm infero-temporal corneal paracentesis incision, and directed towards the superonasal quadrant. The needle was then inserted into the sclera guided by the goniolens, slightly anterior to the nonpigmented trabecular meshwork, and the device was released after the needle appeared in the sub-conjunctival space posteriorly, approximately 2–3 mm from the limbus. Subsequently, the subconjunctival mobility of the implant was checked. Following hydration of the incisions, 0.1 ml of 1% cefuroxime was injected in the anterior chamber along with 4 mg/1 mL of dexamethasone phosphate subtenon (Decadron, Farmaceutici Caber SpA, Pomezia, Italy). Post-surgery care included a 2-week course of topical antibiotic for infection prophylaxis and a six-month regimen of gradually tapering topical corticosteroids.

2.2. Statistical Analysis

As previously reported by Senthil et al., to detect a 0.5-diopter (D) difference in astigmatism after surgery with a power of 80% and a type I error of 0.5, the required sample size was 20 eyes in each cohort [19]. For each patient, one eye underwent XEN surgery and the fellow eye acted as a control. Therefore, 40 eyes of 20 subjects with primary open-angle glaucoma (POAG) were enrolled in the study. Descriptive and exploratory data analyses were conducted. Statistical analysis was performed using IBM SPSS Statistics, version 25 for Windows. Means ± standard deviations (SDs) for continuous variables were estimated or percent distributions were presented. We examined the normality and the homogeneity of the continuous variables under investigation employing the Shapiro-Wilk test. Fisher's test was used to compare categorical variables. Parametric (*t*-test) and non-parametric (Mann–Whitney test) tests were used to compare normally and non-normally distributed variables, respectively. Statistical analyses among groups were performed by Friedman's test and a pairwise signed rank test. In addition, BCVA, astigmatism, and IOP changes were tested for possible correlation using Pearson's test. Visual acuity was converted to logMAR for statistical analysis. A p value of <0.05 was considered statistically significant.

3. Results

3.1. Baseline Characteristics of the Study Population

In this study, 40 eyes of 20 Caucasian patients (12 males and 8 females) with primary open angle glaucoma (POAG) were included. The mean age was 64.3 years (range 44–83 years). The eye that underwent XEN implantation (study group, n = 20) and the fellow eye (control group, n = 20) were analyzed in each patient. In the study group, thirteen eyes (65%) were phakic and seven (35%) were pseudophakic. Eight eyes (40%) had a previous surgery. The control group included twelve phakic (60%) and eight pseudophakic eyes (40%). Eight eyes had a previous surgery (40%). In the study group, sixteen eyes underwent XEN implantation alone (80%) and four eyes underwent combined surgery with phacoemulsification (20%). Demographic data from the patients are summarized in Table 1.

Table 1. Demographic data. The statistical analysis indicated no significant differences between the study and control groups ($p > 0.05$).

	Study Group (n = 20) n (%)	Control Group (n = 20) n (%)	p-Value
Gender			
Male	12 (60%)		
Female	8 (40%)		
Mean Age (SD)	64.3 (11.25)		
Eye			0.75
Right	11 (55%)	9 (45%)	
Left	9 (45%)	11 (55%)	
Previous Ocular Surgery			0.75
Phaco + IOL	7 (35%)	8 (40%)	
PPV	1 (5%)	0 (0%)	
Lens Status			1
Phakic	13 (65%)	12 (60%)	
Pseudophakic	7 (35%)	8 (40%)	
Surgical Procedure			
XEN standalone	16 (80%)		
XEN + Phaco	4 (20%)		

3.2. Intraocular Pressure and Medications

Concerning eyes in the study group, after a follow-up period of 3 months, IOP exhibited a significant decrease from 28.75 ± 7.52 mmHg preoperatively to 14.30 ± 5.42 mmHg ($p < 0.001$), corresponding to a 50.26% reduction. The mean preoperative IOP dropped significantly after stent implantation at all investigated time intervals ($p < 0.05$).

In the control group, the mean preoperative IOP was 17.05 ± 3.68 mmHg, and the mean final IOP after 3 months was not significantly different, 15.65 ± 2.96 mmHg ($p = 0.285$). The mean number of preoperative medications was 2.65 ± 1.04 for the study group and 2.50 ± 0.83 for the control group. Postoperatively, the mean number of medications decreased significantly to 0.20 ± 0.52 ($p < 0.001$) in the study group and was not significantly different in the control group 2.65 ± 0.88 ($p = 0.186$).

3.3. BCVA Examination

In the study eyes, BCVA was 0.45 ± 0.55 logMAR at baseline and improved to 0.33 ± 0.57 logMAR at the final follow-up ($p = 0.029$), while in the control group, it was 0.10 ± 0.09 logMAR at baseline and 0.09 ± 0.09 logMAR ($p = 0.6181$) at the final follow-up.

3.4. Pentacam Parameter Evaluation

In the study group, the mean ACD was 3.37 ± 0.59 mm at baseline and 3.27 ± 0.55 mm, 3.30 ± 0.59 mm, and 3.32 ± 0.51 mm at 1 day, 1 month, and 3 months after surgery, respectively. In comparison, in the control group, the mean ACD was 3.44 ± 0.48 mm at baseline and 3.45 ± 0.46 mm, 3.41 ± 0.46 mm, and 3.38 ± 0.43 mm at 1 day, 1 month, and 3 months of follow up, respectively. In both groups, changes in the mean ACD did not reveal statistically significant differences at any of the follow-up examinations. When comparing the ACD results between the study and control groups, no statistically significant difference was detectable at baseline or at any follow-up visit ($p > 0.05$). Accordingly, in both groups, changes in ACD did not reveal statistically significant differences at any of the follow-up examinations. There was no statistically significant difference between the two groups during follow-up examinations ($p > 0.05$) (Table 2).

Table 2. Baseline and follow-up results for the mean ACD, ACV, astigmatism, and steep during the 3 months of follow up.

		Study Group (n = 20)	Comparison to Baseline p-Value (Pairwise Signed Rank Test)	Control Group (n = 20)	Comparison to Baseline p-Value (Pairwise Signed Rank Test)	Intergroup Comparison p-Value
AC depth (mm)	Baseline	3.37 ± 0.59		3.44 ± 0.48		0.67
	POD 1	3.27 ± 0.55	0.30	3.45 ± 0.46	0.83	0.28
	POD 7	3.25 ± 0.54	0.35	3.38 ± 0.44	0.28	0.41
	POD 14	3.30 ± 0.56	0.40	3.41 ± 0.43	0.22	0.47
	POM 1	3.30 ± 0.59	0.22	3.41 ± 0.46	0.07	0.49
	POM 2	3.23 ± 0.51	0.07	3.29 ± 0.39	0.12	0.66
	POM 3	3.32 ± 0.51	0.43	3.38 ± 0.43	0.11	0.69
AC volume (mm^3)	Baseline	169.30 ± 39.36		170.55 ± 34.81		0.91
	POD 1	161.90 ± 31.57	0.51	171.15 ± 33.40	0.46	0.37
	POD 7	160.60 ± 33.95	0.33	166.05 ± 28.33	0.34	0.58
	POD 14	164.40 ± 39.75	0.43	171.30 ± 33.89	0.51	0.55
	POM 1	165.85 ± 41.31	0.49	171.30 ± 36.51	0.45	0.66
	POM 2	168.05 ± 40.43	0.83	161.95 ± 29.82	0.45	0.64
	POM 3	170.90 ± 35.34	1	171.10 ± 26.52	0.69	0.72
Astigmatism	Baseline	0.94 ± 0.64		0.80 ± 0.52		0.62
	POD 1	0.91 ± 0.44	0.32	0.77 ± 0.46	0.93	0.34
	POD 7	0.89 ± 0.40	0.96	0.73 ± 0.44	0.17	0.23
	POD 14	0.91 ± 0.41	0.53	0.72 ± 0.48	0.09	0.19
	POM 1	0.93 ± 0.41	0.88	0.75 ± 0.52	0.57	0.12
	POM 2	0.87 ± 0.42	0.93	0.75 ± 0.50	0.51	0.24
	POM 3	0.87 ± 0.39	1	0.80 ± 0.56	0.97	0.35
Steep	Baseline	99.3 ± 43.7		97.1 ± 45.5		0.87
	POD 1	91.8 ± 37.9	0.98	104.3 ± 40.3	0.30	0.31
	POD 7	89.3 ± 37.3	0.61	110.7 ± 44.8	0.13	0.10
	POD 14	91.3 ± 37.3	0.69	102.1 ± 43.4	0.08	0.31
	POM 1	88.7 ± 31.4	0.53	107.5 ± 41.6	0.07	0.08
	POM 2	89.5 ± 33.6	0.48	101.2 ± 42.9	0.48	0.34
	POM 3	84.8 ± 31.9	0.77	98.0 ± 40.1	0.92	0.18

Moreover, even the total astigmatism and the steep did not change significantly in both groups. Specifically, in the study group, mean astigmatism was 0.94 ± 0.64 D at baseline and 0.91 ± 0.44 D, 0.89 ± 0.40 D, 0.93 ± 0.41 D, and 0.87 ± 0.39 D at 1 day, 7 days, 1 month, and 3 months after surgery, respectively. In control group, mean astigmatism was 0.80 ± 0.52 D at baseline and 0.77 ± 0.46 D, 0,73 ± 0.44 D, 0.75 ± 0.52, and 0.80 ± 0.56 D at 1 day, 7 days, 1 month, and 3 months of follow up. Similarly, the steep did not show significative changes in both groups [(in the study group, 99.3° ± 43.7° and 84.8° ± 31.9° at baseline and 3 months after surgery, respectively, $p = 0.77$) (in the control group, 97.1° ± 45.5° and 98.0° ± 40.1° at baseline and at 3 months of follow up, respectively, $p = 0.92$)] Further analysis showed no statistically significant intergroup differences at each follow-up visit ($p > 0.05$) (Table 2).

Furthermore, BCVA and astigmatism changes in the two groups were tested for a possible correlation. No significant results at baseline and at 1 month or 3 months of follow up were observed in the study group. Conversely, in the control group, a significant negative correlation was found at the 3-month follow-up (study group baseline: r = 0.15, $p = 0.53$; 1 month: r = −0. 13, $p = 0.58$; 3 months: r = 0.05, $p = 0.83$; and control group baseline: r = −0.37, $p = 0.10$; 1 month: r = −0.32, $p = 0.17$; 3 months: r = −0.47, $p = 0.037$).

Moreover, a possible correlation between ACD and IOP variations was examined and a significant negative correlation was detected in the study group at 1 and 3 months after surgery. For the control group, no significant correlation was observed between IOP and ACD at each follow-up visit (study group baseline: $r = 0.21$, $p = 0.36$; 1 month: $r = -0.49$, $p = 0.027$; 3 months: $r = -0.58$, $p = 0.007$; and control group baseline: $r = -0.06$, $p = 0.79$; 1 month: $r = -0.01$, $p = 0.96$; 3 months: $r = -0.02$, $p = 0.92$).

3.5. Complications and Reoperations

There were no reports of intraoperative complications in the study group. During follow-up period, 11 eyes (55%) did not experience any postoperative complications. The most frequent complication in the remaining eyes (45%, $n = 9$) was numerical hypotony, with 88.89% of these cases resolving at week 2 without intervention. Persistent hypotony occurred in one eye (5%).

Two patients (10%) experienced a proximal ostium obstruction of the XEN, which was successfully treated with a YAG laser. Due to bleb flattening, filtration area fibrosis or distal XEN obstruction, seven eyes (35%) developed a decrease in bleb function, resulting in an IOP elevation. In all of these patients, a needling procedure with MMC injection was performed. The time to needling procedure ranged between 15 and 60 days (mean 30.85 ± 14.15) after XEN implantation

3.6. Surgical Outcomes

In the study group, complete success was achieved in 10 eyes (50%), and overall success in 17 eyes (85%). Qualified success was achieved in seven eyes (35%).

4. Discussion

MIGS has been shown to be both safe and effective at lowering IOP, as well as the number of glaucoma medications, in patients with mild to moderate disease [20]. The findings of our study are consistent with those that have been reported by various authors in the past, highlighting XEN as a valuable tool for reducing and controlling IOP in glaucoma patients [20]. Specifically, a statistically significant drop in IOP of 50.26% was observed during the 3-month follow-up, surpassing or mirroring outcomes from previously published studies. Indeed, various authors have documented the mid- and long-term efficacy of the XEN45 implant, both in terms of lowering IOP and reducing ocular hypotensive medications [21–23]. This holds true whether it is used alone or in conjunction with phacoemulsification surgery, particularly in POAG patients [24].

This procedure demonstrated safety in terms of complications that occurred during and after the operation, which is in line with the findings of other research [25]. The study group did not report any intraoperative complications. Only two patients (10%) encountered XEN device obstruction, which was effectively treated with YAG laser and needling procedures, as previously described by our group [26]. The second and most common complication was numerical hypotony, which was seen in 45% of the cases ($n = 9$). It was resolved in almost all of the cases (88.89%) by the second week without further intervention. Persistent hypotony occurred in one eye, and these transient and self-limited findings are comparable to records reported by other authors [25].

Our research additionally highlighted a significant negative correlation between IOP and ACD within the study group at both 1 and 3 months post-surgery. Similar findings were reported in other glaucoma procedures. Francis et al. observed a variable reduction in axial length, contingent on the degree of IOP reduction and the final postoperative IOP. They highlighted the importance of considering this alteration in axial length when anticipating the intended refractive outcome [27]. Nevertheless, in our study, despite a significant alteration in ACD, no significant changes in BCVA occurred.

In this context, an unexpected lack of significant change in keratometry was observed in both the study group and the control group. This finding contrasts with reports from various authors who documented significant changes in keratometry following various glaucoma procedures. Hugkulstone was the first author to investigate corneal astigmatism after trabeculectomy, describing a steepening of the vertical meridian [28]. However, no correlation was found between the decrease in IOP and changes in BCVA and corneal radii [28]. Other authors have also confirmed alterations in the keratometry index following trabeculectomy [11,12]. Additionally, researchers have studied this parameter in relation to various glaucoma devices. Hammel et al. reported only a transient modification of corneal astigmatism in 19 patients who underwent Ex-PRESS Miniature Glaucoma Implant surgery (Alcon Inc., Geneva, Switzerland), which was correlated with fluctuations in IOP and ACD [29]. More recently, Tzu et al. investigated refractive outcomes after glaucoma drainage device surgery, finding a mean induced astigmatism [30]. However, this study did not differentiate between the trabeculectomy and combined glaucoma drainage device populations [30]. A recent study compared surgically induced astigmatism following trabeculectomy and XEN implantation [9]. The authors showed a significant and comparable surgically induced astigmatism 3 months after surgery, which remained stable during the further follow-up period of 24 months. However, in contrast with this latter study that only analyzed objective and subjective refraction, our data did not show any significant changes in topographical analysis following XEN implantation.

The etiology of induced astigmatism following glaucoma procedures remains incompletely elucidated. Some authors have proposed several hypotheses, including surgically induced wound gape [28], removal of scleral tissue [11], the role of sutures and suture lysis [12], the influence of postoperative intraocular pressure (IOP) [31], and the pressure exerted by the eyelid and bleb on the cornea surface [32]. Moreover, there is insufficient information on the astigmatic effects of other minimally invasive glaucoma surgeries. To the best of our knowledge, this study is first to investigate both keratometry and ACD changes following XEN surgery.

Our findings distinctly highlight that XEN implantation does not lead to changes in keratometry or BCVA outcomes. This procedure involves the use of mitomycin C and the development of a bleb, while not necessitating sutures or structural alterations to the eye for successful outcomes. This suggests that induced astigmatism following glaucoma procedures could likely be attributable to structural changes in the eye and the use of sutures, with mitomycin C and bleb formation playing negligible roles. In light of these findings, the lack of significant induced astigmatism supports the feasibility of combining cataract and XEN implantation surgeries without the risk of unaccurate refractive outcomes.

Nonetheless, our study has several limitations. First, a small sample size was evaluated; this study helps to plan prospective studies with a sufficient sample size to detect possible differences between trabeculectomy and XEN or other device implantation. Moreover, the follow-up time was only 3 months and further studies investigating long-term outcomes are required.

5. Conclusions

The present study revealed that the XEN implantation did not result in a decline in the visual acuity or changes in keratometry or ACD. Patients undergoing XEN implantation could hence be reassured about this aspect. Moreover, this research provides evidence that this surgery is both effective and safe for patients with open-angle glaucoma.

Author Contributions: Conceptualization, F.T. and M.F.; data curation, C.T.; formal analysis, F.L.; investigation, C.T., F.L. and S.K.; methodology, F.T., F.L. and G.D.; supervision, E.P., M.F. and G.G.; writing—original draft, F.T.; writing—review and editing, G.D., E.P., M.F. and G.G. All authors have read and agreed to the published version of the manuscript.

Funding: This research received no specific grant from any public funding agency or from the commercial or not-for-profit sector.

Institutional Review Board Statement: The study was approved by the Local Institutional Review Board (PG/2022/341, 26 January 2022). All procedures were performed in accordance with the principles of the Declaration of Helsinki.

Informed Consent Statement: Written informed consent was obtained from each participant.

Data Availability Statement: The original contributions presented in the study are included in the article, further inquiries can be directed to the corresponding author.

Conflicts of Interest: The authors declare no conflicts of interest.

References

1. Tham, Y.C.; Li, X.; Wong, T.Y.; Quigley, H.A.; Aung, T.; Cheng, C.Y. Global Prevalence of Glaucoma and Projections of Glaucoma Burden through 2040: A Systematic Review and Meta-Analysis. *Ophthalmology* **2014**, *121*, 2081–2090. [CrossRef] [PubMed]
2. European Glaucoma Society. Chapter 3: Treatment Principles and Options. In *European Glaucoma Society Terminology and Guidelines for Glaucoma*, 4th ed.; Supported by the EGS Foundation; European Glaucoma Society: Zug, Switzerland, 2017; Volume 101, pp. 130–195. [CrossRef]
3. Feldman, R.M.; Gross, R.L.; Spaeth, G.L.; Steinmann, W.C.; Varma, R.; Katz, L.J.; Wilson, R.P.; Moster, M.R.; Spiegel, D. Risk Factors for the Development of Tenon's Capsule Cycts after Trabeculectomy. *Ophthalmology* **1989**, *96*, 336–341. [CrossRef] [PubMed]
4. Schwartz, A.L.; Van Veldhuisen, P.C.; Gaasterland, D.E.; Ederer, F.; Sullivan, E.K.; Cyrlin, M.N. The Advanced Glaucoma Intervention Study (AGIS): Encapsulated Bleb after Initial Trabeculectomy. *Am. J. Ophthalmol.* **1999**, *127*, 8–19. [CrossRef] [PubMed]
5. Rulli, E.; Biagioli, E.; Riva, I.; Gambirasio, G.; De Simone, I.; Floriani, I.; Quaranta, L. Efficacy and Safety of Trabeculectomy vs Nonpenetrating Surgical Procedures. *JAMA Ophthalmol.* **2013**, *131*, 1573. [CrossRef] [PubMed]
6. Edmunds, B.; Thompson, J.R.; Salmon, J.F.; Wormald, R.P. The National Survey of Trabeculectomy. III. Early and Late Complications. *Eye* **2002**, *16*, 297–303. [CrossRef] [PubMed]
7. Tunç, Y.; Tetikoglu, M.; Kara, N.; Sagdık, H.M.; Özarpaci, S.; Elçioğlu, M.N. Management of Hypotony and Flat Anterior Chamber Associated with Glaucoma Filtration Surgery. *Int. J. Ophthalmol.* **2015**, *8*, 950–953. [CrossRef] [PubMed]
8. Bormann, C.; Busch, C.; Rehak, M.; Schmidt, M.; Scharenberg, C.; Ziemssen, F.; Unterlauft, J.D. Refractive Changes after Glaucoma Surgery-A Comparison between Trabeculectomy and XEN Microstent Implantation. *Life* **2022**, *12*, 1889. [CrossRef] [PubMed]
9. Pakravan, M.; Alvani, A.; Esfandiari, H.; Ghahari, E.; Yaseri, M. Post-Trabeculectomy Ocular Biometric Changes. *Clin. Exp. Optom.* **2017**, *100*, 128–132. [CrossRef]
10. Cunliffe, I.A.; Dapling, R.B.; West, J.; Longstaff, S. A Prospective Study Examining the Changes in Factors That Affect Visual Acuity Following Trabeculectomy. *Eye* **1992**, *6*, 618–622. [CrossRef]
11. Claridge, K.G.; Galbraith, J.K.; Karmel, V.; Bates, A.K. The Effect of Trabeculectomy on Refraction, Keratometry and Corneal Topography. *Eye* **1995**, *9*, 292–298. [CrossRef]
12. Chan, H.H.L.; Kong, Y.X.G. Glaucoma Surgery and Induced Astigmatism: A Systematic Review. *Eye Vis.* **2017**, *4*, 27. [CrossRef] [PubMed]
13. Yuan, Y.; Zhang, Z.; Zhu, J.; He, X.; Du, E.; Jiang, K.; Zheng, W.; Ke, B. Responses of the Ocular Anterior Segment and Refraction to 0.5% Tropicamide in Chinese School-Aged Children of Myopia, Emmetropia, and Hyperopia. *J. Ophthalmol.* **2015**, *2015*, 612728. [CrossRef] [PubMed]
14. Diagourtas, A.; Papaconstantinou, D.; Vergados, A.; Andreanos, K.; Koutsandrea, C. Objective Documentation of Anterior Chamber Depth Following Trabeculectomy and Its Correlation with Intraocular Pressure and Bleb Functionality. *Medicine* **2018**, *97*, e11824. [CrossRef] [PubMed]
15. Saheb, H.; Ahmed, I.I.K. Micro-Invasive Glaucoma Surgery. *Curr. Opin. Ophthalmol.* **2012**, *23*, 96–104. [CrossRef] [PubMed]
16. Caprioli, J.; Kim, J.H.; Friedman, D.S.; Kiang, T.; Moster, M.R.; Parrish, R.K.; Rorer, E.M.; Samuelson, T.; Tarver, M.E.; Singh, K.; et al. Special Commentary: Supporting Innovation for Safe and Effective Minimally Invasive Glaucoma Surgery. *Ophthalmology* **2015**, *122*, 1795–1801. [CrossRef] [PubMed]
17. Sheybani, A.; Dick, H.B.; Ahmed, I.I.K. Early Clinical Results of a Novel Ab Interno Gel Stent for the Surgical Treatment of Open-Angle Glaucoma. *J. Glaucoma* **2016**, *25*, e691–e696. [CrossRef] [PubMed]
18. Grover, D.S.; Flynn, W.J.; Bashford, K.P.; Lewis, R.A.; Duh, Y.-J.; Nangia, R.S.; Niksch, B. Performance and Safety of a New Ab Interno Gelatin Stent in Refractory Glaucoma at 12 Months. *Am. J. Ophthalmol.* **2017**, *183*, 25–36. [CrossRef] [PubMed]
19. Senthil, S.; Deshmukh, S.; Turaga, K.; Pesala, V.; Bandela, P.; Ganesh, J.; Garudadri, C.; Bharadwaj, S. Surgically Induced Astigmatism and Refractive Outcomes Following Phacotrabeculectomy. *Indian J. Ophthalmol.* **2020**, *68*, 609. [CrossRef] [PubMed]
20. Lavia, C.; Dallorto, L.; Maule, M.; Ceccarelli, M.; Fea, A.M. Minimally-Invasive Glaucoma Surgeries (MIGS) for Open Angle Glaucoma: A Systematic Review and Meta-Analysis. *PLoS ONE* **2017**, *12*, e0183142. [CrossRef]
21. Hengerer, F.H.; Kohnen, T.; Mueller, M.; Conrad-Hengerer, I. Ab Interno Gel Implant for the Treatment of Glaucoma Patients with or without Prior Glaucoma Surgery: 1-Year Results. *J. Glaucoma* **2017**, *26*, 1130–1136. [CrossRef]
22. Schlenker, M.B.; Gulamhusein, H.; Conrad-Hengerer, I.; Somers, A.; Lenzhofer, M.; Stalmans, I.; Reitsamer, H.; Hengerer, F.H.; Ahmed, I.I.K. Efficacy, Safety, and Risk Factors for Failure of Standalone Ab Interno Gelatin Microstent Implantation Versus Standalone Trabeculectomy. *Ophthalmology* **2017**, *124*, 1579–1588. [CrossRef] [PubMed]

23. Reitsamer, H.; Sng, C.; Vera, V.; Lenzhofer, M.; Barton, K.; Stalmans, I. Two-Year Results of a Multicenter Study of the Ab Interno Gelatin Implant in Medically Uncontrolled Primary Open-Angle Glaucoma. *Graefe's Arch. Clin. Exp. Ophthalmol.* **2019**, *257*, 983–996. [CrossRef] [PubMed]
24. Pirani, V.; Virgili, F.; Ramovecchi, V. Short-Term Outcomes of XEN45 Standalone versus Combined with Phacoemulsification in Open-Angle Glaucoma Patients: A Retrospective Study. *J. Clin. Med.* **2023**, *13*, 157. [CrossRef] [PubMed]
25. Wanichwecharungruang, B.; Ratprasatporn, N. 24-Month Outcomes of XEN45 Gel Implant Versus Trabeculectomy in Primary Glaucoma. *PLoS ONE* **2021**, *16*, e0256362. [CrossRef] [PubMed]
26. Tatti, F.; Lixi, F.; Demarinis, G.; Napoli, P.; Fossarello, M. Anterior Segment Optical Coherence Tomography for Cases of High Intraocular Pressure Following XEN Implant for Glaucoma. *J. Glaucoma* **2023**. [CrossRef] [PubMed]
27. Francis, B.A. Changes in Axial Length Following Trabeculectomy and Glaucoma Drainage Device Surgery. *Br. J. Ophthalmol.* **2005**, *89*, 17–20. [CrossRef] [PubMed]
28. Hugkulstone, C.E. Changes in Keratometry Following Trabeculectomy. *Br. J. Ophthalmol.* **1991**, *75*, 217–218. [CrossRef] [PubMed]
29. Hammel, N.; Lusky, M.; Kaiserman, I.; Robinson, A.; Bahar, I. Changes in Anterior Segment Parameters After Insertion of Ex-PRESS Miniature Glaucoma Implant. *J. Glaucoma* **2013**, *22*, 565–568. [CrossRef] [PubMed]
30. Tzu, J.H.; Shah, C.T.; Galor, A.; Junk, A.K.; Sastry, A.; Wellik, S.R. Refractive Outcomes of Combined Cataract and Glaucoma Surgery. *J. Glaucoma* **2015**, *24*, 161–164. [CrossRef]
31. Kook, M.S.; Kim, H.B.; Lee, S.U. Short-Term Effect of Mitomycin-C Augmented Trabeculectomy on Axial Length and Corneal Astigmatism. *J. Cataract Refract. Surg.* **2001**, *27*, 518–523. [CrossRef]
32. Delbeke, H.; Stalmans, I.; Vandewalle, E.; Zeyen, T. The Effect of Trabeculectomy on Astigmatism. *J. Glaucoma* **2016**, *25*, e308–e312. [CrossRef] [PubMed]

Journal of
Clinical Medicine

MDPI

Article

Investigating the Relationship between Telomere-Related Gene Variants and Leukocyte Telomere Length in Optic Neuritis Patients

Monika Duseikaite [1,2,*], Greta Gedvilaite [1,3], Paulius Mikuzis [3], Juste Andrulionyte [3], Loresa Kriauciuniene [1] and Rasa Liutkeviciene [1]

1 Laboratory of Ophthalmology, Institute of Neuroscience, Lithuanian University of Health Sciences, Eivenių Street 2, LT-50161 Kaunas, Lithuania; greta.gedvilaite@lsmuni.lt (G.G.); loresa.kriauciuniene@lsmu.lt (L.K.); rasa.liutkeviciene@lsmu.lt (R.L.)
2 Faculty of Pharmacy, Lithuanian University of Health Sciences, Sukilėlių Pr. 13, LT-50166 Kaunas, Lithuania
3 Medical Faculty, Lithuanian University of Health Sciences, LT-50161 Kaunas, Lithuania; paulius.mikuzis@stud.lsmuni.lt (P.M.); juste.andrulionyte@stud.lsmuni.lt (J.A.)
* Correspondence: monika.duseikaite@lsmu.lt

Abstract: Optic neuritis (ON) is a condition marked by optic nerve inflammation due to various potential triggers. Research indicates a link between telomeres and inflammation, as studies demonstrate that inflammation can lead to increased telomere shortening. **Aim**: We aimed to determine the associations of telomere-related telomeric repeat binding factor 1 (*TERF1*) rs1545827, rs10107605, and telomeric repeat binding factor 2 (*TERF2*) rs251796 polymorphisms and relative leukocyte telomere length (LTL) with the occurrence of ON. **Methods**: In this research, a total of 73 individuals diagnosed with optic neuritis (ON) were studied and the control group included 170 individuals without any health issues. The DNA samples were obtained from peripheral blood leukocytes, which were purified using the DNA salting-out technique. Real-time polymerase chain reaction (RT-PCR) assessed single-nucleotide polymorphisms (SNPs) and relative leukocyte telomere lengths (LTL). The data obtained were processed and analyzed using the "IBM SPSS Statistics 29.0" program. **Results**: Our study revealed the following results: in the male group, *TERF2* rs251796 (AA, AG, and TT) statistically significantly differed between the long and short telomere group, with frequencies of 65.7%, 22.9%, and 2.0% in long telomeres, compared to 35.1%, 56.8%, and 8.1% in the short telomere group ($p = 0.013$). The *TERF2* rs251796 CT genotype, compared to CC, under the codominant genetic model, was associated with 4.7-fold decreased odds of telomere shortening ($p = 0.005$). Meanwhile, CT+TT genotypes, compared to CC under the dominant genetic model, were associated with 3.5-fold decreased odds of telomere shortening ($p = 0.011$). Also, the CT genotype, compared to CC+TT, under the overdominant genetic model, was associated with 4.4-fold decreased odds of telomere shortening ($p = 0.004$). **Conclusions**: The current evidence may suggest a protective role of *TERF2* rs251796 in the occurrence of ON in men.

Keywords: optic neuritis; *TERF1*; *TERF2*; telomeres

1. Introduction

Optic neuritis (ON) is the most common cause of subacute optic neuropathy in young adults [1]. ON, a demyelinating disorder characterized by acute, transient, predominantly monocular vision loss, is intricately linked to multiple sclerosis (MS), serving as the initial manifestation of MS in approximately 15–20% of affected individuals [2]. The occurrence of ON varies between 1 and 5 cases per 100,000 people [3], and its underlying mechanisms are not fully understood. Evidence suggests it is likely an immune-related condition, as indicated by the presence of systemic T-cells during disease onset and the detection of B-cells targeting myelin basic protein in the cerebrospinal fluid of individuals with ON [4].

Studies conducted globally indicate that the prevalence of the disease typically manifests within the age range of 18 to 45 years [5]. Etiologically, ON can be divided into two main forms, typical and atypical [6].

While the aforementioned factors are undeniably linked to optic nerve inflammation, the significance of genetic components remains uncertain, with growing acknowledgment of the role of hereditary or congenital influences on the onset of specific diseases.

Telomeres, consisting of repetitive nucleotide sequences, exhibit a high degree of conservation and comprise both double-stranded and single-stranded segments, which, when bound with shelterin proteins, protect chromosomal ends, thereby preserving genomic stability [7]. The shortening of telomeres with advancing age is a recognized phenomenon, with gradual diminishment contributing to somatic cell aging, programmed cell death, or potentially carcinogenic alterations, all of which can impact an individual's health and life expectancy [8]. The telomeres, structured as histone octamer-composed nucleosomes, are stabilized through specific protein–protein and protein–DNA interactions between shelterin subunits and tandem repeat sequences [9]. This shelterin complex serves to protect chromosomes from end-joining and damage by forming unique T-loop structures [10]. The T-loop formations serve as protective caps at the chromosome ends, shielding them from being identified as breaks within the double-stranded DNA structure, thus maintaining the chromosomes' stability and structural integrity [11]. Telomeric repeat binding factor 1 (TERF1) and telomeric repeat binding factor 2 (TERF2) act as inhibitors of telomerase activity, thereby participating in the control of telomere length [12]. Increased expression of TERF1 and TERF2 leads to the suppression of telomere length and effective telomere replication, potentially resulting in telomere shortening. Conversely, decreased expression may contribute to telomere elongation [13].

Chronic systemic inflammation is a recognized risk factor for various chronic disorders, including cardiovascular diseases, neurodegenerative diseases, autoimmune diseases, and cancers [14]. Numerous molecules known as inflammatory cytokines, such as tumour-necrosis factor-α (TNF-α), IL-1, IL-6 and many others, are produced by various cell types, particularly by macrophages and mast cells. These cytokines have several roles in the inflammatory process, including activation of the endothelium and leukocytes, as well as initiation of the acute-phase response [15]. Previous studies have indicated the relationship between telomere/telomerase dysfunction and inflammatory signaling [16]. Dysregulation of telomere-related genes and dysfunction in telomeres within diseases may lead to persistent, chronic, low-grade inflammation [17]. An interaction exists between inflammation and telomeres, as research indicates that inflammation accelerates telomere shortening, resulting in telomere dysfunction. At the same time, components of telomeres also contribute to the regulation of inflammatory responses [18].

As changes in telomere length are closely related to inflammation, we aimed to investigate whether telomere-associated genes are associated with the occurrence of optic neuritis.

2. Materials and Methods

The research was carried out at the Laboratory of Ophthalmology, Lithuanian University of Health Sciences, with approval from the Kaunas Regional Biomedical Research Ethics Committee (approval number: BE-2-102). Prior to participation, all individuals provided informed consent through a formal Informed Consent Form.

2.1. Study Group

The study included 243 subjects divided into two groups, a reference group (n = 170) and patients with ON (n = 73). The reference group was adjusted by sex and age to the ON group (p = 0.100 and p = 0.940, respectively). Relative leukocyte telomere length (LTL) was determined in all study subjects. There were no statistically significant differences between the reference and optical neuritis groups between relative LTL (p = 0.242). The demographic data of the study subjects are presented in Table 1.

Table 1. Demographic characteristics of the study.

Characteristics		Group		p-Value
		ON Group	Reference Group	
Sex	Males, N (%)	27 (37)	45 (26.5)	0.100
	Females, N (%)	46 (63)	125 (73.5)	
Age median (IQR)		33 (17)	29.5 (22)	0.940
Relative leukocyte telomere length median (IQR)		0.550 (0.698)	0.517 (0.577)	0.242

Mann–Whitney U test was used; ON—optical neuritis; IQR—interquartile range; p-value: significance level (alpha = 0.05).

2.2. DNA Extraction and Genotyping

Peripheral venous blood leukocytes were used for the extraction of genomic DNA using the salting-out technique. The analysis of single nucleotide polymorphisms (SNPs) of *TERF1* (rs1545827 and rs10107605) and *TERF2* (rs251796) was conducted using the real-time polymerase chain reaction (RT-PCR) method. TaqMan® Genotyping assays (Applied Biosystems; Thermo Fisher Scientific, Inc., Waltham, MA, USA) were used according to the manufacturer's protocols by StepOne Plus (Applied Biosystems) to determine SNPs. The assays IDs were C___1869846_10, C___1869856_10, and C___706068_10.

2.3. Relative Leukocyte Telomere Length Measurement

The relative leukocyte telomere length (LTL) was measured using the quantitative real-time PCR method developed by Cawthon (2002) [19]. This involved the analysis of telomeric DNA fragments and the reference gene albumin in duplicate. The RT-PCR analysis to determine relative LTL was conducted using a Rotor-Gene Q quantitative PCR machine (QIAGEN, Hilden, Germany). A reference DNA sample from the same age group was utilized for comparison. Additionally, DNA extracted from the commercial human cell line 1301 with extended telomeres (Sigma Aldrich, St. Louis, MO, USA) that served as a positive control. The primers used were obtained from IDT (Integrated DNA Technologies, Inc., Coralville, IA, USA) and were previously described in detail in our previous study [20].

In our study, we adopted a relative quantitative data analysis approach based on the recommendation by BioRad Laboratories in 2006. To determine the relative leukocyte telomere length (LTL) in peripheral blood leukocytes, we followed the relative analysis method developed by Livak in 2001 (relative LTL = $2^{-\Delta\Delta Ct}$) [21], after validating the PCR amplification efficiency. As specified by BioRad Laboratories in 2006, this approach is appropriate when the amplification efficiency of both telomere fragments and the albumin gene is between 90% and 105%, and the variation in efficiency between them is within 5%.

The ΔCt value for each sample is computed by finding the disparity between the Ct value of the tested telomere fragments and the Ct value of the reference albumin gene using the following equation:

$$\Delta Ct = Ct\ (\text{telomere fragments}) - Ct\ (\text{reference albumin gene})$$

The ΔΔCt value characterizes the distinction between the ΔCt value of the test sample and the ΔCt value of the reference sample, which, similar to the test samples, has a concentration of 20 ng/μL and can be calculated using the following equation:

$$\Delta\Delta Ct = Ct\ (\text{test sample}) - Ct\ (\text{reference sample})$$ [22].

2.4. Statistical Analysis

Statistical analysis was performed using the "IBM SPSS Statistics 29.0" software (Statistical Package for the Social Sciences for Windows, Inc., Chicago, IL, USA). The data are presented in absolute numbers (percentages), median values, and interquartile ranges (IQRs). The demographic characteristics data were compared between the reference and ON groups using the Mann–Whitney U test. The frequencies of *TERF1* rs1545827 and rs10107605 and *TERF2* rs251796 genotypes and alleles are presented in percentages. Binary logistic regression analysis was conducted to assess the relationships between the chosen

SNPs and the occurrence of ON. Various inheritance models and genotype combinations (including codominant, dominant, recessive, overdominant, and additive genetic models) were considered, giving an OR with a 95% confidence interval (CI). The Akaike Information Criterion (AIC) was used to identify the most suitable inheritance model, with the model having the lowest AIC value considered the best fit. A nonparametric Mann–Whitney U test compared different groups when the data distribution was not normal. Statistical significance was proven when the *p*-value was less than 0.05, indicating significant differences and correlations.

2.5. Limitations

Although our research offers valuable insights into telomere dynamics, it is important to acknowledge several limitations. Firstly, despite the participants' age and sex, factors such as smoking, obesity, and stress disorders, which are known to affect telomere length, were not specifically analyzed in our study, leaving the influence of these variables on telomere attrition unexplored. Secondly, despite the fact ON is considered a rare disease, the sample size could be increased. In future studies, it would be beneficial to conduct comprehensive evaluations of lifestyle factors in order to fully understand the complex relationship between environmental influences and the dynamics of telomeres. One more limitation of our study is that the population under investigation appears to be predominantly composed of patients from Lithuania. This homogeneity may not fully reflect the genetic diversity, environmental exposures, and healthcare practices present in the broader global population. Variations in these factors across different geographic regions could potentially influence the associations observed between the *TERF1* and *TERF2* variants and the risk of ON. Therefore, the generalizability of our findings to other populations may be limited, and caution should be exercised when extrapolating the results to diverse ethnic or geographical groups. Despite these limitations, our study highlights the necessity for further research to gain a comprehensive understanding of telomere regulation and its implications for health and disease.

3. Results

The frequencies of genotypes and alleles for the single-nucleotide polymorphisms (SNPs) *TERF1* rs1545827, rs10107605 and *TERF2* rs251796 were analyzed within the study groups. No significant differences were found in the distribution of genotypes and alleles between patients diagnosed with ON and the reference group for the following SNPs: *TERF1* rs1545827, rs10107605, and *TERF2* rs251796 (see Supplementary Material Table S1).

The results of the Hardy–Weinberg equilibrium (HWE) test indicated that the genotypes of *TERF1* rs1545827 and *TERF2* rs251796 in the reference group did not show any significant deviation from HWE ($p > 0.05$) (Table 2). However, we identified that *TERF1* rs10107605 is not in HWE (Table 2). Regarding these findings, we excluded this SNP from the following analysis [23].

Table 2. Analysis of Hardy–Weinberg equilibrium in the reference group.

Gene and SNP	Allele Frequencies		Genotype Distribution	*p*-Value
TERF1 rs1545827	0.60 C	0.40 T	23/89/58	0.223
TERF1 rs10107605	0.89 A	0.11 C	9/21/140	**<0.0001**
TERF2 rs251796	0.70 A	0.30 G	18/66/86	0.324

SNP—single-nucleotide polymorphism; *p*-value—significance level (alpha = 0.05). Statistically significant results are marked in bold.

Binary logistic regression analysis was conducted in patients with ON and the reference group to investigate the associations of *TERF1* rs1545827, and *TERF2* rs251796 with ON occurrence. However, no statistically significant results were found when analyzing associations between ON occurrence and *TERF1* rs1545827 and *TERF2* rs251796 (Supplementary Material Table S2).

The frequencies of genotypes and alleles for the selected SNPs were analyzed within the study groups, stratified by sex. However, there were no statistically significant differences in the distribution of genotypes and alleles between females and males with ON and the reference group for the following SNPs (Supplementary Material Tables S3 and S5).

Binary logistic regression analysis was conducted in patients with ON and the reference group to investigate the associations of selected SNPs with ON occurrence in females and males. However, no statistically significant results were found when analyzing associations between ON occurrence in females and males and *TERF1* rs1545827 and *TERF2* rs251796 (Supplementary material Tables S4 and S6).

The frequencies of genotypes and alleles for the selected SNPs were analyzed within the study groups, stratified by age median. There were no statistically significant differences in the distribution of genotypes and alleles and binary logistic regression analysis between patients with ON and the reference group for the following SNPs: *TERF1* rs1545827 and *TERF2* rs251796 (age $\leq$ 30) (Supplementary Material Tables S7 and S8). The same results were found within the study groups when the study's subjects' age was over 30 years old (all $p > 0.05$) (Supplementary Material Tables S9 and S10).

Relative LTL was measured for 73 patients with ON and 170 reference group subjects. We found no statistically significant difference in relative LTL between the ON group and the reference group (median (IQR): 0.550 (0.698) vs. 0.518 (0.577), $p = 0.242$).

Regarding the median length of the reference groups relative LTL, we performed an analysis for subjects with long telomeres (when relative LTL $\geq$ 0.517) and those with short telomeres (when relative LTL < 0.517). However, no statistically significant differences in the frequencies of genotypes and alleles and binary logistic regression analysis for the selected SNPs were observed between the long and short telomeres (Supplementary Material Tables S11 and S12).

The frequencies of genotypes and alleles for the selected SNPs were analyzed within the study groups, stratified by sex regarding the median length of the reference groups relative LTL. However, there were no statistically significant differences in the distribution of genotypes and alleles and binary logistic regression analysis between females with ON and the reference group for the following SNPs (Supplementary Material Tables S13 and S14). When analyzing the male group, we observed that *TERF2* rs251796 (AA, AG, and TT) statistically significantly differed between the long and short group telomeres in males, with frequencies of 65.7%, 22.9%, and 2.0% in long telomeres, compared to 35.1%, 56.8%, and 8.1% in the short telomere group ($p = 0.013$) (Table 3).

Binary logistic regression analysis was conducted in males according to telomere shortening. The results revealed the following associations: the *TERF2* rs251796 AG genotype, compared to AA, under the codominant genetic model, was associated with 4.7-fold decreased odds of telomere shortening (OR: 0.215; 95% CI: 0.075–0.622; $p = 0.005$). Also, the AG+GG genotype, compared to AA, under the dominant genetic model, is associated with 3.5-fold decreased odds of telomere shortening (OR: 0.283; 95% CI: 0.107–0.746; $p = 0.011$). Lastly, the AG genotype compared to AA+GG, under the overdominant genetic model, is associated with 4.4-fold decreased odds of telomere shortening (OR: 0.226; 95% CI: 0.081–0.628; $p = 0.004$). The results are shown in Table 4.

The frequencies of genotypes and alleles for the selected SNPs were analyzed within the study groups, stratified by age median regarding the median length of the reference groups relative LTL. However, there were no statistically significant differences in the distribution of genotypes and alleles and binary logistic regression analysis between patients with ON and the reference group for the following SNPs (Supplementary Material Tables S15–S18).

Table 3. Frequencies of genotypes and alleles of *TERF1* rs1545827, and *TERF2* rs251796 in the long and short telomere groups in males (T/S median = 0.517).

Gene, SNP	Genotype, Allele	Long Telomeres	Short Telomeres	*p*-Value
TERF1 rs1545827	CC	13 (37.1)	12 (32.4)	0.530
	CT	20 (57.1)	20 (54.1)	
	TT	2 (5.7)	5 (13.5)	
	Total	35 (100)	37 (100)	
	Allele			
	C	46 (65.7)	44 (59.5)	0.438
	T	24 (34.3)	30 (40.5)	
TERF2 rs251796	AA	23 (65.7)	13 (35.1)	**0.013**
	AG	8 (22.9)	21 (56.8)	
	GG	4 (11.4)	3 (8.1)	
	Total	35 (100)	37 (100)	
	Allele			
	A	54 (77.1)	47 (63.5)	0.074
	G	16 (22.9)	27 (36.5)	

p-value: significance level (alpha = 0.05); statistically significant results are marked in bold.

Table 4. Binary logistic regression analysis of *TERF1* rs1545827 and *TERF2* rs251796 in telomere shortening in males.

Model	Genotype/Allele	OR (95% CI)	*p*-Value	AIC
		TERF1 rs1545827		
Codominant	CT vs. CC TT vs. CC	0.923 (0.340–2.509) 0.369 (0.060–2.274)	0.875 0.283	102.445
Dominant	CT+TT vs. CC	0.812 (0.307–2.146)	0.675	101.582
Recessive	TT vs. CC+CT	0.388 (0.070–2.145)	0.278	100.470
Overdominant	CT vs. CC+TT	1.133 (0.447–2.874)	0.792	101.688
Additive	T	0.719 (0.337–1.533)	0.393	101.017
		TERF2 rs251796		
Codominant	AG vs. AA GG vs. AA	0.215 (0.075–0.622) 0.754 (0.146–3.901)	**0.005** 0.736	94.815
Dominant	AG+GG vs. AA	0.283 (0.107–0.746)	0.011	94.921
Recessive	GG vs. AA+AG	1.462 (0.303–7.058)	0.636	101.531
Overdominant	AG vs. AA+GG	0.226 (0.081–0.628)	0.004	92.927
Additive	G	0.521 (0.249–1.094)	0.085	98.624

OR: odds ratio; CI: confidence interval; *p*-value: significance level (alpha = 0.05); AIC: Akaike information criterion; statistically significant results are marked in bold.

4. Discussion

Our study aimed to explore the potential association between genetic variations in telomere maintenance-related genes, telomere length, and ON incidence. To achieve this, we conducted an analysis focusing on the following two polymorphisms located within genes associated with telomerase: *TERF1* rs1545827 and *TERF2* rs251796.

The results were evaluated according to gender and age groups. The relationship between relative LTL and age is the most studied and evidence-based in the literature; it is known that telomeres become shorter with years, and this is related to cellular aging mechanisms [24]. According to the results of our investigation, the frequencies of genotypes and alleles for the selected SNPs were analyzed within the study groups, stratified by age median. There were no statistically significant differences in the distribution of genotypes and alleles and binary logistic regression analysis between patients with ON and the reference group for the following SNPs: *TERF1* rs1545827 and *TERF2* rs251796 (age $\leq$ 30). The same results were found within the study groups when the study's subjects' age was over 30 years old (all $p > 0.05$). Also, the frequencies of genotypes and alleles for the selected SNPs were analyzed within the study groups, stratified by age median regarding the median length of the reference groups relative LTL. However, there were no statistically significant differences in the distribution of genotypes and alleles and binary logistic regression analysis between patients with ON and the reference group for the following SNPs.

Not only does relative LTL rely on age, but it also depends on genetic and environmental factors. Hereditary factors determine about 70% of relative LTL [25]; a sex difference has also been observed in many studies; they determined that women's telomeres are statistically significantly longer than men's [26]. Optic neuritis tends to affect females more than males, with a ratio of around 3:1, regardless of whether individuals are of Caucasian or Oriental descent. Despite this observation, the precise underlying mechanisms remain unclear. It is hypothesized that there may be a sex-specific susceptibility to autoimmune diseases, although further research is needed to clarify this relationship [27]. Kim et al. found that ON onset is later in men than in women (average 49 vs. 41 years of age), neuritic attacks are less frequent at onset (17 vs. 44%) and are less frequent during the course of the disease (0.08 vs. 0.27 per year) in men than in women. Males more often tend to develop an isolated form of myelitis (67 vs. 28%). Visual evoked potential testing showed a shorter latency of P100 in men. Men were also noted to have fewer acute optic neuritis attacks, independent of age at onset of the disease [28].

Bekaert and others reported that telomere attrition in their study proceeded faster in men (30.0 bp per year, $R^2 = 0.062$) compared to women (20.3 bp per year, $R^2 = 0.028$) [29]. During our investigation, the analysis showed that when analyzing the male group, the *TERF2* rs251796 AG genotype, compared to AA, under the codominant genetic model, is associated with 4.7-fold decreased odds of telomere shortening (OR: 0.215; 95% CI: 0.075–0.622; $p = 0.005$). The AG+GG genotype, compared to AA, under the dominant genetic model, is associated with 3.5-fold decreased odds of telomere shortening (OR: 0.283; 95% CI: 0.107–0.746; $p = 0.011$). Lastly, the AG genotype, compared to AA+GG, under the overdominant genetic model, is associated with 4.4-fold decreased odds of telomere shortening (OR: 0.226; 95% CI: 0.081–0.628; $p = 0.004$). The current evidence may suggest a protective role of *TERF2* rs251796 SNP in the occurrence of ON in men. We did not find any statistical significance in the distribution of genotypes and alleles and binary logistic regression analysis between females with ON and the reference group. These results could be due to the small sample size of the women studied and the characteristics of the population. According to The Optic Neuritis Treatment Trial, the majority (77%) of patients with ON are young women. Women are at least twice as likely to develop MS compared with men, yet the latter have been reported to have worse clinical outcomes and faster disease progression [30]. Several factors have been proposed to account for gender differences in MS including sex hormones, genetics, immune biases, and environmental influences [31]. Estrogen, as a sex hormone, has demonstrated efficacy in reducing the severity of experimental autoimmune encephalomyelitis in animal models of central nervous system (CNS) inflammation, as well as in clinical settings where treatment with estrogen derivatives correlated with decreased MRI-measured gadolinium-enhancing lesions in women with relapsing-remitting multiple sclerosis (RRMS) [32]. Additionally, estrogen has exhibited the ability to enhance retinal blood flow and protect the retinal nerve fiber layer (RNFL) in both animal and clinical models of optic nerve injury [33]. In a study involving an experimental model of Leber hereditary optic neuropathy, 17β-estradiol activated mitochondrial biogenesis and improved energetic competence, leading researchers to theorize that the protective effects of estrogen could explain the higher prevalence of Leber hereditary optic neuropathy in men compared to women [34]. While it is plausible that estrogen's neuroprotective benefits may have contributed to the relatively preserved RNFL values observed in women compared to men in a particular study, specific evaluation of sex hormones was not conducted. Thus, further research is needed. Our study did not evaluate environmental factors such as smoking, psychological stress, diet, obesity, or physical activity, which could affect the telomere length in the patients of ON and healthy subjects [35]. In future studies, it would be beneficial to conduct in-depth assessments of lifestyle factors to interpret the relationship between environmental factors and the dynamics of telomeres.

To our knowledge, no studies are currently examining the relative LTL associations with the development of ON. However, several studies have investigated the relationship between MS and relative LTL. In the case of MS, it has been suggested that the reduced telomere length observed in patients with primary progressive MS represents the most advanced stage of the disease, indicating that biological aging contributes to MS progression. This association between shorter telomere length and increased disability and brain atrophy suggests a link between telomere length and disease severity [36]. Additionally, Krysko et al. reported that greater MS aggressiveness operates mechanisms that initiate specific DNA damage, which deactivates telomerase to prolong telomere length, leading to telomere shortening [37].

In the scenario of potential telomere shortening in the future, it remains ambiguous whether this is a precursor or an outcome of ON or MS development. If accelerated telomere shortening occurred before disease manifestation, it could become a risk factor. However, leukocyte telomere length could also indicate the combined effect of oxidative stress and inflammation throughout the progression, severity, and duration of the disease.

Many authors put forward the hypothesis that the shortening of telomeres in chronic inflammatory diseases may result from a prolonged and severe inflammatory process and oxidative stress [38–41]. New significant differences that could explain the changes in telomere length in ON inflammation were not found, but this work may contribute to the hypothesis previously put forward by other authors. However, further research is needed to comprehend the underlying mechanisms and their potential therapeutic implications.

5. Conclusions

To conclude, the current evidence may suggest a protective role of *TERF2* rs251796 in the occurrence of ON in men.

Supplementary Materials: The following supporting information can be downloaded at: https://www.mdpi.com/article/10.3390/jcm13092694/s1, Table S1: Genotype and allele frequencies of single-nucleotide polymorphisms (*TERF1* rs1545827, rs10107605 and *TERF2* rs251796) within ON and reference groups; Table S2: Binary logistic regression analysis within patients with ON and reference group subjects; Table S3: Genotype and allele frequencies of *TERF1* rs1545827 and *TERF2* rs251796 within ON and reference group females; Table S4: Binary logistic regression analysis within females with ON and reference group females; Table S5: Genotype and allele frequencies of *TERF1* rs1545827 and *TERF2* rs251796 within ON and reference group males; Table S6: Binary logistic regression analysis within males with ON and reference group males; Table S7: Genotype and allele frequencies of *TERF1* rs1545827 and *TERF2* rs251796 within ON and reference group subjects (age $\leq$ 30); Table S8: Binary logistic regression analysis within patients with ON and reference group subjects (age $\leq$ 30); Table S9: Genotype and allele frequencies of *TERF1* rs1545827 and *TERF2* rs251796 within ON and reference group subjects (age > 30); Table S10: Binary logistic regression analysis within patients with ON and reference group subjects (age > 30); Table S11: Frequencies of genotypes and alleles of *TERF1* rs1545827 and *TERF2* rs251796 in the long and short telomere groups (T/S median = 0.517); Table S12: Binary logistic regression analysis of *TERF1* rs1545827 and *TERF2* rs251796 in telomere shortening; Table S13: Frequencies of genotypes and alleles of *TERF1* rs1545827 and *TERF2* rs251796 in the long and short telomere groups for females (T/S median = 0.517); Table S14: Binary logistic regression analysis of *TERF1* rs1545827 and *TERF2* rs251796 in telomere shortening in females; Table S15: Frequencies of genotypes and alleles of *TERF1* rs1545827 and *TERF2* rs251796 in the long and short telomere groups for subjects aged ≤ 30 (T/S median = 0.517); Table S16: Binary logistic regression analysis of *TERF1* rs1545827 and *TERF2* rs251796 in telomere shortening for subjects aged ≤ 30; Table S17: Frequencies of genotypes and alleles of *TERF1* rs1545827 and *TERF2* rs251796 in the long and short telomere groups for subjects aged > 30 (T/S median = 0.517); Table S18: Binary logistic regression analysis of *TERF1* rs1545827 and *TERF2* rs251796 in telomere shortening for subjects aged > 30.

Author Contributions: Conceptualization, M.D., G.G., L.K. and R.L.; methodology, M.D. and G.G.; software, M.D.; validation, M.D. and G.G.; formal analysis, M.D., P.M. and J.A.; investigation, M.D., P.M. and J.A.; resources, R.L.; data curation, M.D. and R.L.; writing—original draft preparation, M.D., G.G. and R.L.; writing—review and editing, M.D., G.G. and R.L.; visualization, M.D., R.L. and L.K.; supervision, R.L.; project administration, R.L.; funding acquisition, M.D. All authors have read and agreed to the published version of the manuscript.

Funding: This research received no external funding.

Institutional Review Board Statement: This study was conducted in the Department of Ophthalmology, Hospital of Lithuanian University of Health Sciences and Laboratory of Ophthalmology, Neuroscience Institute, Lithuanian University of Health Sciences. Ethical approval was obtained from the Ethics Committee for Biomedical Research (BE-2-102 (approved 5 November 2019)).

Informed Consent Statement: Informed consent was obtained from all subjects involved in the study.

Data Availability Statement: Data will be sent upon request.

Conflicts of Interest: The authors declare no conflicts of interest.

References

1. Kraker, J.A.; Chen, J.J. An update on optic neuritis. *J. Neurol.* **2023**, *270*, 5113–5126. [CrossRef]
2. Kale, N. Optic neuritis as an early sign of multiple sclerosis. *Eye Brain* **2016**, *8*, 195–202. [CrossRef]
3. Lee, J.Y.; Han, J.; Yang, M.; Oh, S.Y. Population-based incidence of pediatric and adult optic neuritis and the risk of multiple sclerosis. *Ophthalmology* **2020**, *127*, 417–425. [CrossRef]
4. Ma, K.S.; Lee, C.M.; Chen, P.H.; Yang, Y.; Dong, Y.W.; Wang, Y.H.; Wei, J.C.; Zheng, W.J. Risk of Autoimmune Diseases Following Optic Neuritis: A Nationwide Population-Based Cohort Study. *Front. Med.* **2022**, *9*, 903608. [CrossRef]
5. Punytė, V.; Liutkevičienė, R.; Gelžinis, A.; Žemaitienė, R. Optic neuritis. *J. Med. Sci.* **2020**, *8*, 170–175.
6. Morrow, M.J. Ischemic Optic Neuropathy. *Continuum* **2019**, *25*, 1215–1235. [CrossRef]
7. Srinivas, N.; Rachakonda, S.; Kumar, R. Telomeres and Telomere Length: A General Overview. *Cancers* **2020**, *12*, 558. [CrossRef]
8. Shammas, M.A. Telomeres, lifestyle, cancer, and aging. *Curr. Opin. Clin. Nutr. Metab. Care* **2011**, *14*, 28–34. [CrossRef]
9. Alanazi, A.F.R.; Parkinson, G.N.; Haider, S. Structural Motifs at the Telomeres and Their Role in Regulatory Pathways. *Biochemistry* **2024**, *63*, 827–842. [CrossRef]
10. de Lange, T. Shelterin-mediated telomere protection. *Annu. Rev. Genet.* **2018**, *52*, 223–247. [CrossRef]
11. Ruis, P.; Boulton, S.J. The end protection problem-an unexpected twist in the tail. *Genes Dev.* **2021**, *35*, 1–21. [CrossRef]
12. Erdel, F.; Kratz, K.; Willcox, S.; Griffith, J.D.; Greene, E.C.; de Lange, T. Telomere recognition and assembly mechanism of mammalian shelterin. *Cell Rep.* **2017**, *18*, 41–53. [CrossRef]
13. Lin, J.; Countryman, P.; Buncher, N.; Kaur, P.; Longjiang, E.; Zhang, Y.; Gibson, G.; You, C.; Watkins, S.C.; Piehler, J.; et al. Trf1 and Trf2 use different mechanisms to find telomeric DNA but share a novel mechanism to search for protein partners at telomeres. *Nucleic Acids Res.* **2014**, *42*, 2493–2504. [CrossRef]
14. Zhao, H.; Wu, L.; Yan, G.; Chen, Y.; Zhou, M.; Wu, Y.; Li, Y. Inflammation and tumor progression: Signaling pathways and targeted intervention. *Signal Transduct. Target. Ther.* **2021**, *6*, 263. [CrossRef]
15. Medzhitov, R. Origin and physiological roles of inflammation. *Nature* **2008**, *454*, 428–435. [CrossRef]
16. Lin, J.; Epel, E. Stress and telomere shortening: Insights from cellular mechanisms. *Ageing Res. Rev.* **2022**, *73*, 101507. [CrossRef]
17. Chakravarti, D.; Hu, B.; Mao, X.; Rashid, A.; Li, J.; Li, J.; Liao, W.T.; Whitley, E.M.; Dey, P.; Hou, P.; et al. Telomere dysfunction activates Yap1 to drive tissue inflammation. *Nat. Commun.* **2020**, *11*, 4766. [CrossRef]
18. Liu, S.; Nong, W.; Ji, L.; Zhuge, X.; Wei, H.; Luo, M.; Zhou, L.; Chen, S.; Zhang, S.; Lei, X.; et al. The regulatory feedback of inflammatory signaling and telomere/telomerase complex dysfunction in chronic inflammatory diseases. *Exp. Gerontol.* **2023**, *174*, 112132. [CrossRef]
19. Cawthon, R.M. Telomere measurement by quantitative PCR. *Nucleic Acids Res.* **2002**, *30*, e47. [CrossRef]

20. Gedvilaite, G.; Vilkeviciute, A.; Kriauciuniene, L.; Banevičius, M.; Liutkeviciene, R. The relationship between leukocyte telomere length and TERT, TRF1 single nucleotide polymorphisms in healthy people of different age groups. *Biogerontology* **2020**, *21*, 57–67. [CrossRef]
21. Livak, K.J.; Schmittgen, T.D. Analysis of relative gene expression data using real-time quantitative PCR and the $2^{-\Delta\Delta CT}$ Method. *Methods* **2001**, *25*, 402–408. [CrossRef] [PubMed]
22. Gedvilaite, G.; Kriauciuniene, L.; Tamasauskas, A.; Liutkeviciene, R. The Influence of Telomere-Related Gene Variants, Serum Levels, and Relative Leukocyte Telomere Length in Pituitary Adenoma Occurrence and Recurrence. *Cancers* **2024**, *16*, 643. [CrossRef] [PubMed]
23. Wigginton, J.E.; Cutler, D.J.; Abecasis, G.R. A note on exact tests of Hardy-Weinberg equilibrium. *Am. J. Hum. Genet.* **2005**, *76*, 887–893. [CrossRef] [PubMed]
24. Birch, J.; Victorelli, S.; Rahmatika, D.; Anderson, R.K.; Jiwa, K.; Moisey, E.; Ward, C.; Fisher, A.J.; Soyza, A.D.; Passos, J.F. Telomere dysfunction and senescence-associated pathways in bronchiectasis. *Am. J. Respir. Crit. Care Med.* **2016**, *193*, 929–932. [CrossRef] [PubMed]
25. Hjelmborg, J.B.; Dalgård, C.; Möller, S.; Steenstrup, T.; Kimura, M.; Christensen, K.; Kyvik, K.O.; Aviv, A. The heritability of leucocyte telomere length dynamics. *J. Med. Genet.* **2015**, *52*, 297–302. [CrossRef] [PubMed]
26. Gardner, M.; Bann, D.; Wiley, L.; Cooper, R.; Hardy, R.; Nitsch, D.; Martin-Ruiz, C.; Shiels, P.; Sayer, A.A.; Barbieri, M.; et al. Gender and telomere length: Systematic review and meta-analysis. *Exp. Gerontol.* **2014**, *51*, 15–27. [CrossRef] [PubMed]
27. Balcer, L.J. Clinical practice. Optic neuritis. *N. Engl. J. Med.* **2006**, *354*, 1273–1280. [CrossRef]
28. Kim, S.M.; Waters, P.; Woodhall, M.; Kim, Y.J.; Kim, J.A.; Cheon, S.Y.; Lee, S.; Jo, S.R.; Kim, D.G.; Jung, K.C.; et al. Gender effect on neuromyelitis optica spectrum disorder with aquaporin4-immunoglobulin G. *Mult. Scler. J.* **2017**, *23*, 1104–1111. [CrossRef]
29. Bekaert, S.; De Meyer, T.; Rietzschel, E.R.; De Buyzere, M.L.; De Bacquer, D.; Langlois, M.; Segers, P.; Cooman, L.; Van Damme, P.; Cassiman, P.; et al. Telomere length and cardiovascular risk factors in a middle-aged population free of overt cardiovascular disease. *Aging Cell* **2007**, *6*, 639–647. [CrossRef]
30. Costello, F.; Hodge, W.; Pan, Y.I.; Burton, J.M.; Freedman, M.S.; Stys, P.K.; Trufyn, J.; Kardon, R. Sex-specific differences in retinal nerve fiber layer thinning after acute optic neuritis. *Neurology* **2012**, *79*, 1866–1872. [CrossRef]
31. Benson, V.S.; Kirichek, O.; Beral, V.; Green, J. Menopausal hormone therapy and central nervous system tumor risk: Large UK prospective study and meta-analysis. *Int. J. Cancer* **2015**, *136*, 2369–2377. [CrossRef] [PubMed]
32. Gold, S.M.; Voskuhl, R.R. Estrogen treatment in multiple sclerosis. *J. Neurol. Sci.* **2009**, *286*, 99–103. [CrossRef] [PubMed]
33. Deschênes, M.C.; Descovich, D.; Moreau, M.; Granger, L.; Kuchel, G.A.; Mikkola, T.S.; Fick, G.H.; Chemtob, S.; Vaucher, E.; Lesk, M.R. Postmenopausal hormone therapy increases retinal blood flow and protects the retinal nerve fiber layer. *Investig. Ophthalmol. Vis. Sci.* **2010**, *51*, 2587–2600. [CrossRef] [PubMed]
34. Giordano, C.; Montopoli, M.; Perli, E.; Orlandi, M.; Fantin, M.; Ross-Cisneros, F.N.; Caparrotta, L.; Martinuzzi, A.; Ragazzi, E.; Ghelli, A.; et al. Oestrogens ameliorate mitochondrial dysfunction in Leber's hereditary optic neuropathy. *Brain* **2011**, *134 Pt 1*, 220–234. [CrossRef] [PubMed]
35. Espinosa-Otalora, R.E.; Flórez-Villamizar, J.; Esteban-Pérez, C.I.; Forero-Castro, M.; Marín-Suarez, J. Lifestyle Effects on Telomeric Shortening as a Factor Associated with Biological Aging: A Systematic Review. *Nutr. Healthy Aging* **2021**, *6*, 95–103. [CrossRef]
36. Habib, R.; Ocklenburg, S.; Hoffjan, S.; Haghikia, A.; Epplen, J.T.; Arning, L. Association between shorter leukocyte telomeres and multiple sclerosis. *J. Neuroimmunol.* **2020**, *341*, 577187. [CrossRef] [PubMed]
37. Krysko, K.M.; Henry, R.G.; Cree, B.A.; Lin, J.; University of California, San Francisco MS-EPIC Team; Caillier, S.; Santaniello, A.; Zhao, C.; Gomez, R.; Bevan, C.; et al. Telomere length is associated with disability progression in multiple sclerosis. *Ann. Neurol.* **2019**, *86*, 671–682. [CrossRef] [PubMed]
38. Barnes, R.P.; Fouquerel, E.; Opresko, P.L. The impact of oxidative DNA damage and stress on telomere homeostasis. *Mech. Ageing Dev.* **2019**, *177*, 37–45. [CrossRef] [PubMed]
39. Gavia-García, G.; Rosado-Pérez, J.; Arista-Ugalde, T.L.; Aguiñiga-Sánchez, I.; Santiago-Osorio, E.; Mendoza-Núñez, V.M. Telomere Length and Oxidative Stress and Its Relation with Metabolic Syndrome Components in the Aging. *Biology* **2021**, *10*, 253. [CrossRef]
40. Reichert, S.; Stier, A. Does oxidative stress shorten telomeres in vivo? A review. *Biol. Lett.* **2017**, *13*, 20170463. [CrossRef]
41. Kordinas, V.; Ioannidis, A.; Chatzipanagiotou, S. The Telomere/Telomerase System in Chronic Inflammatory Diseases. Cause or Effect? *Genes* **2016**, *7*, 60. [CrossRef] [PubMed]

Journal of
Clinical Medicine

MDPI

Review

Retinal Ganglion Cell Replacement in Glaucoma Therapy: A Narrative Review

Ewa Kosior-Jarecka [1,*] and Andrzej Grzybowski [2]

1 Department of Diagnostics and Microsurgery of Glaucoma, Medical University of Lublin, 20-079 Lublin, Poland
2 Institute for Research in Ophthalmology, Foundation for Ophthalmology Development, 60-836 Poznan, Poland; ae.grzybowski@gmail.com
* Correspondence: ewakosiorjarecka@umlub.pl

Abstract: Glaucoma is a leading cause of irreversible blindness worldwide. It leads to the progressive degeneration of retinal ganglion cells (RGCs), the axons of which form the optic nerve. Enormous RGC apoptosis causes a lack of transfer of visual information to the brain. The RGC loss typical of the central nervous system is irreversible, and when glaucoma progresses, the total amount of RGCs in the retina enormously diminishes. The successful treatment in glaucoma patients is a direct neuroprotection by decreasing the intraocular pressure, which enables RGC protection but does not revive the lost ones. The intriguing new therapy for advanced glaucoma is the possibility of RGC replacement with new healthy cells. In this review article, the strategies regarding RGC replacement therapy are presented with the latest advances in the technique and the obstacles that it meets.

Keywords: glaucoma; retinal ganglion cells; replacement theraphy

1. Introduction

Glaucoma is one of the leading causes of blindness worldwide, which will affect 111.8 million people by 2040 [1,2]. It is a neurodegenerative disorder characterized by selective, progressive degeneration of the retinal ganglion cells (RGCs) and as a result, also the optic nerve (ON) [3]. The glaucomatous degeneration of the ON results in cupping, a characteristic appearance of the optic nerve head (ONH) observed in the eye fundus and the gradual deterioration in the visual field (VF), which leads to irreversible visual loss. The biological background of glaucoma is not fully understood, and the factors contributing to its progression have not yet been sufficiently characterized [4]. Glaucoma remains undiagnosed for many years until the advanced stages of its prolonged asymptomatic course. Additionally, it takes many years from the disease's initial stages to the first typical changes in the visual field. There is some risk factors identified for glaucoma with elevated intraocular pressure (IOP) as the only one that is modifiable. It is highly proven that decreasing the IOP slows down the disease progression. However, an elevated IOP may remain increased for many years in patients, not causing glaucomatous damage and, on the other hand, there are patients with a low IOP and advanced glaucoma [5].

Although the primary site of glaucomatous injury is not fully clear, the disease leads to a progressive degeneration of the RGCs with their somas and dendrites located in the retina and axons forming the optic nerve [6]. The location of the RGCs in the retina is crucial for understanding the possibilities and difficulties facing replacement therapy. The human retina contains six main neural layers, three of which contain cell somas: the outer nuclear layer (ONL), the inner nuclear layer (INL), and the retinal ganglion cell layer (GCL). The ONL contains the rod and cone photoreceptors; the INL comprises three distinct populations of interneurons: the bipolar cells, the horizontal cells and the amacrine cells; the inner layer of the retina (GCL) is where the RGCs are localized [6]. The distinct retinal layers are well distinguishable in the scans obtained via optical coherent tomography (OCT) [Figure 1].

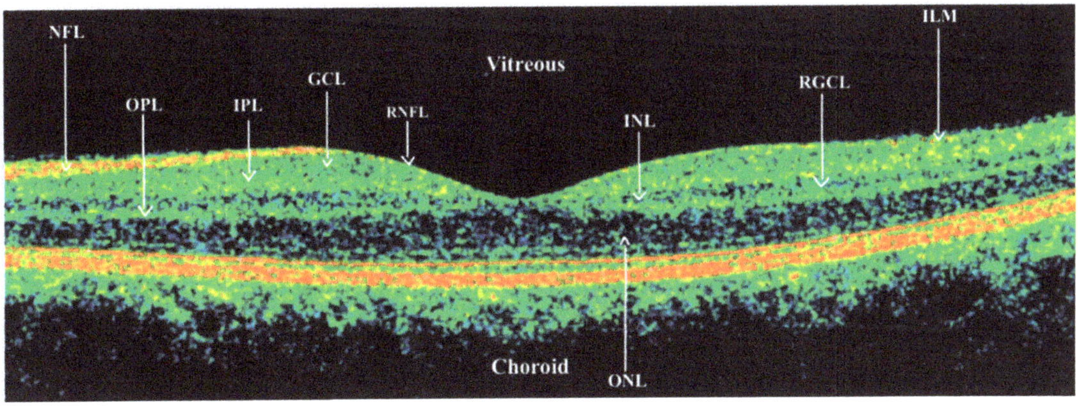

Figure 1. Linear scan obtained using OCT technique from healthy subject in the macular region with marked retinal layers (obtained using Zeiss Cirrus 6000, Carl Zeiss Meditech, Warsaw, Poland). ONL—outer nuclear layer; OPL—outer plexus layer; INL—inner nuclear layer; IPL—inner plexus layer; RGCL—retinal ganglion cell layer; RNFL—retinal nerve fiber layer; ILM—internal limiting membrane.

2. Retinal Ganglion Cells

RGCs are larger than most of the other retinal neurons, and their dendrites obtain inputs from all the preceding retinal neurons initializing the visual pathway. Their large-diameter axons transmit the visual signal to the related areas of the brain, located far away from the RGC somas. In the retina, RGC axons converge toward the center, where they form the ON starting at the ONH; the nerve passes the information to the brain centers, mainly the lateral geniculate nuclei in the thalamus, and to a lesser extent to the suprachiasmatic nuclei, the superior colliculi, and other pretectal nuclei. These highly complex and unique connections develop during RGC axon growth, which enables the forming of synapses toward the appropriate target cells [6].

RGCs function as the only output neurons transporting the visual information from the retina to the specific targets in the brain. However, they are also involved in the early processing of visual information. RGCs extract in parallel different attributes of the image: spatial contrast, flicker, color, fine details, motion, absolute light level, and coarse textures [7,8]. Moreover, RGCs are not a homogeneous population; for example, in mice, up to 40 subtypes of RGCs have been differentiated according to the multiple visual functions. The mechanisms underlying this diversity are still not clearly understood [7,9,10]. Each RGC subtype is responsible for the distinct features of the visual transmission to the central brain targets [11]. Moreover, RGC subtypes differ in their capacities to survive and to regenerate after injury [12,13]. The RGC dysfunction or death during glaucoma may cause irreversible blindness because the surviving RGCs are not able to regenerate [13].

During embryogenesis, RGCs are the first cells arising from retinal progenitor cells (RPCs), which are a multipotent cell type that further differentiate into seven cell subtypes forming the neural retina: cone and rod photoreceptors, horizontal, bipolar, and amacrine interneurons, the cell bodies of radial Müller glia and RGCs [14].

RGCs in Glaucoma Pathogenesis

Since RGCs are thought to be the one of the possible sites of primary injury leading to glaucoma, their repair and replacement have been identified as a crucial target for visual function restoration which could be an effective treatment of the disease. The pathology of glaucoma involves a lot of different cellular processes related to RGCs such as axonal degeneration and the degeneration of dendritic arbors and neuron soma [15]. The degeneration of RGC axons in glaucoma injures the transport of the information to the brain, leading to the loss of the input from the visual pathway in the anterograde direction and the subsequent RGC death, which finally leads to the irreversible loss of vision.

During early glaucoma, a causative harmful factor leads to RGC dysfunction and the activation of the glial cells in the retina and ON. It is believed that at this stage of glaucoma, possible neuroprotective strategies may concentrate on restoring the normal homeostasis between injured RGCs and their environment. As the disease progresses, the subsequent early degenerative events include the remodeling of the cytoskeletal and synaptic structures throughout the RGC projection and increased inflammatory signaling from resident glial cells. At this early stage, possible neuroprotective therapies are thought to repair the damage, which probably remains still reversible at the cellular and molecular level and aim to decrease the level of inflammation to prevent additional damage. Ongoing glaucoma includes the irreversible loss of RGCs and their axons with glial scarring in the ON, which constitutes the obstacle to axonal regeneration. Therefore, at late stages, neuroregenerative and replacement therapies to restore visual function are needed [16].

In some cases, neuroprotective treatment may protect RGCs before the occurrence of apoptosis. The strategy of having a neuroprotective potential has been broadly proven in a plethora of multicenter studies focused on decreasing the IOP. However, RGC regenerative or enhancing strategies with IOP decline or the possible application of direct neurotrophic factors cannot be a viable solution for many patients with advanced glaucoma. In such cases, only cell replacement therapy replenishing the lost RGCs can constitute a treatment option providing vision restoration. However, RGCs are incapable of self-renewal, so the replacement of injured RGCs with healthy cells has always been a proper therapeutic target [17,18].

Therapeutic strategies that support visual restoration have focused on protecting RGCs from degeneration, promoting RGC and axon regeneration after injury, and reestablishing their correct projection relationships [13]. However, every part of this strategy meets obstacles when preserving/restoring RGCs and regenerating their axons are considered using the following approaches: (1) increase the RGC survival or supplement the retina with new RGCs, (2) overcome the inhibitory potential of the optic nerve environment for neurogenesis, (3) enhance/create RGC axon growth, and (4) create the right RGC connections with their typical targets in the brain [19]. Vision restoration at the translational level in clinics has been hindered by several challenges such as the source of the stem cells, differentiation into appropriate cell types, transplantation approaches, survival, and the functional integration of cells into the target retina. Additionally, to establish functional neuronal connectivity, an optimal microenvironment mediated by the trophic factors is crucial. Similarly, the survival of the transplanted cells also depends on a healthy retinal microenvironment [20].

Moreover, the problem with the restoration of vision is that it requires transplanted RGCs to grow normally functioning axons which could extend beyond the ONH, their remyelination by oligodendrocytes, and the proper guidance toward the terminals in the CNS where new synaptic formation should occur. RGCs do not act as an isolated unit; their function relies on cells' both intrinsic and extrinsic factors changing during glaucoma to determine the cell fate. In fact, RGCs rely on numerous cell populations for survival in the visual pathway. The latest research showed that astrocytes straightaway take action to deliver neuroprotection during stress by using alternative metabolic resources [16].

On the other hand, neuroprotective strategies with the application of transplanted cells which defend the endogenous neural tissue have demonstrated encouraging outcomes in animal models of some retinal disorders (reviewed in [21]). Initial studies transplanting hippocampus-derived neural progenitor cells into the retina showed some structural integration. Grafting these cells into mature rodent eyes after iatrogenic retinal scarring or ischemia-reperfusion insult, evolved donor neurite integration and the cellular expression of microtubule-associated protein 2 (MAP2) and glial fibrillary acidic protein (GFAP) [22]. These findings provide initial evidence for the possibility of the therapeutic application of cell transplantation within the inner retina. Since then, studies have been accomplished evaluating the intravitreal transplantation of different cell types, including embryonic stem cells (ESCs), Müller glial-derived cells, mesenchymal stem cells (MSCs), and primary or stem cell-derived RGCs [23]. The possible neuroprotective pathway of action may involve the secretion of trophic factors and/or the modulation of inflammatory processes. Moreover, cell transplantation may improve the endogenous repair mechanisms via the enhancement of inhibitory signals to encourage axonal regeneration and neuritic growth [24].

Although encouraging, the progression from the initial basic research studies to functional and clinically relevant RGC transplantation requires more steps toward a significant increase in the efficacy of the integration of transplanted neurons within the retina [23]. Below, we review the most important achievements in the dynamically evolving field of RGS transplantation. A lot has been achieved; however, still a lot needs to be addressed to apply these results to restore the vision of blind glaucoma patients. Unfortunately, nowadays, there are neither neuroprotective nor axogenic therapies capable of restoring lost visual pathway connectivity in degenerative retinal disease nor translatable techniques to replace the lost RGCs and photoreceptors [25].

3. Source of Cells for Transplantation

The RGC is incapable of self-renewal, so the only possible treatment is the replacement of injured RGCs with healthy cells. One of the crucial questions that endures in cell transplantation is whether to use allogeneic or autologous cell sources for the derivation of cell therapy products.

The first idea that comes to mind is allogeneic RGC transplantation, which has been considered in research isolating RGCs from the retinas of recently deceased persons for transplantation into patients [26]. However, RGC transplantation therapy needs a more sufficient and possibly a more vigorous source of healthy RGCs to become an applicable treatment option [27]. Previous RGC transplantation research has produced diverse outcomes and success (reviewed in [28]), but thus far, unfortunately, has resulted in narrow clinical application. The inconsistency in transplantation efficacy may be the result of the availability and purity of a reliable donor cell source, the diversity in a tested host and graft species, and the mode of cell delivery [28].

In a relatively new branch of studies, allogeneic stem cells can be arranged not to have the Human Leukocyte Antigen (HLA) genes, which make them "cloaked" to the host immunological system. According to this theory, one donor could be the source of blindness-reversing treatments for a lot of patients. These involve stem cells obtained from blastocysts—human embryonic stem cells (hESCs) or induced pluripotent stem cells (iPSCs). Such strategy passes the exam in the case of retinal pigment epithelial (RPE) cells: hESC-derived RPE cells were the first pluripotent stem cell-derived RPE cells transplanted into the eyes of patients [29].

In contrast, autologous cell sources focus on the application of the patient's own cells. First, the patient's own retinal cells with the potential for regeneration could be used. Troeppe et al. showed that adults' retinal stem cells may be found in the pigmented ciliary margin, indicating that they are homologous to the cells found in the ocular germinal zone of other nonmammalian vertebrates [30]. However, there is a lack of evidence showing that they can replace damaged RGCs. In fish and amphibians, similar cells are located in the poorly differentiated ciliary marginal zone and are responsible for providing the recruitment of cells to the growing retina and are involved in the regeneration of the injured retina. In mammals, this region is represented by a limited number of cells localized in the ora serrata [31].

Of the endogenous retinal stem cells, Müller glia were successfully induced to dedifferentiate into RPCs able to transform into multiple retinal phenotypes. Ciliary epithelial-derived stem cells are multipotential and self-renewing retinal RPCs which may be obtained from the pigmented ciliary epithelium of the retina with the potential for differentiation in vitro into photoreceptors. The RPE layer is able to generate the remaining layers to create new retina in some animals and, in humans, contains a tiny group of stem cells that can differentiate into new RPE cells and cells with a neuronal phenotype. Transplantation and manipulation within endogenous retinal stem cells have the capability to cure retinal degeneration; however, their application is probably restricted to RPE and photoreceptor replacement therapies. RGC replacement seems to be much more refractory to such strategies [23].

Studies undertaken on whole eye specimens or on vitreous samples obtained during vitrectomy showed that human non-pigmented ciliary epithelium cells (NPCECs) proliferate within the vitreous base in the proliferative vitreoretinopathy [32]. Too et al. described the spontaneous formation of cells migrating from human equatorial retinal explants obtained during vitrectomy for retinal detachment. These migrating cells, probably derived from human equatorial Müller cells, expressed markers suggesting that they re-entered a cell cycle. Such retinal explants are plentiful in retinal units, which may be a promising source of RPCs [33]. Additionally, some studies have proved that mammalian Muller cells have the ability to reprogram into a proliferative progenitor-like state via the application of diverse intervention methods [34]. Some studies reported that NPCECs can differentiate into ganglion, amacrine, and Muller glia cells [35]. Moreover, NPCECs' secretome may induce RGC differentiation in vitro, and TGF-beta 1 is one of the neurotrophic factors pivotal in this process [36].

Since RGCs differentiate straight from stem cells, it may offer a promising area for research to introduce RGCs derived from stem cells, which constitutes a new attitude with an ample source of RGCs efficiently available for replacement therapy [20]. Stem cells are defined as undifferentiated cells with the ability of proliferating, self-renewal, and reproducing identical multipotent stem cells indefinitely in their undifferentiated state and being able to produce one or more differentiated cell types [27]. They constitute one of the possible therapeutic strategies to be applied if tissue repair and regeneration is required, and one of such cases is glaucoma [37]. The studies on RGC-ablated mouse models showed that stem cells transplanted into the retina could survive, differentiate into an RGC lineage, and to some extent integrate into the GCL to refine the visual function [20]. In addition, the derivation of RGCs from stem cells is a promising modality in restoring vision when the transplanted stem cells are able to express RGC-specific proteins and to develop some of the RGC morphology features [27].

Two types of stem cells may be found in humans: ESCs found in blastocysts and adult stem cells or pluripotent cells that can be found in a wide variety of adult tissues. The stem cells may also be obtained by inducing mature cells to re-differentiate into the pluripotent status via molecular manipulation and are then called iPSCs. Most iPSCs are manufactured via the application of viruses (lentiviruses and retroviruses) carrying the genes responsible for the transcription factors needed in adult cells for modification. These genes will then enable transcription and translation into a protein initializing the mature cell nucleus to acquire an embryonic state [37].

In vivo, the differentiation of stem cells into RGCs is regulated by several transcription factors such as Brn3, Ath5, and Notch. Brn3 and Ath5 play a pivotal part in the differentiation of RGCs, and their levels increase during eye development [38]. Notch is a negative regulator of RGC differentiation with decreased levels during normal eye development. The addition of Brn3, Ath5, and the Notch antagonist is one of the applied strategies to obtain RGCs from stem cells [14]. Additionally, the studies identified various neurotrophic pathways and the differentiation of stem cells into RGCs consisting of fibroblast growth factor, insulin-like growth factor [39], bone morphogenetic protein, nodal, and Wnt signaling pathways [37,40].

The research on stem cell technologies has made rapid progress, from the isolation and culture methods of ESCs to the remarkable improvement of the methods of the differentiation of pluripotent cells into retinal lineages in vitro [6].

3.1. Embryonic Stem Cells

ESCs are capable of indefinite proliferation by following the cycles of the natural development and differentiate into any cell types of all three germ layers (ectoderm, mesoderm, and endoderm). Recent studies have reported the successful production of human RGCs from hESCs [27].

A few groups have attempted to transplant different types of RPCs into rodent eyes with rather poor results because of insufficient survival and limited evidence of functional RGC replacement. In preclinical studies, RPCs obtained from hESCs were able to integrate into the murine GCL and expressed the RGC marker Brn3a, and an increase in ONL thickness was detected [41]. RGCs derived from mice ESCs and transplanted into the eyes of recipient mice, that had performed the previous NMDA-mediated depletion of endogenous RGCs, were able to survive for at least 12 weeks, grow long neurites that laminated within the IP, and formed synaptic structures [42]. HESC-derived RGCs transplanted into rodent eyes have been reported to localize to the GCL. However, these cells were not able to grow neurites and to express RNA binding protein. Recently, a crucial study showed moderate success in transplanting primary mouse RGCs into rodent eyes, describing quite rare instances of mature RGC morphology, visible synaptogenesis, and functional electrophysiologic responses to light despite an insufficient survival rate [23]. In another study on non-human primates, the subretinal transplantation of retinal organoids obtained from hESCs was well tolerated, and the transplanted cells were found to be integrating into the retinal injury site after laser ablation [41].

Despite the vast promises of hESCs' application, the possible risk related to the formation of tumors and ethical arguments regarding the usage of human embryos are the typical concerns that constrain their application at the moment. Moreover, the development of iPSC technology has caused a reduction in the use of hESCs [27].

3.2. Induced Pluripotent Stem Cells

In 2006, Takahashi and Yamanaka [43] published their study in which mouse and adult fibroblasts were successfully reprogrammed into a pluripotent state after the application of specific transcription factors (Oct3/4, Klf4, Sox2, and c-Myc) delivered thanks to transfection mediated by the retroviruses. The cells obtained as the result of this modification, iPSCs, were able to form colonies morphologically similar to ESCs and with the potential for differentiation into three germ layer cell lineages. Since iPSCs could be obtained by reprogramming of the patient's somatic cells, the individual genomic information could be maintained [43,44]. It was a breakthrough in the field of stem cell research since these patient-derived iPSCs may be used as an ideal in vitro model for the studies on genetic diseases, and thus, they may in future have a favorable role in the work on personalized treatment without the need for using embryos [45]. Potential non retinal-derived mature stem cell-derived strategies which have evolved as a cure for retinal degeneration include NSCs and MSCs obtained from either bone marrow, dental pulp, or adipose tissues [25]. There have been many advancements in the technology applied for generating and manipulating iPSCs. The derivation of iPSCs from somatic cells has made them an encouraging therapeutic option in regenerative medicine without the risk of immunological rejection [27]. Additionally, the application of viral vectors to enable the introduction of the reprogramming factors was substituted by non-viral methods, such as plasmid, protein, and miRNA as new vectors to deliver the transcription factors without the possible risk of the subsequent mutagenesis of the recipient cells. Other studies showed that the addition of small molecules, such as valproic acid, butyrate, AZA5-aza-cytidine, vitamin C, MEK inhibitor, transforming growth factor-β receptor inhibitor, ROCK inhibitor, and GSK3β inhibitor could increase the reprogramming efficacy and finally replace the application of certain transcription factors in the methods of obtaining iPSCs [44]. Moreover, the number of reprogramming factors was reduced, making the process more effective and cost-minimal [45].

In recent years, iPSCs have been broadly studied for neurological diseases mainly because of the limited possibilities to study the human brain directly. iPSCs can be directly obtained from patients with specific neurological diseases (such as Parkinson's disease, Alzheimer's disease (AD) [46]. In glaucoma, recent research has shown that human iPSCs have the potential to differentiate into RGCs. For example, in their studies, Li et al. [47] forced human iPSCs to create a three-dimensional (3D) retina [48]. Afterwards, the RGCs were generated from this human iPSC-derived neural retina. Additionally, Tanaka et al. [49] obtained self-induced RGCs with growing axons from human iPSCs. Moreover, lately, there have been reports showing the successes in the production of human RGCs from human pluripotent stem cells and human Tenon's capsule fibroblast-derived iPSCs [27].

On the basis of transcriptome profiles, a few iPSC-RGC subtypes have been distinguished. It was possible to obtain the transcriptomes of all iPSC-RGCs from typical iPSCs without the need for additional gene manipulation, but they may be different during the development or maturation of specific cells. These differences in gene expression may be used as potential biomarkers for the classification of RGC subsets. It is possible that understanding the RGC diversity will help to identify the different RGC subtypes with the possibly different susceptibility to degeneration or an injury during the subsequent stages of glaucoma and/or optic neuropathies, and consequently, the identification of RGC subpopulations susceptible or resistant to ON injury may enable the planning of precise and individual treatment strategies [46].

RGCs differentiated from human iPSCs were reported to survive for 5 months post-transplantation, migrate into the endogenous RGC layer, and extend "wild type like" dendritic arbors into the IPL [42]. Johnson et al. [42] performed electrophysiology in five of six iPSC-RGCs and demonstrated the response to full-field photopic light stimuli. However, the RGC response to the light stimulus is driven by photoreceptors or may come from melanopsin-expressing RGCs themselves. The natures and kinetics of both types of responses significantly differ, with the melanopsin-driven one being much slower in origin and recovery. Surprisingly, in the case of hiPSC-RGCs, the exposure to light created a distinct rise in their firing rate, which declined to the basic values in less than a second after the light was extinguished. Such kinetics are not similar to the typical kinetics of melanopsin-driven responses, so hiPSC-RGC responses should be classified as photoreceptor-driven [28]. The efficiency of transplanted RGC integration suggests normal synaptic connectivity to the inner retinal plexus [42].

Stem cell differentiation is a complex and slow process, and as a consequence, the obtaining of RGC-like cells from stem cells constitutes a real barrier when stem cell-based therapies of glaucoma are considered. To demonstrate this problem, lots of different factors need consideration: more than forty diverse RGC subtypes have been described without clear features enabling one to distinguish them from other types of neurons, but also in vitro-obtained RGCs do not have specific signature characteristics helping to distinguish them from other neurons. Moreover, there are neither definitive proteins or RNAs that are entirely expressed in RGCs nor distinct electrophysiological features to discern RGCs from other neurons. Therefore, a lot of scientific discoveries are required to be made before RGC creation becomes a process that can enable the delivery of effective RGC differentiation methods [28].

Additionally, some ethical concerns regarding the application of iPSCs are pointed out. The usage of iPSCs for research and therapeutical reasons could cause inequity in the access to healthcare, as nowadays the technology to produce and apply these cells remains high-priced and not broadly accessible [45]. Moreover, there are discussions about the limitation of genetic diversity, which jeopardizes the fairness and may hinder the pace of biological breakthroughs. There is also the possibility of the iPSC application in controversial sectors, such as the creation of genetically modified organisms or human cloning [45].

The advantages and disadvantages of the different sources of RGCs are summed up in Table 1.

Table 1. The advantages and disadvantages of the different sources of RGCSs.

Source of RGC	Advantages	Disadvantages
Emryogenic stem cells	• Extensive proliferative and differentiation potential • Follow the natural process of differentiation	• Possible tumor formation risk • Ethical considerations (using human embryos) • Long-life immunomodulation
Induced pluripotent cells	• Pluripotent differentiation ability • Possible cell modifications • No immunomodulation needed after transplantation	• Ethical considerations (human cloning and genetic modification)

3.3. *Two-Dimensional (2D) Cell Culture and Three-Dimensional (3D) Organoid*

The differentiation and the culture of iPSCs resemble the normal development of the eye [44]. At the beginning, the embryoid bodies (EBs) are established with later OV-like structures or neurosphere formation. EBs are cellular aggregates containing a combination of ectodermal, mesodermal, and endodermal cells, which reflect the three germ layers. OV-like structures or neurospheres are proliferative cellular aggregates of neural progenitor cells differentiating later into neurons or glia. Initially, research showed that the dynamic behavior and critical development of the checkpoints in RGC induction are crucial in the confirmation that the RGCs have established a lineage and followed the typical stages of eye development [44]. The most ubiquitous type of cell culture created during the studies is the 2D culturing system, which involves single-layer cell growth on a flat surface [50]. The application of iPSCs in 2D culture may give insights into the processes connected with neurotransmission within the CNS, and the differentiation of particular cells such as astrocytes, neurons, and microglia [51] subsequently enables a better understanding of the molecular and genetic conditions of neurological diseases [52].

Although the 2D type of cell culturing is broadly used and constitutes an important tool in basic science studies, in fact its role in disease modeling is rather limited since it does not correctly reflect the communications between cells, the dynamic situation of the in vivo environment, and organ- and tissue-level complexity in detail. The reason for this is that 2D cultures have the ability, so far, to differentiate into only one cell type in such mono-layer system [45]. It additionally causes an artificial behavior of these cells, such as atypical proliferation and/or differentiation, and decreased cellular interaction compared to in vivo conditions [53,54]. In spite of these above-mentioned limitations, 2D cell culturing constitutes a useful laboratory method, which has been significantly improved in recent years via the techniques for analyzing and characterizing cells, such as high-content imaging and transcriptomics, which in turn enable more detailed studies on the characteristics of cultured cells [45,55,56].

The conventional 2D cultures have been developed for the attachment and proliferation of iPSCs. On the other hand, the three-dimensional (3D) culture system has become more popular, thanks to its capacity to self-organize. Additionally, it does not need so many extrinsic growth factors, and the intrinsic pattern seems to resemble the normal development of the eye. The used 3D culture techniques involve the suspension of the culture and then cell encapsulation in gels and further cell culturing in the scaffolds [44]. Organoids are 3D structures obtained from stem cells or tissue explants that can self-organize into structures similar to specific organs. They can display the complexity of cellular configurations, structural orientations, and actions resembling normal in vivo tissue, comprising various cell types, and may be used to investigate disease modeling, organ development, and drug screening [45]. The 3D culture of iPSCs allows for self-organization of the earliest eye structure. These structures include optic vesicles and optic cups, which finally become retinal lineages with photoreceptors, RPE cells, and RGCs within the structure. Under such culture conditions, different retinal cell types are generated, and later organize into a typical retinal layout. Unfortunately, the large-scale culturing or enrichment of specific retinal cells (i.e., RGCs) still seems to be limited [57]. Early retinal organoids (8–12 weeks after induction) include all the types of retinal cells and layers, which can be found in a typically developing human fetal retina [58].

As in normal human developing retinas, rod photoreceptors are far more frequent than the RGC-like cells. The average number of such RGC-like cells has been evaluated to be 0.1–30% of the total cell count. Moreover, the number of RGC-like cells tends to decline with time, which is comprehensible knowing that early RGCs undergo two apoptosis cycles in normal development. During this period, RGCs are strictly dependent on brain trophic support, which is not present in organoid cultures [59].

The usage of both ESCs and iPSCs has shown the capacity for differentiation into 3D retinal organoids [60,61], and thus, retinal organoid techniques could establish the main approach in transplantation studies [58], as recent research efforts have successfully shown [62,63]. To delineate the contribution of distinct signaling pathways of RGC differentiation, Dorgau et al. [64] studied the influence of Laminin c3 in RGC differentiation in retinal organoids obtained from hPSCs. Other studies evaluated RGCs obtained from 3D retinal organoids as RGC transplantation media [65]. Summarizing, retinal organoids are now a promising direction in the studies, and hopefully, one day, scientists will find solutions for overcoming the problems with RGC replacement strategies, and result in vision restoration methods [58]. However, comprehensive, effective, and safe protocols for organoid manipulation are waiting to be developed to produce RGCs in large quantities and to be applied in human therapies [27].

The viability and gaining the function via transplanted cells are crucial to the success and effectivity of cell transplantation within the transplanted microenvironment [66]. It has been shown that the application of 2D or 3D tissue-engineered scaffolds constitutes an effective strategy to defeat the limitations of cell transplantation since cell suspension seems to have a smaller immune advantage for substrates provided as a whole structure. Additionally, the total differentiation and correct integrity of the supporting material may be mentioned as further advantages of the scaffold application. Tissue-engineered scaffolds may provide a physical base for cell transportation, viability, and integration [67]. So, the scaffold application as a cell transportation mode shows a promising way to achieve success in cell transplant strategies in the therapy of glaucoma and other retinal degenerative disorders [68]. This is because the scaffolds are able to create the natural microenvironment typical for neural tissues, and as a consequence, help in the restoration of broken axonal connections and the RGC replacement [27,69].

4. Application of RGCs to the Donor's Retina

4.1. *Scaffold Material*

All the cell replacement strategies need the transplanted cells to relocate from the distribution site to their final location within the recipient organism. However, RGC replacement therapy encounters specific obstacles: RGCs delivered to the eye need to penetrate within the retina, connect with bipolar and amacrine cells on one site, and connect via axons with the specific targets in the brain [70]. Success critically depends on the survival of the delivered cells, maintenance of their phenotype, and their integration within the proper tissue [70]. The low cell viability and engraftment rates at the transplant location and problems with the maintaining of the injected cells in a targeted area remain the major challenge. It is pivotal to find a scaffold for RGC delivery that additionally enhances regeneration. Without a structural base in the retina, the delivered cells will miss cell–cell and cell–substrate support, which will promote excessive apoptosis. The surviving cells would not have a matrix to be structurally laid out in and would usually migrate from the correct place to nearby host tissue [71]. So, there are attempts to discover an ideal cell-carrier scaffold for transplanted cells which could enhance the ability of RGC delivery, planting newly created dendrites into the IPL, producing axons toward the ONH, and regenerating axons for places a distance away [68]. Moreover, these biopolymeric scaffolds should enhance the guidance of the RGC radial growth from the ONH to the brain [27,72]. An ideal scaffold material would increase the cell viability but disappear within a specific time without inducing an inflammatory reaction harmful for the graft fates [68]. Unfortunately, the studies show that the outer retina environment is unfavorable for the viability of transplanted RGCs [24,27].

Typically, the grafted cells are distributed to the target location in a buffered saline solution (BSS). Questions remain as to whether the cells obtain sufficient chemical and physical stimuli to promote therapeutic success, and whether the cells stay at the target location for enough time to anchor and become integrated within the host tissue [73]. For ocular applications, the biomaterial substitute of BSS should be injectable but simultaneously be able to transform into a solid material in vivo. Lots of hydrogels have such potential; however, only a few can perform spontaneous covalent cross-linking in situ to enable the right control of the degradation rate, gelation, and mechanical behavior [74].

Many biomaterials may help in sustaining the planned cell phenotype, differentiation, and proliferation [75]. However, another discussive and difficult point in RGC replacement attempts is the diversity between the conditions of the in vitro culture and in vivo systems. The cells in the lab grow in the ideal culture conditions to achieve the highest survival rate; after transplantation, in vivo, the cells encounter challenging degenerative conditions. If RGCs undergo successful encapsulation within the gels, they become provided with a 3D protective microenvironment protecting them from the direct exposure to the hostile host tissue conditions [71].

A lot of biopolymer materials, mostly carrying the functional ester group, have been studied as a scaffold for the monolayers obtained from stem cells [76,77], namely polylactic acid (PLA) [78], polylactic-co-glycolic acid (PLGA) [79], polycaprolactone (PCL) [80,81], and polyglycerol sebacate (PGS) [82]. The advantage of the mentioned biopolymers is that they keep differentiated cells able to achieve the management of RGCs' function and structure. The research is focused on scaffold modification to obtain optimal effective RGC growth towards the ONH. Kador et al. [78] obtained a PLA electrospun scaffold imitating the mode of radial RNFL axon paths. PLA-derived scaffolds help to increase the RGC axon growth, improving the regeneration of long-distance connections to the CNS. Lately, Li et al. [83] obtained PLGA-based scaffolds as a base for human RGCs and described that the RGCs had integrated with the scaffolds and exhibited their structural character. This engineered scaffold was able to mimic the RNFL bundles and to present dendritic arbors, grow axons and a neurite plexus, and exhibit electrophysiological features [27].

In addition to the need for the further advances in the world of scaffolds, surface modification techniques are also crucial for the improvement of the clinical success in RGC replacement therapies. The control of cell differentiation is needed to achieve not only anatomical but also functional regeneration. An appropriate biopolymer scaffold should encourage the correct cell differentiation of the RGCs transported to the retina; however, this is feasible only at the surface area of the scaffold at the nodal points of cellular attachment. Specific surface modifications to biomaterial scaffolds were helpful for the viability of delivered cells by imitating their natural microenvironment and, as a result, improving the biocompatibility and enhancement of phenotype expression in comparison to unmodified scaffolds [27,84].

4.2. Intraocular Barriers

The intraocular transplantation of the prepared replacement RGCs for retinal therapy can be obtained via two modes of application, either subretinally or intravitreally, with each approach having its pros and cons. First, subretinal injections put cells nearby the outer layers of the retina and near to abundant blood circulation, which is desired in the case of photoreceptor therapies. On the other hand, intravitreal injections have an easier technique, familiar to every vitreoretinal surgeon, and enable the straight access to the inner retinal layers. Most studies into intraocular grafts are related to subretinal approaches, partially because of being focused on the degenerative diseases of photoreceptors [42]. However, in the case of inner retinal disease with glaucoma as an example, intravitreal injections constitute probably the more applicable approach than subretinal injections.

Unfortunately, the studies regarding subretinal application described both cellular factors and ECM molecules as inhibitory to graft migration. However, it remains elusive whether they have the same role after intravitreal placement of the graft [42].

The subretinal injection typically used in photoreceptor transplantation seems to be less effective in RGC replacement strategies because the transplanted RGCs need to pass the whole retina with its many layers to target the RGCL and then grow axons toward the RNFL. On the contrary, intravitreal transplantation enables a straighter approach to the internal layers of the retina. However, it causes new problems with the distribution of the injected cells into a large three-dimensional vitreous cavity and behind physical barriers not existing when using the subretinal way of cell administration [85]. Additionally, for the transplantation of RGCs into the eye, intravitreal injection is the most favored way of administration as it does not disrupt the blood–retinal barrier, and it avoids systemic exposure. However, in the large vitreous space, the control of the distribution of the injected RGCs to a targeted retinal layer remains laborious, and the donor cells may sometimes be found at the posterior lens capsule and ciliary body [28]. It was reported that only about 1% of RGCs administered into the vitreous cavity usually find the targeted retina, and unfortunately, most of them remain outside of the neural tissue [42].

Prior studies have reported that the ILM constitutes the main barrier inhibiting the integration of transplanted RGCs to the retina. The ILM is a basement membrane mostly comprising laminin, collagen IV, and other ECM proteins [70]. Other studies have shown that rather more reactive gliosis than the ILM may result in the failure of the RGCs' implantation via the vitreous approach [86].

Lately, the ILM has attracted more clinical interest with an increase in the recognition of its role as a barrier which may impede the breakthroughs with novel transplanting ophthalmic strategies. The ILM may hamper retinal targeting due to intravitreally delivered gene therapy vectors but also the retinal integration of cell transplants. The ILM also constitutes a barrier to intravitreally injected nanoparticles and antibodies [23]. Intravitreally transplanted cells are blocked at the level of the ILM surface without approaching the host retina.

Zhang et al. provided the straight proof that recognizes the ILM as a crucial barrier hampering transplanted human RGCs from integration [86]. Using organotypic mouse retinal explants with transplanted hES-RGCs, they found that hES-RGCs encountering an unbroken ILM were not able to grow neurites toward the recipient retinal parenchyma. On the contrary, transplanted RGCs integrated neurites into the IPL in areas where the ILM was mechanically broken. Localization of the RGC dendrites to the IPL is a prerequisite for the further development of working synaptogenesis with amacrine and bipolar cells. An intact ILM seems to create a pivotal barrier to hES-RGC neurite ingrowth in the retina, as the mechanical disruption or enzymatic degradation of ILM proteins caused the visible improvement of the retinal neurite ingrowth. So, it seems that novel methods enabling grafted RGC neurites to cross the ILM is basic to the improvement of RGC replacement success [87].

The ILM's thickness increases with aging and in the course of some diseases such as diabetes as an example [88], which may cause a greater problem with engraftment in patients with age-related optic neuropathies such as glaucoma. The administration of enzymes degrading the ILM may not be obligatory in human patients since the surgical technique of the ILM peeling is a broadly used and safe maneuver in vitreoretinal surgery. On the other hand, the intravitreal application of proteolytic enzymes may be toxic to the adjacent tissue when applied at the concentrations necessary for the clinical digestion of the ILM [85].

The studies on retinal development show that the interactions of neurons with the components of the ECM is obligatory for their growth, maturation, and polarization. Therefore, although the enzymatic disruption or mechanical removal of the ILM improves RGCs' migration and further neurite implantation into the retina, the ECM molecular pathways seem to be necessary to achieve the real functional integration requiring donor cell polarization, dendrite stratification, and axon pathfinding. Such approach shows that it may be more important to manipulate cell–ILM interactions, rather than to anatomically eliminate the ILM.

Neurons communicate with the ILM through a group of cell surface receptors. The integrin class is the major family of RGC superficiality that is operated by ECM laminins. The removal of integrins or their downstream Cas adaptor proteins in RGCs may effectively result in RGCL disturbance with RGC ectopic migration through the ILM [89]. Therefore, genetic modification in the integrin pathways in donor RGCs may enhance their migration through the ILM and improve their integration after transplantation [85].

5. Paracrine Factors

When planning an optimal cell replacement approach, the unique microenvironment existing within the glaucomatous host retinas needs consideration. Retinas changed during glaucoma may on the one hand have a better ability to accept donor hiPSC-RGCs compared to healthy mature retinas [28]. On the other hand, and theoretically more probably, the paracrine environment in the donor retina may be full of potentially toxic substances which may harm the newly transplanted RGCs.

On the other hand, the paracrine effects of stem cells may offer a new all-encompassing approach to the treatment of neurodegenerative diseases [90]. The paracrine effects of MSCs comprise the production of trophic factors, cytokine neurotrophins, and signaling molecules, which may be helpful for the restoration process by promoting angiogenesis and tissue regeneration, but also via the inhibition of apoptosis and fibrosis. They also change the immune response and the inflammatory process, and the major hypothesis explaining the neuroprotective effects of hMSC focuses on their involvement in the modulation of neuroinflammation, a key process initializing RGC regeneration [91].

Human bone-marrow MSCs are currently authorized for allogeneic and autologous application in humans, and their usage has been previously studied in some clinical trials in traumatology, cardiology, and ophthalmology (ocular surface). However, MSCs have not yet been approved for intravitreal injections. Some initial studies showed that the intravitreal application of MSCs is well tolerated and safe in rabbits, and the cells are bioavailable in the vitreous space [90]. The intravitreal application of MSCs in mice models of different ocular disorders, e.g., retinal degeneration, retinal ischemia, retinitis pigmentosa, and also glaucoma, show that the agents produced by the MSCs have beneficial neuroprotective effects. Bone MSCs constitute an optimal source of cells for the therapy of retinal degenerative disorders and can be obtained in response to tissue injury and repair to strive for paracrine neurotrophic influence [92].

Additionally, some factors which could be involved in the modification of the paracrine environment during RGC replacement therapy are discussed. For example, the α-crystallin proteins necessary for maintaining lens transparency are additionally produced in the case of a light-induced injury to the retina, but also during the wound healing process after a retinal tear. Their expression also correlates with an increased RGC survival following optic nerve axotomy [92]. Nath et al. showed that supplementation with recombinant αA-crystallin protein promotes the endurance of primary RGCs after metabolic injury [93]. The other paracrine factor with a suggested neurotrophic and neuroprotective role is VEGF. The studies reported that VEGF is produced by RGCs to enhance their own vitality [94]. Additionally, Müller glia have been reported to produce different trophic agents with the capacity to influence the various stages of the formation of retinal neuronal connection during the differentiation, synaptogenesis, and neuroprotection of photoreceptors and RGCs in the retina [93].

The molecular pathways beneficial for RGC survival and axon regeneration have been studied via the evaluation of the behavior of endogenous RGCs evolving during experimental stress [95]. For example, intrinsic mTOR and CNTF/JAK/STAT signaling improves the RGC endurance and regeneration of axons [96,97]. Insulin signaling [98], the overexpression of Lin28 [99], the production of thrombospondin-1 [100], the deletion of

PTEN and SOCS3 [101–103], and the blockage of KLF [104] in RGCs may promote axonal regeneration in different models of traumatic optic neuropathy. On the other hand, over 40 negative intrinsic factors influencing RGC regeneration have been found up today [105]. RGC-extrinsic signaling molecules with oncomodulin may additionally improve the axon regeneration in glaucoma models [85,106].

Finally, donor RGCs may be genetically modified to produce neuroprotective factors and change the recipient microenvironment to improve the endogenous cell vitality and decrease ongoing functional and structural injury. Moreover, the intrinsic molecular signaling in donor cells could be changed to improve their own protective mechanisms to resist the harmful conditions in the host [92].

6. RGC Axons

RGC replacement provides a possible therapy to restore the vision loss due to glaucoma. The promising results of photoreceptor transplantation studies initially proved that vision restoration may be achievable via mammalian retinal cell replacement [23]. However, RGC transplantation causes many more possible troubles compared to photoreceptor transplantation, as the transplanted cells need to connect via dendrites with bipolar or amacrine cells and grow their axons through the retina to the ONH and finally meet their postsynaptic targets in the CNS [68]. New RGC axons must penetrate deep into the brain to reach the visual cortex of the cerebrum passing the thalamus centers.

Relying on the type and presence of regenerative stimuli, some axons are able to grow sufficiently toward their targets. However, in many cases, the axons do not elongate but take way back toward the soma. Since functional regeneration needs connections between axons and their related targets, there is a need to define the cellular and molecular factors regulating this process in adulthood [107]. At the time of the primary creation formation of visual projections, RGC axons grow fast in vitro or in vivo, and RGCs can regenerate devastated axons in vivo, but mainly for small distances. The axonal ability for regeneration and growth is absent from the early postnatal period at the moment when RGCs enhance dendritic growth and synaptic inputs expand, which is triggered by the contacts between RGCs and amacrine cells [108].

On the other hand, some studies have described that during regeneration, axons follow astrocytes [107]. In the ON, the astrocytes consist predominantly of the fibrous type, which can be further divided into three subtypes according to their morphology: the transverse subtype, with processes projecting perpendicular to the ON; the longitudinal subtype, with processes projecting parallel to the ON; and the random subtype, with processes projecting in both directions [107]. The studies show that during regeneration, RGC axons just follow their closest astrocyte type. Then, these axons travel stochastically in all different directions, in parallel or perpendicular to the ON. In regenerative therapies with the application of CNTF, many RGC axons travel in diverse directions. Other studies have described that some RGCs can extend toward the CNS more efficiently with the microenvironment enriched with different types of regenerative paracrine agents [108].

Despite the common proofs that RGCs can regenerate axons through a peripheral nerve environment, the regeneration of the mature ON is not thought to be possible because of the strong growth-inhibiting influence of CNS myelin. Berry et al. [109] claimed a diverse point of view regarding the peripheral nerve grafting experiments and proposed that Schwann cell-derived trophic agents may be the primary cause. His team studied if grafting an autologous part of a peripheral nerve into the posterior part of the eye bulb could enhance mature rodent RGCs to grow axons through the ON. In fact, the implants caused visible axon growth, showing for the first time that the ON was not a definitive barrier to regeneration in the case of adequate RGC stimulation [108]. Recent studies have reported that a combination of genetic stimulation and modification of the signaling pathway enhances the regenerative processes in the ON before RGCs find their targets in the CNS. The additive application of ephrin molecules, cell-adhesion molecules, proteoglycans, and semaphorin can help the RGC axons to reach the optic chiasm [110]. Moreover, the application of cadherin, ephrin, and the Wnt signaling pathway molecules can stimulate synapse formation and guide them toward brain centers [107].

Unfortunately, the delivery of NTF has no proven efficacy in enhancing the long-term neuroprotection, which is probably caused by the need for regular administration, and additionally, it applies in combination which may cause the receptor down-regulation after therapy. The application of cells releasing NTF naturally or those which have been modified to release glial cell line-derived NTF and CNFT does not improve the situation. On the contrary, the resolution of this down-regulation problem may be achieved via the application of a virus to enhance the expression of BDNF and its receptor TrkB in RGCs which have been proved to have a neuroprotective action in the case of laser-induced glaucoma [111].

Extracellular vesicles (EVs) are membranous microvesicles containing proteins, RNA, or a whole organelle in specific cases [29]. They are secreted by the cells to play important extra- and intercellular roles in many processes such as immune modulation, cellular communication, physiological regulation, and biomolecular transport [112]. Exosomes are a EV subclass related to disease induction and regeneration. The protective effect of intravitreal injection of MSC-derived exosomes in an experimental model of ON injury was reported to have better RGC vitality and axonal regeneration [113,114]. Additionally, Mead and Tomarev have analyzed the potential of MSC-derived agents, cells, and engineered MSCs to improve the injured retina. EVs derived from human BM-MSCs significantly protected RGCs and diminished RNFL thinning in two rodent models of glaucoma via the EV secreted by BM-MSCs and the miRNAs contained within [115]. The delivery of miRNAs via Schwann cell-derived exosomes into neuronal cultures enhanced neuritogenesis, and the possible miRNAs involved were miR-21, miR18a miR-222, and miR182. The capacity of miRNA to decrease the level and action of a plethora of mRNA makes them a probable candidate for RGC neuroprotective therapy, especially in that they can be easily applied to the vitreous cavity to achieve a rapid and focused influence on RGCs [111].

Though a lot of information was obtained from diverse studies of the endogenous RGC axon regeneration processes regarding molecular pathways engaged in the reestablishment of efferent connections [110], the factors inhibiting donor RGCs from dendrite growth toward the IPL and synapsing with amacrine and bipolar cells still remain unclear. The ILM is thought to be a possible candidate for being such an obstacle.

hES-RGC neurites after reaching the retinal microenvironment do not uniquely grow toward the IPL. The specific agents that drive the RGC dendrite pattern of laminar growth during the normal development to and within the IPL involve molecular cues and activity-dependent refinement [116]. Spontaneous electrophysiological activity in organotypic retinal explants is modest, additionally diminishing gradually, so it may have only modest, if any, potential IPL-guided dendrite localization reinforced by neuronal activity [117] During development, RGC dendrites target pre-patterned IPL afferents [118]. Sublamination within the IPL is driven by the presence of the specific expression of cell surface receptors and their binding to localized lamina-specific ligands, including integrins, plexins, and cadherins which play a pivotal part in correct dendritic guidance and outgrowth [119]. It is highly probably that the control of specific surface receptor expression may help to navigate hES-RGC dendrites toward their correct targets where afferent synaptogenesis would hopefully happen. It remains elusive whether ligand expression remains present within the mature IPL, but the identification of typical dendritic stratification by transplanted RGCs shows that at least a part of the crucial signaling pathway is visible [23].

7. Summary

The in vivo transplantation of stem cell-derived RGCs or exogenous primary RGCs is a highly needed strategy in clinics, providing a chance for the improvement of visual acuity for patients with advanced glaucoma. Unfortunately, basic research and clinical trials remain a field in its infancy. However, the early transplantation studies showed light-evoked electrophysiological responses from donor RGCs [32] and an increase in the visually dependent behavior in studied animal subjects, indicating the principal direction for the clinical potential of RGC transplantation. There are several studies regarding RGC axon regeneration and efferent connectivity after injury; however, there is only scant progress in the specific methods to improve the donor cell vitality, guide RGCs toward the targeted retinal layers, or achieve the afferent synaptogenesis of grafted RGCs [85]. On the other hand, there are a plethora of glaucoma patients for whom RGC replacement therapy is the only way to restore their vision. The possibility of renewing the ability to see for our blind patients makes the RGC replacement therapy a matter of great importance.

There are a few challenges to be addressed in the transplantation of stem cells in the therapy of glaucoma before clinical implementation. First is the source of cells: stem cell application causes ethical concerns and potential tumorigenic worries. The application of iPS, on the other hand, does not solve the potential genetic involvement in glaucoma pathogenesis. Additionally, the introduction of the cells into the host retina needs improvement, not only the process of transplantation but also the integration into the proper layer and reaching the brain target. However, despite the many challenges, there is no doubt that stem cell therapy constitutes the most promising approach for advanced glaucoma patients.

Funding: This research received no external funding.

Conflicts of Interest: The authors declare no conflict of interest.

References

1. Quigley, H.A.; Broman, A.T. The number of people with glaucoma worldwide in 2010 and 2020. *Br. J. Ophthalmol.* **2006**, *90*, 262–267. [CrossRef] [PubMed]
2. Tham, Y.C.; Li, X.; Wong, T.Y.; Quigley, H.A.; Aung, T.; Cheng, C.Y. Global prevalence of glaucoma and projections of glaucoma burden through 2040: A systematic review and meta-analysis. *Ophthalmology* **2014**, *121*, 2081–2090. [CrossRef] [PubMed]
3. Quigley, H.A. The contribution of the sclera and lamina cribrosa to the pathogenesis of glaucoma: Diagnostic and treatment implications. *Prog. Brain Res.* **2015**, *220*, 59–86.
4. Quigley, H.A. Glaucoma. *Lancet* **2011**, *377*, 1367–1377. [CrossRef]
5. Weinreb, R.N.; Aung, T.; Medeiros, F.A. The pathophysiology and treatment of glaucoma: A review. *JAMA* **2014**, *311*, 1901–1911. [CrossRef]
6. Miltner, A.M.; La Torre, A. Retinal Ganglion Cell Replacement: Current Status and Challenges Ahead. *Dev. Dyn.* **2019**, *248*, 118–128. [CrossRef]
7. Kim, U.S.; Mahroo, O.A.; Mollon, J.D.; Yu-Wai-Man, P. Retinal Ganglion Cells-Diversity of Cell Types and Clinical Relevance. *Front. Neurol.* **2021**, *12*, 661938. [CrossRef]
8. Sanes, J.R.; Masland, R.H. The types of retinal ganglion cells: Current status and implications for neuronal classification. *Annu. Rev. Neurosci.* **2015**, *38*, 221–246. [CrossRef] [PubMed]
9. Nguyen-Ba-Charvet, K.T.; Rebsam, A. Neurogenesis and Specification of Retinal Ganglion Cells. *Int. J. Mol. Sci.* **2020**, *21*, 451. [CrossRef]
10. Masri, R.A.; Percival, K.A.; Koizumi, A.; Martin, P.R.; Grünert, U. Survey of retinal ganglion cell morphology in marmoset. *J. Comp. Neurol.* **2019**, *527*, 236–258. [CrossRef]
11. Baden, T.; Berens, P.; Franke, K.; Román Rosón, M.; Bethge, M.; Euler, T. The functional diversity of retinal ganglion cells in the mouse. *Nature* **2016**, *529*, 345–350. [CrossRef] [PubMed]
12. Tran, N.M.; Shekhar, K.; Whitney, I.E.; Jacobi, A.; Benhar, I.; Hong, G.; Yan, W.; Adiconis, X.; Arnold, M.E.; Lee, J.M.; et al. Single-Cell Profiles of Retinal Ganglion Cells Differing in Resilience to Injury Reveal Neuroprotective Genes. *Neuron* **2019**, *104*, 1039–1055.e12. [CrossRef]
13. Yuan, F.; Wang, M.; Jin, K.; Xiang, M. Advances in Regeneration of Retinal Ganglion Cells and Optic Nerves. *Int. J. Mol. Sci.* **2021**, *22*, 4616. [CrossRef]
14. Olmos-Carreño, C.L.; Figueres-Oñate, M.; Scicolone, G.E.; López-Mascaraque, L. Cell Fate of Retinal Progenitor Cells: In Ovo UbC-StarTrack Analysis. *Int. J. Mol. Sci.* **2022**, *23*, 12388. [CrossRef]
15. Sieving, P.A.; Caruso, R.C.; Tao, W.; Coleman, H.R.; Thompson, D.J.; Fullmer, K.R.; Bush, R.A. Ciliary neurotrophic factor (CNTF) for human retinal degeneration: Phase I trial of CNTF delivered by encapsulated cell intraocular implants. *Proc. Natl. Acad. Sci. USA* **2006**, *103*, 3896–3901. [CrossRef]
16. Wareham, L.K.; Risner, M.L.; Calkins, D.J. Protect, Repair, and Regenerate: Towards Restoring Vision in Glaucoma. *Curr. Ophthalmol. Rep.* **2020**, *8*, 301–310. [CrossRef]

17. Ferrari, M.P.; Mantelli, F.; Sacchetti, M.; Antonangeli, M.I.; Cattani, F.; D'Anniballe, G.; Sinigaglia, F.; Ruffini, P.A.; Lambiase, A. Safety and pharmacokinetics of escalating doses of human recombinant nerve growth factor eye drops in a double-masked, randomized clinical trial. *BioDrugs* **2014**, *28*, 275–283. [CrossRef]
18. Yap, T.E.; Donna, P.; Almonte, M.T.; Cordeiro, M.F. Real-time imaging of retinal ganglion cell apoptosis. *Cells* **2018**, *7*, 60. [CrossRef]
19. Moore, D.L.; Goldberg, J.L. Four steps to optic nerve regeneration. *J. Neuroophthalmol.* **2010**, *30*, 347–360. [CrossRef]
20. Divya, M.S.; Rasheed, V.A.; Schmidt, T.; Lalitha, S.; Hattar, S.; James, J. Intraocular Injection of ES Cell-Derived Neural Progenitors Improve Visual Function in Retinal Ganglion Cell-Depleted Mouse Models. *Front. Cell Neurosci.* **2017**, *11*, 295. [CrossRef]
21. Gagliardi, G.; Ben M'Barek, K.; Goureau, O. Photoreceptor cell replacement in macular degeneration and retinitis pigmentosa: A pluripotent stem cell-based approach. *Prog. Retin. Eye Res.* **2019**, *71*, 1–25. [CrossRef] [PubMed]
22. Young, M.J.; Ray, J.; Whiteley, S.J.; Klassen, H.; Gage, F.H. Neuronal differentiation and morphological integration of hippocampal progenitor cells transplanted to the retina of immature and mature dystrophic rats. *Mol. Cell Neurosci.* **2000**, *16*, 197–205. [CrossRef] [PubMed]
23. Zhang, X.; Tenerelli, K.; Wu, S.; Xia, X.; Yokota, S.; Sun, C.; Galvao, J.; Venugopalan, P.; Li, C.; Madaan, A.; et al. Cell transplantation of retinal ganglion cells derived from hESCs. *Restor. Neurol. Neurosci.* **2020**, *38*, 131–140. [CrossRef]
24. Johnson, T.V.; Bull, N.D.; Martin, K.R. Identification of barriers to retinal engraftment of transplanted stem cells. *Investig. Ophthalmol. Vis. Sci.* **2010**, *51*, 960–970. [CrossRef]
25. Mead, B.; Berry, M.; Logan, A.; Scott, R.A.; Leadbeater, W.; Scheven, B.A. Stem cell treatment of degenerative eye disease. *Stem Cell Res.* **2015**, *14*, 243–257. [CrossRef]
26. Laha, B.; Stafford, B.K.; Huberman, A.D. Regenerating optic pathways from the eye to the brain. *Science* **2017**, *356*, 1031–1034. [CrossRef]
27. Behtaj, S.; Öchsner, A.; Anissimov, Y.G.; Rybachuk, M. Retinal Tissue Bioengineering, Materials and Methods for the Treatment of Glaucoma. *Tissue Eng. Regen. Med.* **2020**, *17*, 253–269. [CrossRef] [PubMed]
28. Vrathasha, V.; Nikonov, S.; Bell, B.A.; He, J.; Bungatavula, Y.; Uyhazi, K.E.; Murthy Chavali, V.R. Transplanted human induced pluripotent stem cells- derived retinal ganglion cells embed within mouse retinas and are electrophysiologically functional. *iScience* **2022**, *25*, 105308. [CrossRef]
29. Fortress, A.M.; Miyagishima, K.J.; Reed, A.A.; Temple, S.; Clegg, D.O.; Tucker, B.A.; Blenkinsop, T.A.; Harb, G.; Greenwell, T.N.; Ludwig, T.E.; et al. Stem cell sources and characterization in the development of cell-based products for treating retinal disease: An NEI Town Hall report. *Stem Cell Res. Ther.* **2023**, *14*, 53. [CrossRef]
30. Tropepe, V.; Coles, B.L.; Chiasson, B.J.; Horsford, D.J.; Elia, A.J.; McInnes, R.R.; van der Kooy, D. Retinal stem cells in the adult mammalian eye. *Science* **2000**, *287*, 2032–2036. [CrossRef]
31. Grigoryan, E.N. Cell Sources for Retinal Regeneration: Implication for Data Translation in Biomedicine of the Eye. *Cells* **2022**, *11*, 3755. [CrossRef] [PubMed]
32. Ducournau, Y.; Boscher, C.; Adelman, R.A.; Guillaubey, C.; Schmidt-Morand, D.; Mosnier, J.F.; Ducournau, D. Proliferation of the ciliary epithelium with retinal neuronal and photoreceptor cell differentiation in human eyes with retinal detachment and proliferative vitreoretinopathy. *Graefes Arch. Clin. Exp. Ophthalmol.* **2012**, *250*, 409–423. [CrossRef] [PubMed]
33. Too, L.K.; Shen, W.; Mammo, Z.; Osaadon, P.; Gillies, M.C.; Simunovic, M.P. Surgical retinal explants as a source of retinal progenitor cells. *Retina* **2021**, *41*, 1986–1993. [CrossRef]
34. Rueda, E.M.; Hall, B.M.; Hill, M.C.; Swinton, P.G.; Tong, X.; Martin, J.F.; Poché, R.A. The Hippo Pathway Blocks Mammalian Retinal Müller Glial Cell Reprogramming. *Cell Rep.* **2019**, *27*, 1637–1649.e6. [CrossRef] [PubMed]
35. Lamba, D.; Reh, T.A. Regenerative medicine for diseases of the retina. In *Regenerative Medicine for Diseases of the Retina. Principles of Regenerative Medicine*; Academic Press: Cambridge, MA, USA, 2008.
36. Walshe, T.E.; Leach, L.L.; D'Amore, P.A. TGF-b signalling is required for maintenance of retinal ganglion cell differentiation and survival. *Neuroscience* **2011**, *189*, 123–131. [CrossRef]
37. Rizkiawan, D.E.; Evelyn, M.; Tjandra, K.C.; Setiawan, B. Utilization of Modified Induced Pluripotent Stem Cells as the Advance Therapy of Glaucoma: A Systematic Review. *Clin. Ophthalmol.* **2022**, *16*, 2851–2859. [CrossRef]
38. Davis, D.M.; Dyer, M.A. Retinal progenitor cells, differentiation, and barriers to cell cycle reentry. *Curr. Top. Dev. Biol.* **2010**, *93*, 175–188.
39. Lechner, J.; Medina, R.J.; Lois, N.; Stitt, A.W. Advances in cell therapies using stem cells/progenitors as a novel approach for neurovascular repair of the diabetic retina. *Stem Cell Res. Ther.* **2022**, *13*, 388. [CrossRef]
40. Gill, K.P.; Hung, S.S.; Sharov, A.; Lo, C.Y.; Needham, K.; Lidgerwood, G.E.; Jackson, S.; Crombie, D.E.; Nayagam, B.A.; Cook, A.L.; et al. Enriched retinal ganglion cells derived from human embryonic stem cells. *Sci. Rep.* **2016**, *6*, 30552. [CrossRef]
41. Mathew, B.; Ravindran, S.; Liu, X.; Torres, L.; Chennakesavalu, M.; Huang, C.C.; Feng, L.; Zelka, R.; Lopez, J.; Sharma, M.; et al. Mesenchymal stem cell-derived extracellular vesicles and retinal ischemia-reperfusion. *Biomaterials* **2019**, *197*, 146–160. [CrossRef]
42. Johnson, T.V.; Calkins, D.J.; Fortune, B.; Goldberg, J.L.; La Torre, A.; Lamba, D.A.; Meyer, J.S.; Reh, T.A.; Wallace, V.A.; Zack, D.J.; et al. The importance of unambiguous cell origin determination in neuronal repopulation studies. *iScience* **2023**, *26*, 106361. [CrossRef] [PubMed]
43. Takahashi, K.; Yamanaka, S. Induction of pluripotent stem cells from mouse embryonic and adult fibroblast cultures by defined factors. *Cell* **2006**, *126*, 663–667. [CrossRef]

44. Ji, S.L.; Tang, S.B. Differentiation of retinal ganglion cells from induced pluripotent stem cells: A review. *Int. J. Ophthalmol.* **2019**, *12*, 152–160.
45. Silva-Pedrosa, R.; Salgado, A.J.; Ferreira, P.E. Revolutionizing Disease Modeling: The Emergence of Organoids in Cellular Systems. *Cells* **2023**, *12*, 930. [CrossRef] [PubMed]
46. Gudiseva, H.V.; Vrathasha, V.; He, J.; Bungatavula, D.; O'Brien, J.M.; Chavali, V.R.M. Single Cell Sequencing of Induced Pluripotent Stem Cell Derived Retinal Ganglion Cells (iPSC-RGC) Reveals Distinct Molecular Signatures and RGC Subtypes. *Genes* **2021**, *12*, 2015. [CrossRef]
47. Li, J.Y.; Christophersen, N.S.; Hall, V.; Soulet, D.; Brundin, P. Critical issues of clinical human embryonic stem cell therapy for brain repair. *Trends Neurosci.* **2008**, *31*, 146–153. [CrossRef]
48. Zhong, X.; Gutierrez, C.; Xue, T.; Hampton, C.; Vergara, M.N.; Cao, L.H.; Peters, A.; Park, T.S.; Zambidis, E.T.; Meyer, J.S.; et al. Generation of three-dimensional retinal tissue with functional photoreceptors from human iPSCs. *Nat. Commun.* **2014**, *5*, 4047. [CrossRef] [PubMed]
49. Tanaka, T.; Yokoi, T.; Tamalu, F.; Watanabe, S.; Nishina, S.; Azuma, N. Generation of retinal ganglion cells with functional axons from human induced pluripotent stem cells. *Sci. Rep.* **2015**, *5*, 8344. [CrossRef]
50. Chaubey, A.; Ross, K.J.; Leadbetter, R.M.; Burg, K.J. Surface patterning: Tool to modulate stem cell differentiation in an adipose system. *J. Biomed. Mater. Res. B Appl. Biomater.* **2008**, *84*, 70–78. [CrossRef]
51. Jung-Klawitter, S.; Opladen, T. Induced pluripotent stem cells (iPSCs) as model to study inherited defects of neurotransmission in inborn errors of metabolism. *J. Inherit. Metab. Dis.* **2018**, *41*, 1103–1116. [CrossRef]
52. Logan, S.; Arzua, T.; Canfield, S.G.; Seminary, E.R.; Sison, S.L.; Ebert, A.D.; Bai, X. Studying Human Neurological Disorders Using Induced Pluripotent Stem Cells: From 2D Monolayer to 3D Organoid and Blood Brain Barrier Models. *Compr. Physiol.* **2019**, *9*, 565–611. [PubMed]
53. Fontoura, J.C.; Viezzer, C.; Dos Santos, F.G.; Ligabue, R.A.; Weinlich, R.; Puga, R.D.; Antonow, D.; Severino, P.; Bonorino, C. Comparison of 2D and 3D cell culture models for cell growth, gene expression and drug resistance. *Mater. Sci. Eng. C Mater. Biol. Appl.* **2020**, *107*, 110264. [CrossRef] [PubMed]
54. Li, D.W.; He, F.L.; He, J.; Deng, X.; Liu, Y.L.; Liu, Y.Y.; Ye, Y.J.; Yin, D.C. From 2D to 3D: The morphology, proliferation and differentiation of MC3T3-E1 on silk fibroin/chitosan matrices. *Carbohydr. Polym.* **2017**, *178*, 69–77. [CrossRef] [PubMed]
55. Yang, H.; Shao, N.; Holmström, A.; Zhao, X.; Chour, T.; Chen, H.; Itzhaki, I.; Wu, H.; Ameen, M.; Cunningham, N.J.; et al. Transcriptome analysis of non human primate-induced pluripotent stem cell-derived cardiomyocytes in 2D monolayer culture vs. 3D engineered heart tissue. *Cardiovasc. Res.* **2021**, *117*, 2125–2136. [CrossRef]
56. Kim, B.C.; Kwack, K.H.; Chun, J.; Lee, J.H. Comparative Transcriptome Analysis of Human Adipose-Derived Stem Cells Undergoing Osteogenesis in 2D and 3D Culture Conditions. *Int. J. Mol. Sci.* **2021**, *22*, 7939. [CrossRef]
57. Lee, J.; Choi, S.H.; Kim, Y.B.; Jun, I.; Sung, J.J.; Lee, D.R.; Kim, Y.I.; Cho, M.S.; Byeon, S.H.; Kim, D.S.; et al. Defined Conditions for Differentiation of Functional Retinal Ganglion Cells from Human Pluripotent Stem Cells. *Investig. Ophthalmol. Vis. Sci.* **2018**, *59*, 3531–3542. [CrossRef]
58. Singh, R.K.; Binette, F.; Seiler, M.; Petersen-Jones, S.M.; Nasonkin, I.O. Pluripotent Stem Cell-Based Organoid Technologies for Developing Next-Generation Vision Restoration Therapies of Blindness. *J. Ocul. Pharmacol. Ther.* **2021**, *37*, 147–156. [CrossRef]
59. Pereiro, X.; Miltner, A.M.; La Torre, A.; Vecino, E. Effects of Adult Müller Cells and Their Conditioned Media on the Survival of Stem Cell-Derived Retinal Ganglion Cells. *Cells* **2020**, *9*, 1759. [CrossRef]
60. Clevers, H. Modeling development and disease with organoids. *Cell* **2016**, *165*, 1586–1597. [CrossRef]
61. Luo, Z.; Zhong, X.; Li, K.; Xie, B.; Liu, Y.; Ye, M.; Li, K.; Xu, C.; Ge, J. An optimized system for effective derivation of three-dimensional retinal tissue via wnt signaling regulation. *Stem Cells* **2018**, *36*, 1709–1722. [CrossRef]
62. Ito, S.I.; Onishi, A.; Takahashi, M. Chemically-induced photoreceptor degeneration and protection in mouse iPSC-derived three-dimensional retinal organoids. *Stem Cell Res.* **2017**, *24*, 94–101. [CrossRef] [PubMed]
63. Lakowski, J.; Welby, E.; Budinger, D.; Di Marco, F.; Di Foggia, V.; Bainbridge, J.W.B. Isolation of human photoreceptor precursors via a cell surface marker panel from stem cell-derived retinal organoids and fetal retinae. *Stem Cells* **2018**, *36*, 709–722. [CrossRef] [PubMed]
64. Dorgau, B.; Felemban, M.; Sharpe, A.; Bauer, R.; Hallam, D.; Steel, D.H.; Lindsay, S.; Mellough, C.; Lako, M. Laminin γ3 plays an important role in retinal lamination, photoreceptor organisation and ganglion cell differentiation. *Cell Death Dis.* **2018**, *9*, 615. [CrossRef] [PubMed]
65. Kobayashi, W.; Onishi, A.; Tu, H.Y.; Takihara, Y.; Matsumura, M.; Tsujimoto, K.; Inatani, M.; Nakazawa, T.; Takahashi, M. Culture systems of dissociated mouse and human pluripotent stem cell-derived retinal ganglion cells purified by two-step immunopanning. *Investig. Ophthalmol. Vis. Sci.* **2018**, *59*, 776–787. [CrossRef] [PubMed]
66. West, E.L.; Pearson, R.A.; MacLaren, R.E.; Sowden, J.C.; Ali, R.R. Cell transplantation strategies for retinal repair. *Prog. Brain Res.* **2009**, *175*, 3–21.
67. Tomita, M.; Lavik, E.; Klassen, H.; Zahir, T.; Langer, R.; Young, M.J. Biodegradable polymer composite grafts promote the survival and differentiation of retinal progenitor cells. *Stem Cells* **2005**, *23*, 1579–1588. [CrossRef]
68. Kador, K.E.; Montero, R.B.; Venugopalan, P.; Hertz, J.; Zindell, A.N.; Valenzuela, D.A.; Uddin, M.S.; Lavik, E.B.; Muller, K.J.; Andreopoulos, F.M.; et al. Tissue engineering the retinal ganglion cell nerve fiber layer. *Biomaterials* **2013**, *34*, 4242–4250. [CrossRef]
69. Zhang, N.; Yan, H.; Wen, X. Tissue-engineering approaches for axonal guidance. *Brain Res. Rev.* **2005**, *49*, 48–64. [CrossRef]

70. Dromel, P.C.; Singh, D.; Andres, E.; Likes, M.; Kurisawa, M.; Alexander-Katz, A.; Spector, M.; Young, M. A bioinspired gelatin-hyaluronic acid-based hybrid interpenetrating network for the enhancement of retinal ganglion cells replacement therapy. *NPJ Regen. Med.* **2021**, *6*, 85. [CrossRef]
71. Dromel, P.C.; Singh, D.; Alexander-Katz, A.; Kurisawa, M.; Spector, M.; Young, M. Mechano-Chemical Effect of Gelatin- and HA-Based Hydrogels on Human Retinal Progenitor Cells. *Gels* **2023**, *9*, 58. [CrossRef]
72. Zhang, D.; Ni, N.; Chen, J.; Yao, Q.; Shen, B.; Zhang, Y.; Zhu, M.; Wang, Z.; Ruan, J.; Wang, J.; et al. Electrospun SF/PLCL nanofibrous membrane: A potential scaffold for retinal progenitor cell proliferation and differentiation. *Sci. Rep.* **2015**, *5*, 14326. [CrossRef] [PubMed]
73. Murikipudi, S.; Methe, H.; Edelman, E.R. The effect of substrate modulus on the growth and function of matrix-embedded endothelial cells. *Biomaterials* **2013**, *34*, 677–684. [CrossRef] [PubMed]
74. Parhi, R. Cross-linked hydrogel for pharmaceutical applications: A review. *Adv. Pharm. Bull.* **2017**, *7*, 515–530. [CrossRef] [PubMed]
75. Young, M.J. Stem cells in the mammalian eye: A tool for retinal repair. *APMIS* **2005**, *113*, 845–857. [CrossRef] [PubMed]
76. Trese, M.; Regatieri, C.V.; Young, M.J. Advances in retinal tissue engineering. *Materials* **2012**, *5*, 108–120. [CrossRef]
77. Yao, J.; Tao, S.L.; Young, M.J. Synthetic polymer scaffolds for stem cell transplantation in retinal tissue engineering. *Polymers* **2011**, *3*, 899–914. [CrossRef]
78. Kador, K.E.; Alsehli, H.S.; Zindell, A.N.; Lau, L.W.; Andreopoulos, F.M.; Watson, B.D.; Goldberg, J.L. Retinal ganglion cell polarization using immobilized guidance cues on a tissue-engineered scaffold. *Acta Biomater.* **2014**, *10*, 4939–4946. [CrossRef]
79. Warnke, P.H.; Alamein, M.; Skabo, S.; Stephens, S.; Bourke, R.; Heiner, P.; Liu, Q. Primordium of an artificial Bruch's membrane made of nanofibers for engineering of retinal pigment epithelium cell monolayers. *Acta Biomater.* **2013**, *9*, 9414–9422. [CrossRef]
80. Sharifi, F.; Patel, B.B.; Dzuilko, A.K.; Montazami, R.; Sakaguchi, D.S.; Hashemi, N. Polycaprolactone microfibrous scaffolds to navigate neural stem cells. *Biomacromolecules* **2016**, *17*, 3287–3297. [CrossRef]
81. Xiang, P.; Wu, K.C.; Zhu, Y.; Xiang, L.; Li, C.; Chen, D.L.; Chen, F.; Xu, G.; Wang, A.; Li, M.; et al. A novel Bruch's membrane-mimetic electrospun substrate scaffold for human retinal pigment epithelium cells. *Biomaterials* **2014**, *35*, 9777–9788. [CrossRef]
82. Redenti, S.; Neeley, W.L.; Rompani, S.; Saigal, S.; Yang, J.; Klassen, H.; Langer, R.; Young, M.J. Engineering retinal progenitor cell and scrollable poly(glycerol-sebacate) composites for expansion and subretinal transplantation. *Biomaterials* **2009**, *30*, 3405–3414. [CrossRef] [PubMed]
83. Li, K.; Zhong, X.; Yang, S.; Luo, Z.; Li, K.; Liu, Y.; Cai, S.; Gu, H.; Lu, S.; Zhang, H.; et al. HiPSC-derived retinal ganglion cells grow dendritic arbors and functional axons on a tissue-engineered scaffold. *Acta Biomater.* **2017**, *54*, 117–127. [CrossRef] [PubMed]
84. Nazari, H.; Zhang, L.; Zhu, D.; Chader, G.J.; Falabella, P.; Stefanini, F. Stem cell-based therapies for age-related macular degeneration: The promises and the challenges. *Prog. Retin. Eye Res.* **2015**, *48*, 1–39. [CrossRef] [PubMed]
85. Zhang, K.Y.; Aguzzi, E.A.; Johnson, T.V. Retinal Ganglion Cell Transplantation: Approaches for Overcoming Challenges to Functional Integration. *Cells* **2021**, *10*, 1426. [CrossRef] [PubMed]
86. Zhang, K.Y.; Tuffy, C.; Mertz, J.L.; Quillen, S.; Wechsler, L.; Quigley, H.A.; Zack, D.J.; Johnson, T.V. Role of the Internal Limiting Membrane in Structural Engraftment and Topographic Spacing of Transplanted Human Stem Cell-Derived Retinal Ganglion Cells. *Stem Cell Rep.* **2021**, *16*, 149–167. [CrossRef]
87. Venugopalan, P.; Wang, Y.; Nguyen, T.; Huang, A.; Muller, K.J.; Goldberg, J.L. Transplanted neurons integrate into adult retinas and respond to light. *Nat. Commun.* **2016**, *7*, 10472. [CrossRef]
88. Saravia, M. Persistent diffuse diabetic macular edema. The role of the internal limiting membrane as a selective membrane: The oncotic theory. *Med. Hypotheses* **2011**, *76*, 858–860. [CrossRef]
89. Riccomagno, M.M.; Sun, L.O.; Brady, C.M.; Alexandropoulos, K.; Seo, S.; Kurokawa, M.; Kolodkin, A.L. Cas adaptor proteins organize the retinal ganglion cell layer downstream of integrin signaling. *Neuron* **2014**, *81*, 779–786. [CrossRef]
90. Labrador-Velandia, S.; Alonso-Alonso, M.L.; Di Lauro, S.; García-Gutierrez, M.T.; Srivastava, G.K.; Pastor, J.C.; Fernandez-Bueno, I. Mesenchymal stem cells provide paracrine neuroprotective resources that delay degeneration of co-cultured organotypic neuroretinal cultures. *Exp. Eye Res.* **2019**, *185*, 107671. [CrossRef]
91. Teixeira-Pinheiro, L.C.; Toledo, M.F.; Nascimento-Dos-Santos, G.; Mendez-Otero, R.; Mesentier-Louro, L.A.; Santiago, M.F. Paracrine signaling of human mesenchymal stem cell modulates retinal microglia population number and phenotype in vitro. *Exp. Eye Res.* **2020**, *200*, 108212. [CrossRef]
92. Liu, Y.; Lee, R.K. Cell transplantation to replace retinal ganglion cells faces challenges—The Switchboard Dilemma. *Neural Regen. Res.* **2021**, *6*, 1138–1143.
93. Nath, M.; Sluzala, Z.B.; Phadte, A.S.; Shan, Y.; Myers, A.M.; Fort, P.E. Evidence for Paracrine Protective Role of Exogenous αA-Crystallin in Retinal Ganglion Cells. *eNeuro* **2022**, *9*, ENEURO.0045-22.2022. [CrossRef]
94. Froger, N.; Matonti, F.; Roubeix, C.; Forster, V.; Ivkovic, I.; Brunel, N.; Baudouin, C.; Sahel, J.A.; Picaud, S. VEGF is an autocrine/paracrine neuroprotective factor for injured retinal ganglion neurons. *Sci. Rep.* **2020**, *10*, 12409. [CrossRef]
95. Williams, P.R.; Benowitz, L.I.; Goldberg, J.L.; He, Z. Axon Regeneration in the Mammalian Optic Nerve. *Annu. Rev. Vis. Sci.* **2020**, *6*, 195–213. [CrossRef] [PubMed]
96. Duan, X.; Qiao, M.; Bei, F.; Kim, I.-J.; He, Z.; Sanes, J.R. Subtype-Specific Regeneration of Retinal Ganglion Cells following Axotomy: Effects of Osteopontin and mTOR Signaling. *Neuron* **2015**, *85*, 1244–1256. [CrossRef]

97. Leibinger, M.; Andreadaki, A.; Diekmann, H.; Fischer, D. Neuronal STAT3 activation is essential for CNTF- and inflammatory stimulation-induced CNS axon regeneration. *Cell Death Dis.* **2013**, *4*, e805. [CrossRef] [PubMed]
98. Agostinone, J.; Alarcon-Martinez, L.; Gamlin, C.; Yu, W.Q.; Wong, R.O.L.; Di Polo, A. Insulin signalling promotes dendrite and synapse regeneration and restores circuit function after axonal injury. *Brain* **2018**, *141*, 1963–1980. [CrossRef]
99. Zhang, Y.; Williams, P.R.; Jacobi, A.; Wang, C.; Goel, A.; Hirano, A.A.; Brecha, N.C.; Kerschensteiner, D.; He, Z. Elevating Growth Factor Responsiveness and Axon Regeneration by Modulating Presynaptic Inputs. *Neuron* **2019**, *103*, 39–51. [CrossRef]
100. Bray, E.R.; Yungher, B.J.; Levay, K.; Ribeiro, M.; Dvoryanchikov, G.; Ayupe, A.C.; Thakor, K.; Marks, V.; Randolph, M.; Danzi, M.C.; et al. Thrombospondin-1 Mediates Axon Regeneration in Retinal Ganglion Cells. *Neuron* **2019**, *103*, 642–657. [CrossRef]
101. Park, K.K.; Liu, K.; Hu, Y.; Smith, P.D.; Wang, C.; Cai, B.; Xu, B.; Connolly, L.; Kramvis, I.; Sahin, M.; et al. Promoting axon regeneration in the adult CNS by modulation of the PTEN/mTOR pathway. *Science* **2008**, *322*, 963–966. [CrossRef]
102. Smith, P.D.; Sun, F.; Park, K.K.; Cai, B.; Wang, C.; Kuwako, K.; Martinez-Carrasco, I.; Connolly, L.; He, Z. SOCS3 deletion promotes optic nerve regeneration in vivo. *Neuron* **2009**, *64*, 617–623. [CrossRef] [PubMed]
103. Sun, F.; Park, K.K.; Belin, S.; Wang, D.; Lu, T.; Chen, G.; Zhang, K.; Yeung, C.; Feng, G.; Yankner, B.A.; et al. Sustained axon regeneration induced by co-deletion of PTEN and SOCS3. *Nature* **2011**, *480*, 372–375. [CrossRef]
104. Moore, D.L.; Blackmore, M.G.; Hu, Y.; Kaestner, K.H.; Bixby, J.L.; Lemmon, V.P.; Goldberg, J.L. KLF family members regulate intrinsic axon regeneration ability. *Science* **2009**, *326*, 298–301. [CrossRef]
105. Lindborg, J.A.; Tran, N.M.; Chenette, D.M.; DeLuca, K.; Foli, Y.; Kannan, R.; Sekine, Y.; Wang, X.; Wollan, M.; Kim, I.J.; et al. Optic nerve regeneration screen identifies multiple genes restricting adult neural repair. *Cell Rep.* **2021**, *34*, 108777. [CrossRef]
106. Yin, Y.; Henzl, M.T.; Lorber, B.; Nakazawa, T.; Thomas, T.T.; Jiang, F.; Langer, R.; Benowitz, L.I. Oncomodulin is a macrophage-derived signal for axon regeneration in retinal ganglion cells. *Nat. Neurosci.* **2006**, *9*, 843–852. [CrossRef] [PubMed]
107. Ribeiro, M.; Levay, K.; Yon, B.; Ayupe, A.C.; Salgueiro, Y.; Park, K.K. Neural Cadherin Plays Distinct Roles for Neuronal Survival and Axon Growth under Different Regenerative Conditions. *eNeuro* **2020**, *7*, ENEURO.0325-20.2020. [CrossRef]
108. Benowitz, L.I.; He, Z.; Goldberg, J.L. Reaching the brain: Advances in optic nerve regeneration. *Exp. Neurol.* **2017**, *287*, 365–373. [CrossRef]
109. Berry, M.; Carlile, J.; Hunter, A. Peripheral nerve explants grafted into the vitreous body of the eye promote the regeneration of retinal ganglion cell axons severed in the optic nerve. *J. Neurocytol.* **1996**, *25*, 147–170. [CrossRef] [PubMed]
110. de Lima, S.; Koriyama, Y.; Kurimoto, T.; Oliveira, J.T.; Yin, Y.; Li, Y.; Gilbert, H.Y.; Fagiolini, M.; Martinez, A.M.; Benowitz, L. Full-length axon regeneration in the adult mouse optic nerve and partial recovery of simple visual behaviors. *Proc. Natl. Acad. Sci. USA* **2012**, *109*, 9149–9154. [CrossRef]
111. Mead, B.; Cullather, E.; Nakaya, N.; Niu, Y.; Kole, C.; Ahmed, Z.; Tomarev, S. Viral delivery of multiple miRNAs promotes retinal ganglion cell survival and functional preservation after optic nerve crush injury. *Exp. Eye Res.* **2020**, *197*, 108071. [CrossRef]
112. Rudraprasad, D.; Rawat, A.; Joseph, J. Exosomes, extracellular vesicles and the eye. *Exp. Eye Res.* **2022**, *214*, 108892. [CrossRef] [PubMed]
113. Mead, B.; Tomarev, S. Bone Marrow-Derived Mesenchymal Stem Cells-Derived Exosomes Promote Survival of Retinal Ganglion Cells Through miRNA-Dependent Mechanisms. *Stem Cells Transl. Med.* **2017**, *6*, 1273–1285. [CrossRef] [PubMed]
114. Cui, Y.; Liu, C.; Huang, L.; Chen, J.; Xu, N. Protective effects of intravitreal administration of mesenchymal stem cell-derived exosomes in an experimental model of optic nerve injury. *Exp. Cell Res.* **2021**, *407*, 112792. [CrossRef] [PubMed]
115. Mead, B.; Amaral, J.; Tomarev, S. Mesenchymal Stem Cell-Derived Small Extracellular Vesicles Promote Neuroprotection in Rodent Models of Glaucoma. *Investig. Ophthalmol. Vis. Sci.* **2018**, *59*, 702–714. [CrossRef] [PubMed]
116. Tian, N. Developmental mechanisms that regulate retinal ganglion cell dendritic morphology. *Dev. Neurobiol.* **2011**, *71*, 1297–1309. [CrossRef]
117. Alarautalahti, V.; Ragauskas, S.; Hakkarainen, J.J.; Uusitalo-Järvinen, H.; Uusitalo, H.; Hyttinen, J.; Kalesnykas, G.; Nymark, S. Viability of Mouse Retinal Explant Cultures Assessed by Preservation of Functionality and Morphology. *Investig. Ophthalmol. Vis. Sci.* **2019**, *60*, 1914–1927. [CrossRef]
118. Mumm, J.S.; Williams, P.R.; Godinho, L.; Koerber, A.; Pittman, A.J.; Roeser, T.; Chien, C.B.; Baier, H.; Wong, R.O. In vivo imaging reveals dendritic targeting of laminated afferents by zebrafish retinal ganglion cells. *Neuron* **2006**, *52*, 609–621. [CrossRef]
119. Liu, J.; Reggiani, J.D.S.; Laboulaye, M.A.; Pandey, S.; Chen, B.; Rubenstein, J.L.R.; Krishnaswamy, A.; Sanes, J.R. Tbr1 instructs laminar patterning of retinal ganglion cell dendrites. *Nat. Neurosci.* **2018**, *21*, 659–670. [CrossRef]

Journal of
Clinical Medicine

MDPI

Article

Fundus Blood Flow in Patients with Sellar Lesions with Optic Nerve Bending and Chiasmal Compression

Yoichiro Shinohara [1,*], Rei Yamaguchi [2], Masahiko Tosaka [2], Soichi Oya [2] and Hideo Akiyama [1]

[1] Department of Ophthalmology, Gunma University Graduate School of Medicine, Gunma 371-8511, Japan
[2] Department of Neurosurgery, Gunma University Graduate School of Medicine, Gunma 371-8511, Japan; rei.yamaguchi@gunma-u.ac.jp (R.Y.); sooya-gnm@gunma-u.ac.jp (S.O.)
* Correspondence: shinohara@gunma-u.ac.jp; Tel.: +81-27-220-8338; Fax: +81-27-220-3841

Abstract

Background/objectives: Optic nerve bending and chiasmal compression impair vision in patients with sellar lesions; however, their effect on optic nerve head (ONH) blood flow remains unclear. This study used laser speckle flowgraphy to examine the relationship between clinical features and ONH blood flow in patients with optic nerve bending and chiasmal compression. **Methods**: This retrospective study included 32 eyes (16 eyes with and 16 without optic nerve bending on the contralateral side) from 16 patients with sellar lesions. The best-corrected visual acuity (BCVA), simple visual field impairment score (SVFIS), optic nerve head mean blur rate (ONH-MBR), and six-segmented macular ganglion cell layer + inner plexiform layer (GCL + IPL) thickness were examined. **Results**: Preoperative BCVA and SVFIS in eyes with optic nerve bending were significantly worse than those in eyes without bending, and significantly correlated with the optic nerve-canal bending angle (ONCBA). After tumor resection, BCVA and SVFIS significantly improved in both groups. Preoperative ONH-MBR was significantly lower in bending eyes but increased significantly post-treatment in both groups. Preoperative ONH-MBR correlated with ONCBA, while postoperative ONH-MBR correlated with nasal GCL + IPL thickness. **Conclusions**: Optic nerve bending and chiasmal compression showed reduced blood flow to the ONH. These changes in blood flow may be associated with GCL + IPL thickness and optic nerve bending angle.

Keywords: optic nerve bending; sellar lesions; laser speckle flowgraphy; pituitary neuroendocrine tumor; ganglion cell; optical coherence tomography

1. Introduction

Pituitary neuroendocrine tumor (PitNET) and other tumors in the suprasellar and sellar regions can cause visual field defects, including bilateral hemianopsia, due to the compression of the optic chiasm by the tumor [1]. Many sellar tumors originate from the pituitary gland and pituitary stalk, progressing upward from the midline skull base [2], compressing the crossing fibers of the optic chiasm. The prevalence of PitNET ranges from 7.0 to 41.3 per 100,000 individuals, with an incidence of 0.65 to 2.34 per 100,000, and approximately 70% of patients with PitNET experience visual symptoms [3,4]. As the tumor grows, visual field defects caused by the compression of the optic chiasm may progress, resulting in visual impairment [5,6]. Other types of tumors in sellar regions, such as craniopharyngioma, Rathke's cleft cyst, and meningioma, have different growth patterns and therefore show some variation in the pattern of compression on the optic chiasm, but they often cause hemianopia [7–9]. However, in clinical practice, patients with sellar tumors may lack bilateral hemianopsia despite having severe visual impairment. We previously investigated patients with sellar lesions who had visual impairment using magnetic resonance imaging (MRI), and reported that optic nerve bending at the canal entrance may contribute to visual loss [10]. We also reported that eyes with decreased ganglion cell layer + inner plexiform layer (GCL + IPL) thickness due to optic nerve bending caused by sellar tumors showed little improvement in visual acuity, even after tumor resection [11]. Recently, another group reported that optic nerve bending from sellar tumors is linked to visual impairment [12]. Therefore, a detailed understanding of the pathophysiological characteristics of optic nerve bending is essential for elucidating the mechanisms and characteristics of visual dysfunction in sellar tumors and for determining the optimal treatment timing. Optic nerve compression and bending from sellar lesions can lead to demyelination and impaired blood flow in the optic nerve. Some reports have examined retinal vascular density in PitNET compressing the optic chiasm using optical coherence tomography angiography (OCTA) and predicted postoperative visual prognosis [13–15]. Although compression of the optic chiasm by brain tumors can induce loss of ganglion cells and cause changes in the microvascular structure of the retina [16], it remains unclear whether sellar tumors affect fundus blood flow. Laser speckle flowgraphy (LSFG) is a noninvasive method for evaluating fundus blood flow with good reproducibility, and is useful in various diseases, such as glaucoma [17], ocular ischemic syndrome [18], and ischemic optic neuropathy [19]. In this study, we evaluated the characteristics of fundus blood flow in tumors of the sellar region. We analyzed changes in fundus blood flow before and after tumor resection and investigated the association between fundus blood flow and clinical parameters.

2. Materials and Methods

This study followed the guidelines of the Declaration of Helsinki and was approved by the Institutional Review Board of Gunma University Graduate School of Medicine (HS2022-200). An opt-out informed consent protocol was used for this study.

We retrospectively reviewed 54 patients with sellar tumors who underwent endoscopic transsphenoidal tumor resection at Gunma University Hospital between July 2021 and April 2024 and underwent complete ophthalmological examinations both preoperatively and postoperatively. Among these, we analyzed 16 cases (32 eyes) with optic nerve bending in only 1 eye and no optic nerve bending in the other eye. MRI of the sellar and suprasellar lesions in all patients was performed using a 1.5-T or 3-T MRI system. The presence or absence of optic nerve bending was determined using the method reported previously [6], based on the sagittal optic nerve-canal bending angle (ONCBA) measured by MRI before tumor resection surgery. ONCBA refers to the angle created between the optic nerve within the optic canal and the optic nerve in the intracranial subarachnoid space at the entrance of the optic canal. ONCBA was obtained by two neurosurgeons measuring the extent of this bending on sagittal MRI. Each evaluation was conducted by neurosurgeons with over 20 years of experience in pituitary tumor MRI interpretation and surgery. Disagreements were resolved by consensus. Optic nerve bending (large ONCBA) was defined as ONCBA $\geq 45°$, and non-optic nerve bending (moderate ONCBA) was defined as ONCBA $< 45°$, as previously reported [6]. The exclusion criteria were a history of glaucoma or evident glaucomatous optic neuropathy, high myopia (spherical equivalent < -6 diopters), presence of retinal diseases, severe cataract, and poor visualization of the optic nerve on MRI.

All patients underwent ophthalmologic examinations, including measurement of best-corrected visual acuity (BCVA), intraocular pressure refraction, slit-lamp biomicroscopy, color fundus photography (Canon CX-1; Canon Inc., Tokyo, Japan), GCL + IPL thickness using Cirrus high-definition optical coherence tomography (HD-OCT) (Carl Zeiss Meditec, Dublin, CA, USA), visual field testing, and LSFG in both eyes with and without optic nerve bending before and 1 month after tumor resection surgery. BCVA was recorded as the logarithm of the minimum angle of resolution (logMAR) units. The Cirrus HD-OCT ganglion cell analysis algorithm segmentally divided the macula into six regions: the superior, superior nasal, inferior nasal, inferior, inferior temporal, and superior temporal sectors, and subsequently quantifies the combined thickness of GCL + IPL [20]. Visual field testing was conducted using the Goldmann test, and impairment was quantified using the previously reported simple visual field impairment score (SVFIS) [21]. The Goldman perimetry chart was categorized into 12 regions, with lines connecting the upper and lower parts and the nasal and temporal sides within 5°, 5–30°, and >30° of the centers. Points were added if any scotomas were present in each area, including the expansion of physiological scotomas. If the peripheral visual field was narrowed by >10° from the normal range, peripheral visual field impairment was added. Thus, 0 points indicated no visual field impairment, and 12 points indicated visual field impairment in all areas. The evaluation of blood flow in the optic nerve head (ONH) was based on the measurement of the mean blur rate (MBR) using an LSFG-NAVI device (Softcare Co., Ltd., Fukutsu, Japan) with a dilated pupil. Mydrin-P (0.5% tropicamide + phenylephrine hydrochloride) was used to dilate the pupils. LSFG uses a diode laser with a wavelength of 830 nm to illuminate the circulating erythrocytes. The reflected light generated a speckle pattern, which was subsequently utilized to calculate blood flow values, known as the MBR. An elliptical region was manually delineated around the ONH to define the region of interest (ROI) in the composite ocular blood flow map generated by LSFG-NAVI. An experienced operator determined the ROI with elliptical bands of ONH margins in all participants to ensure that the ONH was not over- or under-covered, referring to the fundus photographs. Regarding ONH measurements, the software (LSFG ANALYZER, ver.3.7.0.4; commercially available product) automatically categorized the ROI into large vascular and tissue regions and determined the MBR in three regions: the vascular region ONH (mean of vascular area; MV), tissue region ONH (mean of tissue area; MT), and overall ONH (mean of all area; MA). MV represents the flow in large vessels supplying the retina, MT represents tissue blood flow in the ONH, and MA is a combination of both values.

For statistical analyses, data are presented as the mean ± standard deviation or median (interquartile range). The Mann–Whitney U test or unpaired *t*-test was conducted to compare the BCVA, SVFIS, GCL + IPL thickness measurements, and optic nerve head mean blur rate (ONH-MBR) between the bending and non-bending eyes, as appropriate. The Wilcoxon signed-rank test was conducted to compare changes in BCVA, SVFIS, GCL + IPL thickness, and ONH-MBR before and 1 month after tumor resection. The correlations between BCVA, SVFIS, GCL + IPL thickness, ONH-MBR, and ONCBA were analyzed using Spearman's correlation coefficient. A significance level of $p < 0.05$ was set. Statistical analyses were performed using GraphPad Prism, version 10 (GraphPad Software Inc., La Jolla, CA, USA).

3. Results

Table 1 shows the demographic and clinical characteristics of patients with sellar tumors.

Nine patients had a PitNET, three had a craniopharyngioma, one had a Rathke's cleft cyst, and three had a meningioma. Among the patients with sellar and suprasellar tumors, the average age was 58.9 ± 10.7 years, with 11 men (68.8%) and 5 women (31.3%). The mean

ONCBA was 60.2 ± 9.7° in the bending eyes and 27.1 ± 11.7° in non-bending eyes ($p < 0.0001$). Preoperative and postoperative BCVAs were 0.15 (0.01 to 0.75) and −0.08 (−0.08 to 0.00) in the bending eyes and −0.08 (−0.08 to 0.03) and −0.08 in the non-bending eyes (Figure 1a). At preoperative examination, the BCVA of the bending eyes was significantly worse than that of the non-bending eyes ($p = 0.003$). The postoperative BCVA was significantly improved compared with the preoperative BCVA in the bending and non-bending eyes ($p = 0.003$ and $p = 0.03$, respectively; Figure 1a). Spearman's correlation (r = 0.43, $p = 0.013$) showed that ONCBA positively correlated with preoperative BCVA in 32 eyes of 16 patients (Figure 1b).

Table 1. Systemic characteristics of patients with sellar tumors.

	Participant (n = 16)		
	Optic Nerve Bending (+)	**Optic Nerve Bending (−)**	***p*-Value**
Number of eyes (n)	16	16	
Age (years)	58.9 ± 10.7		
Male–Female (n)	11:5		
Right eye (n)	8	8	1
ONCBA (°)	60.2 ± 9.7	27.1 ± 11.7	<0.0001
Pathology			
Pituitary neuroendocrine tumor	9		
Craniopharyngioma	3		
Rathke's cleft cyst	1		
Meningioma	3		

ONCBA: optic nerve-canal bending angle.

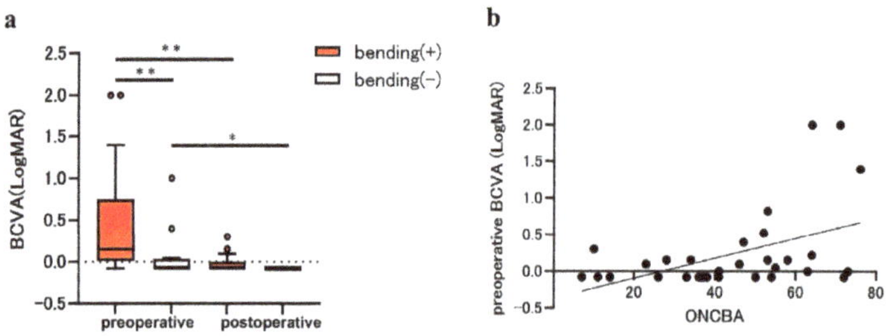

Figure 1. Evaluation of best-corrected visual acuity (BCVA) in eyes with the sellar lesion. The parameters for eyes with optic nerve bending (red bars) and eyes without optic nerve bending (white bars) were compared before and after the tumor resection. (**a**) Comparison of BCVA in eyes with and without optic nerve bending pre- and post-tumor resection. The preoperative BCVA in eyes with optic nerve bending was significantly worse than that in those without optic nerve bending (** $p < 0.01$). The postoperative BCVA was significantly improved in eyes with and without optic nerve bending (** $p < 0.01$ and * $p < 0.05$). (**b**) Graphs showing the correlation between the optic nerve-canal bending angle (ONCBA) and preoperative BCVA in 32 eyes of 16 patients. The ONCBA was positively correlated with preoperative BCVA (r = 0.43, $p = 0.013$).

Preoperative and postoperative SVFIS were 5.00 (3.25 to 9.25) and 2.00 (0.25 to 4.00) in the bending eyes and 4.00 (2.00 to 4.00) and 1.50 (0.00 to 2.00) in the non-bending eyes (Figure 2a). In the preoperative examination, the SVFIS was significantly worse in the bending eyes than in the non-bending eyes ($p = 0.03$). Postoperative SVFIS was significantly improved relative to preoperative SVFIS in the bending ($p = 0.0011$; Figure 2a) and non-bending ($p = 0.004$; Figure 2a) eyes. Spearman's correlation (r = 0.56, $p < 0.001$) showed that ONCBA was positively correlated with the preoperative SVFIS in 32 eyes of 16 patients (Figure 2b).

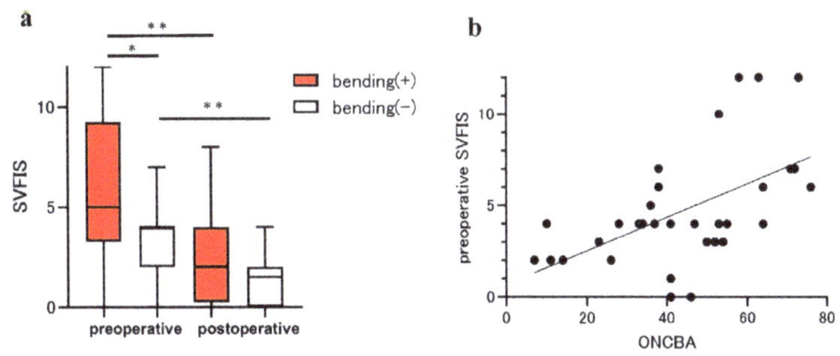

Figure 2. Assessment of visual field using the simple visual field impairment score (SVFIS) in patients with sellar and suprasellar tumors. The parameters for eyes with optic nerve bending (red bars) and eyes without optic nerve bending (white bars) were compared before and after the tumor resection. (**a**) Comparison of SVFIS between eyes with and without optic nerve bending pre- and post-surgery. The preoperative SVFIS of eyes with optic nerve bending was significantly higher than that in those without optic nerve bending (* $p < 0.05$). Postoperative SVFIS was significantly improved in eyes with and without optic nerve bending (** $p < 0.01$). (**b**) Graphs showing the correlation between the optic nerve-canal bending angle (ONCBA) and preoperative SVFIS in 32 eyes of 16 patients. The ONCBA was positively correlated with preoperative SVFIS (r = 0.56, $p < 0.001$).

The MBR parameters of the ONH in both groups are shown in Figure 3. The preoperative MA, MV, and MT of the optic nerve bending group were 22.2 ± 3.5, 45.2 ± 10.0, and 10.1 ± 1.9, respectively, and those of the non-bending group were 25.5 ± 4.8, 51.2 ± 11.2, and 12.0 ± 3.3, respectively. In addition, the postoperative MA, MV, and MT for the optic nerve bending group were 25.9 ± 4.6, 52.6 ± 10.6, and 12.0 ± 2.4, respectively; for the non-optic nerve bending group, they were 28.0 ± 5.5, 57.1 ± 10.0, and 13.2 ± 2.9, respectively (Figure 3a–c). The preoperative MA of the optic nerve bending group was significantly lower than that of the non-optic nerve bending group ($p = 0.04$; Figure 3a). The postoperative MA, MV, and MT in the optic nerve bending group were significantly increased after tumor resection (all $p < 0.001$; Figure 3a–c). Furthermore, the postoperative MA, MV, and MT in the non-optic nerve bending group were significantly increased after tumor resection ($p < 0.001$, MA; $p = 0.006$ and $p = 0.002$, MV and MT; Figure 3a–c).

In preoperative examination, GCL + IPL thicknesses in the bending and non-bending eyes were 67.0 ± 14.2 μm and 72.6 ± 7.9 μm in the superior sector, 66.1 ± 13.6 μm and 69.9 ± 9.8 μm in the superior nasal sector, 64.3 ± 11.6 μm and 68.0 ± 9.2 μm in the inferior nasal sector, 65.9 ± 12.7 μm and 71.2 ± 7.1 μm in the inferior sector, 75.5 ± 10.2 μm and 78.8 ± 7.4 μm in the inferior temporal sector, and 72.3 ± 11.9 μm and 77.7 ± 6.6 μm in the superior temporal sector, respectively. In postoperative examination, GCL + IPL thicknesses in the bending and non-bending eyes were 68.5 ± 9.1 μm and 72.1 ± 7.2 μm in the superior sector, 66.9 ± 10.7 μm and 69.1 ± 9.6 μm in the superior nasal sector, 64.8 ± 10.3 μm and 67.3 ± 8.9 μm in the inferior nasal sector, 67.7 ± 8.4 μm and 71.1 ± 6.7 μm in the inferior sector, 75.4 ± 9.0 μm and 78.2 ± 7.1 μm in the inferior temporal sector, and 73.3 ± 9.4 μm and 77.3 ± 6.3 μm in the superior temporal sector, respectively. No significant differences were observed between the optic nerve bending and non-bending groups in any sector of the GCL + IPL before and after tumor resection. In both bending eyes and non-bending eyes, the thickness of GCL + IPL in the nasal sectors was thinner than that in the temporal sectors both preoperatively and postoperatively. The postoperative SVFIS showed a negative correlation with preoperative GCL + IPL in five sectors aside from the inferior temporal sector (r = −0.65, $p < 0.001$, superior; r = −0.55, $p = 0.001$, superior nasal; r = −0.51, $p = 0.003$, inferior nasal; r = −0.53, $p = 0.002$, inferior; r = −0.17, $p = 0.34$, inferior temporal; and r = −0.38, $p = 0.03$, superior temporal sector).

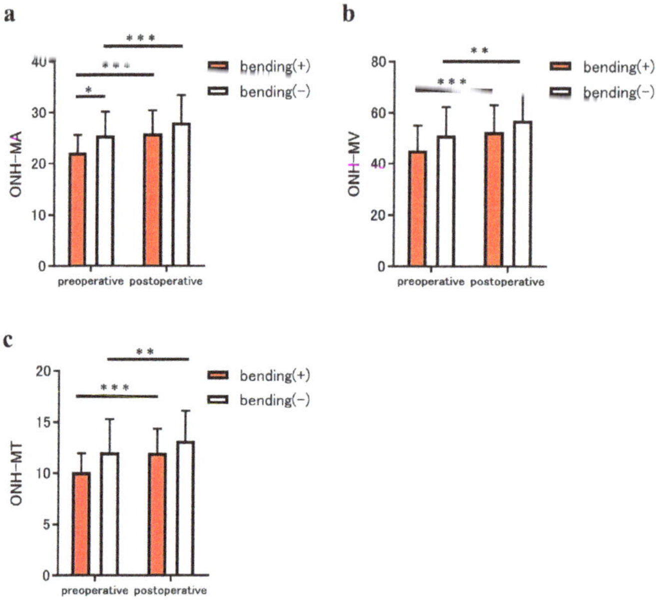

Figure 3. Comparison of the mean blur rate (MBR) measured using laser speckle flowgraphy (LSFG) between eyes in patients with the sellar and suprasellar tumor. The graphs show the optic nerve head (ONH)-MBR of the overall region (MA) (**a**), vessel region (MV) (**b**), and tissue region (MT) (**c**), measured using LSFG. The parameters for eyes with optic nerve bending (red bars) and eyes without optic nerve bending (white bars) were compared before and after the tumor resection. The ONH-MA in eyes with optic nerve bending was significantly lower than that in eyes without bending (* $p < 0.05$). In addition, the preoperative ONH-MA, MV, and MT in eyes with optic nerve bending increased significantly after tumor resection (all *** $p < 0.001$). Similarly, the ONH-MA, MV, and MT of eyes without optic nerve bending increased significantly after tumor resection (*** $p < 0.001$, MA; ** $p < 0.01$, MV and MT).

We further investigated the relationship between the blood flow in the optic nerve head (ONH-MA), measured using LSFG, and other parameters (ONCBA, GCL + IPL, BCVA, and SVFIS). The correlations between the preoperative ONH-MA and other parameters are shown in Table 2.

Table 2. Association between preoperative optic disc blood mean blur rate (all areas) and other measurements in eyes with sellar tumors.

	R	*p*-Value
ONCBA	−0.56	<0.001
Preoperative examination		
GCL + IPL		
Superior	−0.10	0.59
Superior nasal	−0.07	0.72
Inferior nasal	−0.06	0.75
Inferior	−0.10	0.60
Inferior temporal	−0.18	0.33
Superior temporal	−0.22	0.23
BCVA (LogMAR)	−0.16	0.38
SVFIS	−0.18	0.33

ONCBA—optic nerve-canal bending angle; GCL + IPL—ganglion cell layer + inner plexiform layer; BCVA—best-corrected visual acuity; SVFIS—simple visual field impairment score.

Preoperative ONH-MA was negatively correlated with ONCBA (r = −0.56, $p < 0.001$). The correlations between postoperative ONH-MA and other parameters are shown in Table 3.

Table 3. Association between postoperative optic disc blood mean blur rate (all areas) and other measurements in eyes with sellar tumors.

	R	p-Value
ONCBA	−0.27	0.14
Postoperative examination		
GCL + IPL		
Superior	0.39	0.03
Superior nasal	0.49	0.005
Inferior nasal	0.42	0.02
Inferior	0.35	0.047
Inferior temporal	0.13	0.47
Superior temporal	0.16	0.39
BCVA (LogMAR)	−0.01	0.97
SVFIS	−0.10	0.59

ONCBA—optic nerve-canal bending angle; GCL + IPL—ganglion cell layer + inner plexiform layer; BCVA—best-corrected visual acuity; SVFIS—simple visual field impairment score.

Postoperative ONH-MA positively correlated with the thickness of the GCL + IPL in the superior (r = 0.39, $p = 0.03$), superior nasal (r = 0.49, $p = 0.005$), inferior nasal (r = 0.42, $p = 0.02$), and inferior regions (r = 0.35, $p = 0.047$). A representative case of a patient with craniopharyngioma and optic nerve bending in the left eye is shown in Figure 4.

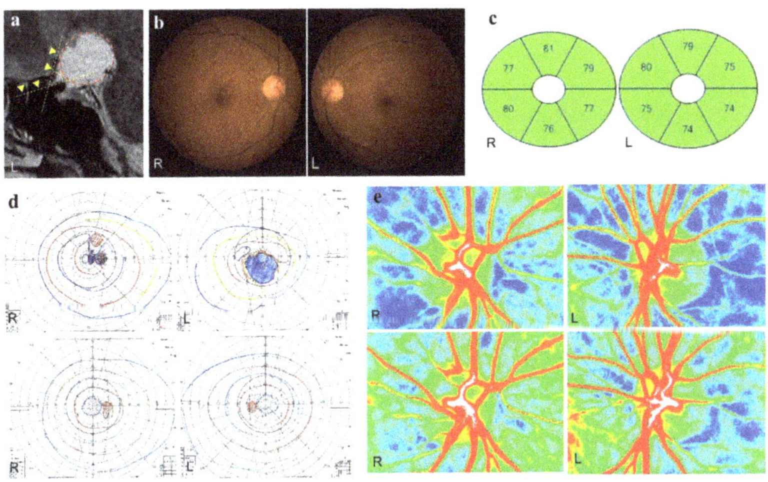

Figure 4. A representative case of craniopharyngioma. A 57-year-old woman has optic nerve bending in her left eye caused by craniopharyngioma. Preoperative and postoperative best-corrected visual acuities (BCVAs; logarithm of the minimum angle of resolution units) are 0.30 and −0.08 in the right eye and 2.0 and −0.08 in the left eye, respectively. (**a**) Sagittal T2-weighted magnetic resonance images before surgery. The optic nerve-canal bending angle (ONCBA) (yellow dotted lines) is formed by the optic nerve in the optic canal and the optic nerve in the intracranial subarachnoid space at the optic canal's exit. The yellow arrowheads indicated the optic nerve. A circle surrounding red dots indicates the tumor. The ONCBAs of this case are 10° in the right eye and 63° in the left eye. (**b**) Color

fundus photograph of both eyes showing the normal appearance at the preoperative visit. (**c**) The thickness of the ganglion cell layer (GCL) + inner plexiform layer (IPL) in both eyes after tumor resection is within the normal range. (**d**) Goldmann perimetry before and after tumor resection. A central scotoma is detected in both eyes before tumor resection. The preoperative SVFIS score for the left eye is lower than that for the right eye (4 points for the right eye; 12 points for the left eye) (**upper** panels). After tumor resection, the central scotoma has disappeared in both eyes, and the SVFIS score is 0 for both eyes (**lower** panels). (**e**) Laser speckle flowgraphy (LSFG) images of the optic nerve head (ONH) before and after tumor resection. The preoperative optic nerve head-mean blur rate (OHN-MBR) of the overall region (MA), vessel region (MV), and tissue region (MT) are 23.1, 46.3 and 11.9 in the right eye, and 22.2, 37.2 and 9.3 in the left eye, respectively (**upper** panels). Postoperative MA, MV and MT for the right eye are 27.9, 54.9 and 12.0; for the left eye, they are 29.6, 55.0 and 11.3, respectively (**bottom** panels).

4. Discussion

We retrospectively analyzed the clinical features of sellar tumors with and without optic nerve bending, focusing on changes in fundus blood flow before and after tumor resection. In eyes with sellar tumors causing optic nerve bending, the ONH blood flow, measured using LSFG, was lower than that in the eyes without optic nerve bending, and significantly improved after tumor resection in both groups. Furthermore, preoperative ONH blood flow was associated with ONCBA, whereas postoperative ONH blood flow was associated with nasal GCL + IPL thickness.

Our group previously reported that sellar tumors can severely impair vision by compressing the optic chiasm and bending the optic nerve, as measured by the sagittal angle at the optic canal entrance on MRI [10]. Although visual impairment due to optic nerve bending is a relatively new concept, another group has recently reported that optic nerve bending is related to visual impairment [12]. This study showed that ONCBA is associated with BCVA and visual field defects. To treat sellar lesions, tumor resection is required before irreversible visual impairment occurs. Optic nerve bending may serve as a key indicator for determining the need for tumor resection. The optic nerve at the entrance of the optic canal is mainly supplied with blood from the superior pituitary artery and does not receive blood from the ophthalmic artery, making it more susceptible to ischemia than the blood-rich optic chiasm [22]. In addition, the optic nerve undergoes demyelination 2 days after compression [23]. Continued compression of the optic nerve can slowly cause irreversible visual impairment despite partial remyelination [23]. Optic nerve bending at the entrance of the optic canal in the narrow peripheral optic nerve may cause more damage to the entire optic nerve than optic chiasm compression in the relatively strong and large optic chiasm [10]. Therefore, optic nerve bending is more likely to cause ischemia and stronger demyelination than optic chiasm compression, and is also more likely to cause severe visual impairment.

LSFG can non-invasively and efficiently evaluate ocular blood flow and has been reported to be useful in differentiating between open-angle glaucoma, optic neuritis, and ischemic optic neuropathy [24]. No prior reports have observed fundus blood flow using LSFG in patients with sellar tumors. This study showed that postoperative ONH blood flow is associated with nasal GCL + IPL thickness. Furthermore, the ONH blood flow improved after tumor resection in the optic nerve bending and non-bending eyes. The nasal GCL + IPL thickness was reduced in patients with PitNET compared to normal participants [25]. This is because compression of the optic chiasm by the tumor damages the crossing fibers, causing retrograde damage to the retinal ganglion cells. A prior OCTA study found reduced retinal vascular density in regions where the retinal ganglion cell layer had thinned, consistent with optic chiasm compression from PitNET [16]. This mechanism involves tumor-induced optic chiasm compression, leading to ganglion cell damage, reduced metabolic activity, and lower retinal nutritional demand [26]. In response, blood flow to the retina decreases, causing changes in the vascular structure of the corresponding area of the retina [27]. One month after tumor resection, the transient functional impairment of retinal ganglion cells caused by optic nerve bending and chiasm compression resolved. Therefore, postoperative ONH blood flow may be related to the original damage to retinal ganglion cells. The improvement in ONH blood flow observed even in eyes without optic nerve bending may be due to the removal of optic chiasm compression by tumor resection. A study that observed the superficial and deep retinal capillary plexus in eyes with PitNET using OCTA reported a significant increase in retinal vascular density after tumor resection [13]. Despite differences between OCTA and LSFG, these findings suggest that sellar lesions cause changes in fundus blood flow and retinal vascular structure before and after surgery. Although postoperative ophthalmic evaluation in this study was performed only 1 month after surgery, GCL + IPL thickness changes due to retrograde degeneration may change for more than 3 months after optic nerve decompression [28,29]. Long-term observation of sellar lesions with optic nerve bending and chiasm compression may reveal further changes in ONH blood flow as well as GCL + IPL thickness. In addition, GCL + IPL thinning in optic nerve-bending eyes was reported to be associated with poor postoperative BCVA [11]. This study showed a correlation between preoperative GCL + IPL thickness in five sectors and postoperative SVFIS. In the treatment of sellar lesions, GCL + IPL thickness may be an important predictor of postoperative visual function.

This study showed that the preoperative ONH blood flow was associated with ON-CBA. Optic nerve bending causes reversible retinal ganglion cell axonal dysfunction in the short term; therefore, a preoperative decrease in ONH blood flow may reflect retinal ganglion cell dysfunction. In addition, the optic nerve around the entrance of the optic canal is adjacent to the internal carotid artery (ICA) and ophthalmic arteries. PitNET, regardless of whether or not stroke is present, may cause direct compression of the ICA [30,31]. Previous studies suggest a link between optic nerve bending angle and tumor size [10,11], indicating that severe bending may anatomically affect the arterial system around the optic nerve. However, because the MRI methods used in this study did not identify any changes in the vascular structure caused by the tumor, further investigation of the MRI method is required to clarify this hypothesis.

This study has several limitations, including its retrospective, single-center design and relatively small sample size. To generalize the results of this study, further evaluation of a larger number of cases at multiple institutions is needed. Moreover, this study did not examine the period from the onset of visual impairment to ophthalmological evaluation. The time from the onset of optic nerve bending and optic chiasm compression may affect visual impairment and GCL + IPL thickness, but it was challenging to identify the onset time in this study. This study includes patients with four different types of tumors (PitNET, craniopharyngiomas, meningiomas, and Rathke's cleft cysts). These tumors differ in their growth patterns, rates, and tissue characteristics, and may have different effects on the optic nerves and surrounding vasculature. However, since they are common in terms of sellar lesions with optic nerve bending and optic chiasm compression, the effect on the results of this study is minimized.

In conclusion, sellar tumors with optic nerve bending and chiasmal compression reduce optic blood flow, which improves after tumor resection. The preoperative optic blood flow was associated with the bending angle of the optic nerve, and postoperative optic blood flow was associated with nasal GCL + IPL thickness. LSFG may be used to evaluate the fundus hemodynamics of PitNET and other sellar regions.

Author Contributions: The authors contributed to the study as follows: Conceptualization, Y.S.; Methodology, Y.S., R.Y. and M.T.; Validation, Y.S. and R.Y.; Formal Analysis, Y.S.; Investigation, Y.S.; Resources, Y.S., R.Y. and M.T.; Data Curation, Y.S., R.Y., M.T. and H.A.; Writing—Original Draft Preparation, Y.S.; Writing—Review and Editing, Y.S., S.O. and H.A.; Visualization, Y.S., S.O. and H.A.; Supervision, M.T., S.O. and H.A.; Project Administration, Y.S.; Funding Acquisition, Y.S. All authors have read and agreed to the published version of the manuscript.

Funding: This work was supported by JSPS KAKENHI, Grant Number 22K16941 (Y.S.).

Institutional Review Board Statement: This study followed the guidelines of the Declaration of Helsinki and were approved by the Institutional Review Board of Gunma University Graduate School of Medicine (HS2022-200). An opt-out informed consent protocol was used for this study.

Informed Consent Statement: An opt-out informed consent protocol was used for this study.

Data Availability Statement: All data relevant to this study are presented in the published manuscript. Additional data supporting the study's conclusions can be obtained by contacting the corresponding author.

Acknowledgments: The authors thank the optometrists at Gunma University for their assistance in acquiring the data used in this study.

Conflicts of Interest: The authors declare no competing interests.

Abbreviations

The following abbreviations are used in this manuscript:

PitNET	Pituitary Neuroendocrine Tumor.
MRI	Magnetic Resonance Imaging.
GCL + IPL	Ganglion Cell Layer plus Inner Plexiform Layer.
OCTA	Optical Coherence Tomography Angiography.
LSFG	Laser Speckle Flowgraphy.
ONCBA	Optic Nerve-Canal Bending Angle.
BCVA	Best-Corrected Visual Acuity.
OCT	Optical Coherence Tomography.
SVFIS	Simple Visual Field Impairment Score.
ONH	Optic Nerve Head.
MBR	Mean Blur Rate.
ROI	Region of Interest.
MV	Mean of Vascular Area.
MT	Mean of Tissue Area.
MA	Mean of All Areas.
ICA	Internal Carotid Artery.

References

1. Ju, D.G.; Jeon, C.; Kim, K.H.; Park, K.A.; Hong, S.D.; Seoul, H.J.; Shin, H.J.; Nam, D.H.; Lee, J.I.; Kong, D.S. Clinical Significance of Tumor-Related Edema of Optic Tract Affecting Visual Function in Patients with Sellar and Suprasellar Tumors. *World Neurosurg.* **2019**, *132*, e862–e868. [CrossRef] [PubMed]
2. Hawkes, R.; Holland, G.; Moore, W.; Corston, R.; Kean, D.; Worthington, B. The application of NMR imaging to the evaluation of pituitary and juxtasellar tumors. *Am. J. Neuroradiol.* **1983**, *4*, 221–222. [PubMed]
3. Ntali, G.; Wass, J.A. Epidemiology, clinical presentation and diagnosis of non-functioning pituitary adenomas. *Pituitary* **2018**, *21*, 111–118. [CrossRef]
4. Ferrante, E.; Ferraroni, M.; Castrignanò, T.; Menicatti, L.; Anagni, M.; Reimondo, G.; Del Monte, P.; Bernasconi, D.; Loli, P.; Faustini-Fustini, M.; et al. Non-functioning pituitary adenoma database: A useful resource to improve the clinical management of pituitary tumors. *Eur. J. Endocrinol.* **2006**, *155*, 823–829. [CrossRef] [PubMed]
5. Monteiro, M.L.; Zambon, B.K.; Cunha, L.P. Predictive factors for the development of visual loss in patients with pituitary macroadenomas and for visual recovery after optic pathway decompression. *Can. J. Ophthalmol.* **2010**, *45*, 404–408. [CrossRef]

6. Wang, H.; Sun, W.; Fu, Z.; Si, Z.; Zhu, Y.; Zhai, G.; Zhao, G.; Xu, S.; Pang, Q. The pattern of visual impairment in patients with pituitary adenoma. *J. Int. Med. Res.* **2008**, *36*, 1064–1069. [CrossRef]
7. Prieto, R.; Pascual, J.M.; Barrios, L. Optic chiasm distortions caused by craniopharyngiomas: Clinical and magnetic resonance imaging correlation and influence on visual outcome. *World Neurosurg.* **2015**, *83*, 500–529. [CrossRef]
8. El-Mahdy, W.; Powell, M. Transsphenoidal management of 28 symptomatic Rathke's cleft cysts, with special reference to visual and hormonal recovery. *Neurosurgery* **1998**, *42*, 7–16; discussion 16–17. [CrossRef]
9. Fahlbusch, R.; Schott, W. Pterional surgery of meningiomas of the tuberculum sellae and planum sphenoidale: Surgical results with special consideration of ophthalmological and endocrinological outcomes. *J. Neurosurg.* **2002**, *96*, 235–243. [CrossRef]
10. Yamaguchi, R.; Tosaka, M.; Miyagishima, T.; Osawa, T.; Horiguchi, K.; Honda, F.; Yoshimoto, Y. Sagittal bending of the optic nerve at the entrance from the intracranial to the optic canal and ipsilateral visual acuity in patients with sellar and suprasellar lesions. *J. Neurosurg.* **2019**, *134*, 180–188. [CrossRef]
11. Shinohara, Y.; Todokoro, D.; Yamaguchi, R.; Tosaka, M.; Yoshimoto, Y.; Akiyama, H. Retinal ganglion cell analysis in patients with sellar and suprasellar tumors with sagittal bending of the optic nerve. *Sci. Rep.* **2022**, *12*, 11092. [CrossRef]
12. Teramoto, S.; Tahara, S.; Goto, H.; Kodama, T.; Watada, H.; Kondo, A. Investigation of predictors of latent visual impairment in patients with sellar lesions. *J. Neurosurg.* **2024**, *142*, 1349–1356. [CrossRef]
13. Ergen, A.; Kaya Ergen, S.; Gunduz, B.; Subasi, S.; Caklili, M.; Cabuk, B.; Anik, I.; Ceylan, S. Retinal vascular and structural recovery analysis by optical coherence tomography angiography after endoscopic decompression in sellar/parasellar tumors. *Sci. Rep.* **2023**, *13*, 14371. [CrossRef] [PubMed]
14. Toumi, E.; Almairac, F.; Mondot, L.; Themelin, A.; Decoux-Poullot, A.G.; Paquis, P.; Chevalier, N.; Baillif, S.; Nahon-Esteve, S.; Martel, A. Benefit of Optical Coherence Tomography-Angiography in Patients Undergoing Transsphenoidal Pituitary Adenoma Surgery: A Prospective Controlled Study. *Diagnostics* **2024**, *14*, 1747. [CrossRef] [PubMed]
15. Tang, Y.; Jia, W.; Xue, Z.; Yuan, L.; Qu, Y.; Yang, L.; Wang, L.; Ma, X.; Wang, M.; Meng, L.; et al. Prognostic value of radial peripapillary capillary density for visual field outcomes in pituitary adenoma: A case-control study. *J. Clin. Neurosci.* **2022**, *100*, 113–119. [CrossRef]
16. Lee, G.I.; Park, K.A.; Oh, S.Y.; Kong, D.S. Analysis of Optic Chiasmal Compression Caused by Brain Tumors Using Optical Coherence Tomography Angiography. *Sci. Rep.* **2020**, *10*, 2088. [CrossRef]
17. Kiyota, N.; Shiga, Y.; Omodaka, K.; Pak, K.; Nakazawa, T. Time-Course Changes in Optic Nerve Head Blood Flow and Retinal Nerve Fiber Layer Thickness in Eyes with Open-angle Glaucoma. *Ophthalmology* **2021**, *128*, 663–671. [CrossRef]
18. Shinohara, Y.; Kashima, T.; Akiyama, H.; Shimoda, Y.; Li, D.; Kishi, S. Evaluation of Fundus Blood Flow in Normal Individuals and Patients with Internal Carotid Artery Obstruction Using Laser Speckle Flowgraphy. *PLoS ONE* **2017**, *12*, e0169596. [CrossRef]
19. Maekubo, T.; Chuman, H.; Nao, I.N. Laser speckle flowgraphy for differentiating between nonarteritic ischemic optic neuropathy and anterior optic neuritis. *Jpn. J. Ophthalmol.* **2013**, *57*, 385–390. [CrossRef]
20. Mwanza, J.C.; Durbin, M.K.; Budenz, D.L.; Sayyad, F.E.; Chang, R.T.; Neelakantan, A.; Godfrey, D.G.; Carter, R.; Crandall, A.S. Glaucoma diagnostic accuracy of ganglion cell-inner plexiform layer thickness: Comparison with nerve fiber layer and optic nerve head. *Ophthalmology* **2012**, *119*, 1151–1158. [CrossRef]
21. Yamaguchi, R.; Tosaka, M.; Shinohara, Y.; Todokoro, D.; Mukada, N.; Miyagishima, T.; Akiyama, H.; Yoshimoto, Y. Analysis of visual field disturbance in patients with sellar and suprasellar lesions. Relationship with magnetic resonance imaging findings and sagittal bending of the optic nerve. *Acta Neurol. Belg.* **2022**, *122*, 1031–1041. [CrossRef] [PubMed]
22. van Overbeeke, J.; Sekhar, L. Microanatomy of the blood supply to the optic nerve. *Orbit* **2003**, *22*, 81–88. [CrossRef] [PubMed]
23. Clifford-Jones, R.E.; McDonald, W.I.; Landon, D.N. Chronic optic nerve compression. An experimental study. *Brain* **1985**, *108*, 241–262. [CrossRef] [PubMed]
24. Yamaguchi, C.; Kiyota, N.; Himori, N.; Omodaka, K.; Tsuda, S.; Nakazawa, T. Differentiating optic neuropathies using laser speckle flowgraphy: Evaluating blood flow patterns in the optic nerve head and peripapillary choroid. *Acta Ophthalmol.* **2025**, *103*, e49–e57. [CrossRef]
25. Akashi, A.; Kanamori, A.; Ueda, K.; Matsumoto, Y.; Yamada, Y.; Nakamura, M. The detection of macular analysis by SD-OCT for optic chiasmal compression neuropathy and nasotemporal overlap. *Investig. Ophthalmol. Vis. Sci.* **2014**, *55*, 4667–4672. [CrossRef]
26. Kiryu, J.; Asrani, S.; Shahidi, M.; Mori, M.; Zeimer, R. Local response of the primate retinal microcirculation to increased metabolic demand induced by flicker. *Investig. Ophthalmol. Vis. Sci.* **1995**, *36*, 1240–1246.
27. Suzuki, A.C.F.; Zacharias, L.C.; Preti, R.C.; Cunha, L.P.; Monteiro, M.L.R. Circumpapillary and macular vessel density assessment by optical coherence tomography angiography in eyes with temporal hemianopia from chiasmal compression. Correlation with retinal neural and visual field loss. *Eye* **2020**, *34*, 695–703. [CrossRef]
28. Moon, C.H.; Hwang, S.C.; Ohn, Y.H.; Park, T.K. The time course of visual field recovery and changes of retinal ganglion cells after optic chiasmal decompression. *Invest. Ophthalmol. Vis. Sci.* **2011**, *52*, 7966–7973. [CrossRef]

29. Moon, C.H.; Hwang, S.C.; Kim, B.T.; Ohn, Y.H.; Park, T.K. Visual prognostic value of optical coherence tomography and photopic negative response in chiasmal compression. *Invest. Ophthalmol. Vis. Sci.* **2011**, *52*, 8527–8533. [CrossRef]
30. Rey-Dios, R.; Payner, T.D.; Cohen-Gadol, A.A. Pituitary macroadenoma causing symptomatic internal carotid artery compression: Surgical treatment through transsphenoidal tumor resection. *J. Clin. Neurosci.* **2014**, *21*, 541–546. [CrossRef]
31. Teramoto, S.; Tahara, S.; Kondo, A.; Morita, A. Key Factors Related to Internal Carotid Artery Stenosis Associated with Pituitary Apoplexy. *World Neurosurg.* **2021**, *149*, e447–e454. [CrossRef]

MDPI AG
Grosspeteranlage 5
4052 Basel
Switzerland
Tel.: +41 61 683 77 34

Journal of Clinical Medicine Editorial Office
E-mail: jcm@mdpi.com
www.mdpi.com/journal/jcm

www.ingramcontent.com/pod-product-compliance
Lightning Source LLC
Chambersburg PA
CBHW062054220926
51850CB00010B/2769
9783725853335